Practical Endocrinology and Diabetes in Children

Practical Endocrinology and Diabetes in Children

Fourth Edition

Malcolm D.C. Donaldson MD, FRCP, FRCPCH, DCH

Honorary Senior Research Fellow
Glasgow University School of Medicine
Honorary Consultant Paediatrician
Royal Hospital for Children
Glasgow, UK

John W. Gregory MBChB, MD, FRCP, DCH, FRCPCH

Professor in Paediatric Endocrinology & Honorary Consultant
Division of Population Medicine, School of Medicine
Cardiff University
Cardiff, Heath Park, Cardiff, UK

Guy Van Vliet MD

Staff Endocrinologist
CHU Sainte-Justine and Professor of Pediatrics
University of Montreal
Montreal, QC, Canada

Joseph I. Wolfsdorf MB, BCh, MA, DCH, FCP, FAAP

Attending Physician in Endocrinology
Boston Children's Hospital Chair in Endocrinology
Professor of Pediatrics, Harvard Medical School
Boston, Massachusetts, U.S.A.

Guest chapter "An Endocrinologist's Guide to Genetics in the Age of Genomics" contributed by

Johnny Deladoëy MD, PhD

Staff Endocrinologist
CHU Sainte-Justine and Associate Professor of Pediatrics
University of Montreal
Montreal, QC, Canada

WILEY Blackwell

Malcolm Donaldson, John Gregory, Guy Van Vliet and Joseph Wolfsdorf would like to dedicate this fourth edition to their long-suffering wives: Julia, Katrin, Chantal, and Gail, with love and thanks for their support.

Contents

Preface to the Fourth Edition

It was Dr Joseph Raine, Consultant Paediatrician at The Whittington Hospital in London, who recognized the gap between the large detailed endocrine reference books and short reviews of topics in paediatric endocrinology and diabetes. *Practical Endocrinology and Diabetes in Children* was Joe's brainchild, aiming to provide a practical, concise and up-to-date account of paediatric endocrinology and diabetes in a readable, user-friendly and portable format.

The first edition of the book featured an all-British cast of co-editors – Joe Raine, Malcolm Donaldson, John Gregory, and Martin Savage. Following its debut and favourable reception, the need to appeal to a wider readership was recognized, and Raymond Hintz (1939–2014) from Stanford University in California was invited to help with the second edition in 2007. For the third edition in 2011, Guy Van Vliet from Montreal in Canada joined the team to replace Martin Savage, further reinforcing the book's transatlantic credentials. Joe Raine has decided to stand down before this fourth edition and in his place Joseph Wolfsdorf from Harvard University has joined the team, taking on the diabetes and hypoglycaemia chapters.

Despite the addition of two North American editors, the book remains rooted in UK practice but with increasing North American and global emphasis. The accumulation of more data to impart, particularly in the field of diabetes, has resulted in a slightly longer book but it nevertheless retains the spirit of user-friendliness and conciseness of Joe Raine's original vision.

As with previous editions, space has been given to describe the practical management of diabetes in detail. The trend towards consensus guidelines over the past decade is reflected in this new edition and at the end of each chapter there are sections on when to contact a specialist centre, controversial areas, transition, potential pitfalls, and future developments.

At the end of the chapters there are also four to five interesting cases which illustrate diagnostic difficulties and management choices. These 'grey cases' are intended to be helpful for those studying for postgraduate examinations.

The book is aimed primarily at paediatricians in general hospitals and at junior paediatric staff with an interest in paediatric endocrinology and diabetes. Nurses working in paediatric endocrinology wards, diabetic nurse specialists, and medical students should also find it useful. Three of the four editors (MD, JG, GVV) have been on the teaching faculty of the European Society for Paediatric Endocrinology (ESPE) Winter School. This experience has made us conscious of the practical difficulties encountered by doctors in resource-limited countries and we hope that the text of our book reflects this awareness.

Finally, we are delighted to welcome Johnny Deladoëy from Montreal, Canada, who has contributed a guest chapter on genomics for the paediatric endocrinologist, in recognition of the importance of the area to modern practice, and the need for trainees and clinicians to have a basic working knowledge of molecular diagnosis.

MDCD, JWG, GVV, JIW
December 2018

Acknowledgements

The authors would like to thank Dr David Neumann, Faculty of Medicine in Hradec Kralove and University Hospital Hradec, Czech Republic, Ms Karen Smith, Department of Biochemistry, Glasgow Royal Infirmary, Dr Jane McNeilly, Department of Biochemistry, Royal Hospital for Children, Glasgow, Dr Robert Lindsay, British Heart Foundation Cardiovascular Research Centre, Glasgow, Dr Heather Maxwell, Department of Nephrology, Royal Hospital for Children, Glasgow, Dr Jarod Wong, Glasgow University School of Medicine, Dr Avril Mason, Royal Hospital for Children, Glasgow, Dr Esther Kinning, West of Scotland Department of Medical Genetics, Glasgow, Dr Judith Simpson, Neonatal Department, Queen Elizabeth Hospital, Glasgow, Dr Renuka Dias, Birmingham Children's Hospital, Professor Michael Preece, Institute of Child Health, London, Professor Tim Cole, UCL Institute of Child Health, London, Professor Peter Hindmarsh, University College London Hospitals and Great Ormond Street Hospital for Children, London, Professor Martin Savage, London Clinic Centre for Endocrinology, Queen Mary, University of London, Professor Juliane Léger, Hôpital Universitaire Robert Debré, Paris, Professor Marc Nicolino, Hôpital Mère-Enfant de Lyon, France, Dr Asmahane Ladjouze, CHU Bab El Oued, Algiers, Algeria, Dr Philippe Campeau Medical Genetics Service, Hôpital Sainte-Justine, Montréal, Canada, and Dr Nina Ma, Boston Children's Hospital, USA, for their help and advice with different sections of the book.

Abbreviations

ACEI	angiotensin converting enzyme inhibitor
ACMG	American College of Medical Genetics
ACR	albumin:creatinine ratio
ACTH	adrenocorticotrophic hormone
AER	albumin excretion rate
AFP	alpha-foetoprotein
AHO	Albright's hereditary osteodystrophy
AIRE	autoimmune regulator
AIS	androgen insensitivity syndrome
ALD	adrenoleukodystrophy
ALS	acid-labile subunit
ALT	alanine amino transferase
AME	apparent mineralocorticoid excess
AMH	anti-Müllerian hormone
APECED	autoimmune polyendocrinopathy with endocrinopathy and cutaneous ectodermal dystrophy
AR	androgen receptor
ARB	angiotensin receptor blocker
ARDS	adult respiratory distress syndrome
ATA	American Thyroid Association
ATD	anti-thyroid drug
ATP	adenosine triphosphate
AVP	arginine-vasopressin
β-hCG	β-human chorionic gonadotrophin
BDR	background diabetic retinopathy
BMI	body mass index
BOHB	beta-hydroxybutyrate
BP	blood pressure
CAH	congenital adrenal hyperplasia
CAI	central adrenal insufficiency
CAIS	complete androgen insensitivity syndrome
cAMP	cyclic adenosine monophosphate
CBG	cortisol binding globulin
CDC	Centers for Disease Control and Prevention
CDGA	constitutional delay in growth and adolescence
CF	cystic fibrosis
CFRD	cystic fibrosis-related diabetes
CGH	comparative genomic hybridization
CGM	continuous glucose monitoring

cGy	centi-Gray units
CNS	central nervous system
CPEG	Canadian Pediatric Endocrine Group
CPP	central precocious puberty
CRH	corticotrophin-releasing hormone
CRP	C-reactive protein
CSII	continuous subcutaneous insulin infusion
CT	computerized tomography
CVD	cardiovascular disease
CYP	cytochrome P450
DAX-1	dosage-sensitive sex reversal adrenal hypoplasia critical region on chromosome X, gene 1
DCCT	Diabetes Control and Complications Trial
DDAVP	desamino-D-arginine-vasopression
DEND	developmental delay, epilepsy, diabetes mellitus
DEXA	dual X-ray absorptiometry
DHEAS	dehydroepiandrosterone sulphate
dHPLC	denaturing high-performance liquid chromatography
DHT	dihydrotestosterone
DI	diabetes insipidus
DIDMOAD	diabetes insipidus, diabetes mellitus, optic atrophy, and deafness
DIT	diiodotyrosine
DKA	diabetic ketoacidosis
DMD	Duchenne muscular dystrophy
DME	diabetic macular oedema
DNA	deoxyribonucleic acid
DNE	diabetes nurse educator
DNS	diabetes nurse specialist
DOC	deoxycorticosterone
DSD	differences in sex development
DUOX2	dual oxidase 2 enzymes
DXA	dual X-ray absorptiometry
DZ	dizygotic
ECF	extracellular fluid
ENaC	epithelial sodium channel
EPP	ectopic posterior pituitary
ER	endoplasmic reticulum

ESPE	European Society for Paediatric Endocrinology		JIA	juvenile idiopathic arthritis
ESR	erthyrocyte sedimentation rate		K	potassium
FASD	foetal alcohol spectrum disorder		LDL	low-density lipoprotein
FBC	full blood count		LDLR	low-density lipoprotein receptor
FFA	free fatty acids		LH	luteinizing hormone
FGD	familial glucocorticoid deficiency		MAF	minimum allele frequency
FGFR3	fibroblast growth factor receptor-3		MASS	mitral valve prolapse, aortic enlargement, skin and skeletal
FISH	fluorescent in situ hybridization		MC-1R	melanocortin-1 receptor
FNA	fine needle aspiration		MDI	multiple daily injections
FSH	follicle-stimulating hormone		MEN	multiple endocrine neoplasia
FT3	free triiodothyronine		MHC	major histocompatibility complex
FT4	free thyroxine		MIT	monoiodotyrosine
GABA	gamma-aminobutyric acid		MKRN3	Makorin ring finger protein 3
GAD	glutamic acid decarboxylase		MODY	maturity onset diabetes of the young
GC	guanine-cytosine		MPH	mid-parental height
GH	growth hormone		MR	mineralocorticoid receptor
GHBP	growth hormone binding protein		MRAP	melanocortin 2 receptor accessory protein
GHD	growth hormone deficiency			
GHRH	growth hormone releasing hormone		MRI	magnetic resonance imaging
GI	glycaemic index		MTC	medullary thyroid carcinoma
GNAS	G-protein stimulatory alpha subunit		MZ	monozygotic
GnRH	gonadotrophin-releasing hormone		NAFLD	non-alcoholic fatty liver disease
GP	general practitioner		NASH	non-alcoholic steatohepatitis
GSD 0	glycogen synthase deficiency		NC-21-OHD	non-classical 21-hydroxylase deficiency
GSD 1	glucose-6-phosphatase deficiency		NCHS	National Center for Health Statistics
HbA1c	glycosylated haemoglobin		NF	neurofibromatosis
hCG	human chorionic gonadotrophin		NGS	next generation sequencing
HDL	high-density lipoprotein		NHS	National Health Service
hGH	human growth hormone		NIS	sodium iodide symporter
HGVS	Human Genome Variation Society		NPH	neutral protamine Hagedorn
HHS	hyperglycaemic hyperosmolar state		OGTT	oral glucose tolerance test
HLA	human leukocyte antigen		PAIS	partial androgen insensitivity syndrome
HMG-CoA	3-hydroxy-3-methylglutaryl coenzyme A		PALS	paediatric advanced life support
H-P	hypothalamo-pituitary		PCOS	polycystic ovarian syndrome
HSD	hydroxysteroid dehydrogenase		PCR	polymerase chain reaction
IA2	insulinoma-associated antigen-2		PDR	proliferative diabetic retinopathy
	17-OHP 17-hydroxyprogesterone		PG	plasma glucose
1GF-1	insulin-like growth factor 1		PGA	polyglandular autoimmune
im	intramuscular		PHA	pseudohypoaldosteronism
IGFBP	insulin-like growth factor-binding protein		PHV	peak height velocity
			PNDM	permanent neonatal diabetes mellitus
INS	insulin gene locus		POMC	proopiomelanocortin
IQ	intelligence quotient		POR	P450-oxidoreductase
ISCN	International System for Human Cytogenetic Nomenclature		PPARγ	peroxisome proliferator-activated receptor gamma
ISPAD	International Society for Pediatric and Adolescent Diabetes		PPGL	phaeochromocytoma and paraganglioma
ISS	idiopathic short stature		PTH	parathyroid hormone
ITT	insulin-tolerance test		PTHrP	parathyroid hormone-related peptide
IUGR	intrauterine growth restriction		PTU	propylthiouracil
IV	intravenous		PUVA	psoralen plus ultraviolet A

PWS	Prader–Willi Syndrome	T3	triiodothyronine
RCPCH	Royal College of Paediatrics and Child Health	T4	thyroxine
		TBG	thyroid-binding globulin
RET	receptor tyrosine	TDD	total daily dose
RFLP	restriction length polymorphisms	td	three times a day
RNA	ribonucleic acid	TFT	thyroid function tests
sc	subcutaneous	Tg	thyroglobulin
SDS	standard deviation score	TH	transient hypothyroxinaemia
SED	spondylo-epiphyseal dysplasia	TNDM	transient neonatal diabetes mellitus
SF-1	steroidogenic factor 1	TPO	thyroid peroxidase
SGA	small for gestational age	TRH	thyrotrophin-releasing hormone
SHBG	sex hormone-binding globulin	TSH	thyroid-stimulating hormone
SHOX	Short Stature Homeobox	TSHR	thyroid-stimulating hormone receptor
SIADH	syndrome of inappropriate antidiuretic hormone secretion	TZD	thiazolidinedione
		U&E	urea and electrolytes
SMBG	self-monitoring of blood glucose	UIC	urinary iodine concentration
SOD	septo-optic dysplasia	UPD	uniparental disomy
SRY	sex-determining region of the Y chromosome	VO$_2$	peak oxygen consumption
		WBC	white blood cells
StAR	steroidogenic acute regulatory (protein) T3 triiodothyronine	WES	whole exome sequencing
		WHO	World Health Organization
SV 21-OHD	simple virilizing 21-hydroxylase deficiency	ZnT8A	zinc transporter 8
SW 21-OHD	salt-wasting 21 hydroxylase deficiency		

1

Diabetes Mellitus

Definition

Diabetes mellitus is a heterogeneous disorder characterized by abnormal metabolism of carbohydrate, fat and protein with persistent fasting or postprandial hyperglycaemia resulting from defects in insulin secretion or insulin action (Skyler et al. 2017). It is diagnosed in one of four ways (see Table 1.1) (American Diabetes 2018). A fasting plasma glucose (PG) of 5.6–6.9 mmol/L (100–125 mg/dL) is considered prediabetes, whereas <5.6 mmol/L (<100 mg/dL) is normal. The oral glucose tolerance test (OGTT) is not recommended for routine clinical use. When classic symptoms are present, the diagnosis is usually straightforward and an OGTT is seldom needed; however, an OGTT may be indicated when mild hyperglycaemia is discovered without symptoms (e.g. in the sibling of a child with diabetes or in children with disorders such as cystic fibrosis (CF) that predispose to diabetes and may be asymptomatic in the early stages).

The incidental discovery of hyperglycaemia without classic symptoms does not necessarily indicate new onset diabetes, especially in young children with an acute illness, who may experience 'stress hyperglycaemia'. The risk of eventually developing diabetes may be increased in some children with incidental or stress hyperglycaemia, especially those with immunologic, metabolic, or genetic markers for type 1 diabetes, and consultation with a paediatric endocrinologist is indicated.

Diabetes mellitus is classified on the basis of its pathogenesis (Table 1.2); it may be the result of severe insulin deficiency or insulin resistance or, more commonly, a combination of milder defects in insulin secretion and action (American Diabetes Association 2018). This chapter primarily focuses on type 1 diabetes, which is the commonest form of diabetes in children. Other causes of diabetes are discussed in Sections 1.21 and 1.24.

Incidence

The incidence of type 1 diabetes in children varies considerably across the world with the Scandinavian countries having the highest incidence; in Finland, 60

Practical Endocrinology and Diabetes in Children, Fourth Edition. Malcolm D.C. Donaldson, John W. Gregory, Guy Van Vliet, and Joseph I. Wolfsdorf.
© 2019 John Wiley & Sons Ltd. Published 2019 by John Wiley & Sons Ltd.

Table 1.1 Criteria for the diagnosis of diabetes mellitus.

1 Fasting plasma glucose ≥126 mg/dL (7 mmol/L)

or

2 Two-hour plasma glucose ≥200 mg/dL (11.1 mmol/L) during an oral glucose tolerance test (OGTT)[b]

or

3 Haemoglobin A_{1c} ≥6.5% (48 mmol/mol)

or

4 In a patient with classic hyperglycaemia symptoms or hyperglycaemic crisis, a random plasma glucose ≥200 mg/dL (11.1 mmol/L).

Definitions are based on venous plasma glucose levels. Glucose meters are useful for screening in clinics and physicians' offices, but the diagnosis of diabetes mellitus must be confirmed by measurement of venous plasma glucose on an analytic instrument in a clinical chemistry laboratory. In the absence of unequivocal hyperglycaemia, criteria 1 – 3 should be confirmed by repeat testing on a different day.
[a] Fasting is defined as no caloric intake for at least eight hours.
[b] OGTT should be performed using a glucose load containing the equivalent of 75 g anhydrous glucose dissolved in water.
[c] Haemoglobin A1c test should be performed in a laboratory using a method certified by the National Glycohemoglobin Standardization Program (www. ngsp.org).

Table 1.2 Protocol for and interpretation of the oral glucose tolerance test.

Indications
Confirmation of the diagnosis of diabetes mellitus in uncertain cases and diagnosis of impaired glucose tolerance

Preparation
Perform in the morning after fasting overnight for at least eight hours

Procedure
1 Pretest – plasma glucose sample

2 0 minute – administer oral glucose 1.75 g/kg (up to a maximum of 75 g) diluted with water (consume over 5–10 min.)

3 +2 hours – plasma glucose sample

Interpretation
1 Fasting plasma glucose >7.0 mmol/L (126 mg/dL) or 2 h concentration >11.1 mmol/L (200 mg/dL) are diagnostic of diabetes

2 2 h plasma glucose concentration >7.8 mmol/L (140 mg/dL) and <11.1 mmol/L (200 mg/dL) is impaired glucose tolerance

3 Fasting plasma glucose 6.1–6.9 mmol/L (100–125 mg/ dL) is impaired fasting glucose

An OGTT should be performed after at least three days of adequate carbohydrate consumption (≥150 g per 1.73 m²) and is performed using 1.75 g/kg anhydrous glucose dissolved in water for individuals ≤43 kg and 75 g for weight >43 kg.

new cases per 100 000 children under 15 years of age. The United Kingdom, Canada, the US, and Australia also have high incidences with more than 20 cases per 100 000 children, whereas Asia and Sub-Saharan Africa have much lower rates (China and India 0.1 cases per 100 000 people each year) (Patterson et al. 2014). The reasons for these large variations are unclear but may include genetic factors given the evidence of variations in the incidence of diabetes in different ethnic groups (e.g. in the US, the incidence is higher in non-Hispanic white than African-American or Hispanic youth). However, this difference cannot solely be attributed to genetic factors. In Europe, the risk of type 1 diabetes differs substantially in people who are genetically close but separated by socio-economic borders. Furthermore, over the past 30 years, the worldwide incidence has steadily increased across all age groups in parallel with an increased standard of living. A European population-based registry showed a 3.9% annual increase in the incidence of type 1 diabetes in children <15 years between 1989 and 2003 (5.4% in the 0–4 year age group) and the US

population-based SEARCH for Diabetes in Youth study has shown that the prevalence in people <20 years increased by 21% between 2001 and 2009.

With some exceptions, type 1 diabetes incidence is related to geographic distance north of the equator, and the onset of disease appears to be higher in autumn and winter than in spring and summer. Table 1.3 presents the American Diabetes Association Classification of Diabetes.

Type 1 diabetes is a chronic autoimmune disease caused by an incompletely understood complex interaction between risk-conferring genes and environmental factors resulting over time (years) in immune-mediated, selective destruction and loss of function of pancreatic β-cell mass. This leads to insulin deficiency, symptoms from hyperglycaemia, and lifelong insulin dependence (Insel et al. 2015). Symptoms occur when approximately two-thirds of the pancreatic islets are devoid of ß-cells.

Table 1.3 The American Diabetes Association classification of diabetes.

Type 1 diabetes caused by autoimmune-mediated ß-cell destruction (and idiopathic forms of β-cell dysfunction) usually leading to severe or absolute insulin deficiency

Type 2 diabetes caused by progressive loss of insulin secretion on a background of insulin resistance.

   Other specific causes of diabetes
   Monogenic diabetes syndromes such as neonatal diabetes and maturity-onset diabetes of the young (MODY)
   Diseases of the exocrine pancreas (such as cystic fibrosis)
   Drug- or chemical-induced diabetes such as with glucocorticoid use, drugs used for treatment of HIV/AIDS, or after organ transplantation

Gestational diabetes mellitus diabetes diagnosed in the second or third trimester of pregnancy that was not clearly overt diabetes prior to gestation

Although 90% of patients with type 1 diabetes do *not* have a family history of the disease, development of type 1 diabetes is strongly influenced by genetic factors. Children born into families with type 1 diabetes have different lifetime risks depending on whether the mother (6%), father (12%), or a sibling (5–10% by age 20 years) has the disease (Pociot and Lernmark 2016). If a twin develops type 1 diabetes, the lifetime risk for the non-affected dizygotic twin is 6–10%, whereas that for a monozygotic twin is approximately 60%.

Type 1 diabetes is a polygenic disorder; more than 50 susceptibility loci that contribute to the likelihood of developing type 1 diabetes have been identified. The major histocompatibility complex (MHC) region encoding the human leukocyte antigen (HLA) on chromosome 6p21 (the *IDDM1* locus) contributes about 50% of the genetic risk. The insulin gene locus (*INS*) is the second most important susceptibility locus, contributing about 10% of genetic susceptibility. Each of the loci identified through genome-wide association studies has a slight individual effect on the total genetic risk for progression to type 1 diabetes, and gene variants collectively explain ~80% of type 1 diabetes heritability (Pociot and Lernmark 2016).

Most of the loci associated with risk of type 1 diabetes are thought to involve immune responses (Concannon et al. 2009), supporting the notion that genetic influences involve mechanisms that collectively contribute to aberrant immune responsiveness.

Genetic susceptibility might also influence responses to environmental stimuli, modify viral responses or physiological pathways. For most of the genetic loci, however, the molecular mechanism of action remains unknown.

Newborn screening has been used to identify children at increased genetic risk who have been followed for the appearance of autoantibodies against ß-cell autoantigens: insulin, glutamic acid decarboxylase (GAD), insulinoma-associated antigen-2 (IA2), and zinc transporter 8 (ZnT8A) that are known to be strongly associated with an increased risk for type 1 diabetes. These autoantibodies can appear as early as age six months, with a peak incidence in the second year of life in genetically susceptible individuals, i.e. they are present months to years before the onset of symptoms. Children who develop two or more islet autoantibodies have a markedly increased likelihood of eventually developing type 1 diabetes, and 100% of those who develop a third and, often, a fourth autoantibody develop clinical type 1 diabetes when followed for 20 years (Ziegler et al. 2013). At the time of diagnosis, more than 90% of individuals with type 1 diabetes have at least one autoantibody, and the presence of autoantibodies against ß-cell autoantigens is a key feature distinguishing type 1 from type 2 diabetes.

Type 1 diabetes is also associated with other autoimmune disorders, most commonly autoimmune thyroiditis. At the time of diagnosis, about 25% of children have thyroid autoantibodies, which predict thyroid dysfunction (most commonly hypothyroidism); Graves' disease occurs in ~0.5% of patients with type 1 diabetes. Addison's disease, likewise, occurs in approximately 0.5% of patients with type 1 diabetes. Coeliac disease is another immune-mediated disorder that occurs with increased frequency in patients with type 1 diabetes, and biopsy-confirmed coeliac disease occurs in 3.5% of individuals with type 1 diabetes compared with 0.3–1% in the general population.

Environment

The increase in incidence described above can only be explained by changes in environment or lifestyle and it is notable that migrants tend to acquire the same risk of type 1 diabetes as the native population in their new area of residence (Rewers and Ludvigsson 2016). Studies of prospective birth cohorts are attempting to identify potential triggers of islet autoimmunity and the natural history of progression to diabetes. Putative triggers include infections, diet, and toxins that affect children in utero, perinatally, or during early childhood. See Rewers and Ludvigsson (2016) for a review of this topic.

Vaccines

There has been speculation that vaccines might trigger autoimmunity; however, no association has been detected with islet autoimmunity or type 1 diabetes, and a recent meta-analysis concluded that childhood vaccines do not increase the risk of type 1 diabetes (Morgan et al. 2016).

Idiopathic type 1 diabetes

Some forms of type 1 diabetes have no known aetiology. Most patients with idiopathic type 1 diabetes are of African or Asian ancestry. They have permanent insulinopenia and are prone to episodic ketoacidosis, but have no evidence of beta-cell autoimmunity (negative islet autoantibodies). This form of diabetes is strongly inherited but not HLA-associated. Between episodes, patients exhibit varying degrees of insulin deficiency and may intermittently need insulin replacement.

Biochemistry

Insulin is an anabolic hormone that acts on liver, fat, and skeletal muscle to increase glucose uptake, oxidation, and storage, and to decrease glucose production. Insulin also inhibits lipolysis and thereby limits the availability of fatty acids for oxidation and inhibits ketogenesis. Insulin is secreted in two major patterns – basal and in response to food (prandial). Basal secretion produces relatively constant, low plasma insulin levels that restrain lipolysis and hepatic glucose production (from glycogenolysis and gluconeogenesis). The blood glucose concentration is the dominant stimulus for insulin secretion. After a meal, in parallel with the rise in plasma glucose, circulating insulin concentrations rise rapidly, facilitating the entry of glucose into cells via glucose-specific transporters, particularly in skeletal muscle and adipose tissue. Insulin stimulates glycogen synthesis in the liver and skeletal muscle, inhibits hepatic gluconeogenesis, and stimulates fat storage and protein synthesis. Conversely, during fasting, plasma glucose concentrations and insulin secretion decrease, leading to reduced glucose uptake in muscle and adipose tissue, increased lipolysis, and stimulation of hepatic glucose production (from glycogenolysis and gluconeogenesis (Figure 1.1).

In type 1 diabetes, insulin deficiency results in hyperglycaemia and when the plasma glucose concentration exceeds the renal threshold for glucose reabsorption (~180 mg/dL or 10 mmol/L) osmotic diuresis occurs, causing polyuria and polydipsia. Insulin deficiency also causes increased lipolysis with the production of excess free fatty acids and ketoacids (beta-hydroxybutyrate (BOHB) and acetoacetate) leading to hyperketonaemia and ketonuria. When fluid losses exceed intake, particularly when nausea and vomiting occur (typical symptoms of ketosis), dehydration develops. The accumulation of ketoacids in the blood causes metabolic acidosis, which results in compensatory rapid, deep breathing (Kussmaul respiration). Acetone, formed from acetoacetate, accounts for the characteristic smell of the breath (described as the odour of nail polish remover or rotten fruit). Accompanying the lack of insulin is an increase in the levels of stress or counter-regulatory hormones (glucagon, catecholamines, cortisol, and growth hormone) whose metabolic actions are opposite to those of insulin. Thus, a lack of insulin together with increased concentrations of counter-regulatory hormones leads to progressive hyperglycaemia, hyperfattyacidemia, and ketosis and eventually ketoacidosis. Progressive dehydration, acidosis, and hyperosmolality cause decreased consciousness and lead to coma and death if untreated.

Clinical presentation

History

At diagnosis, typical symptoms have usually been present for only a few days to about two weeks or longer especially in type 2 diabetes:

- Polyuria (may cause secondary nocturnal enuresis)
- Polydipsia
- Weight loss
- Anorexia or hyperphagia
- Lethargy
- Constipation
- Infection (especially perineal candidiasis)
- Blurred vision
- Muscle cramps

Although most school-aged children report polyuria and polydipsia, these symptoms may be less obvious in the very young child (e.g. an infant in diapers) in whom the other less characteristic symptoms, especially perineal candidiasis, may predominate.

Clinical manifestations of diabetic ketoacidosis (DKA) include:

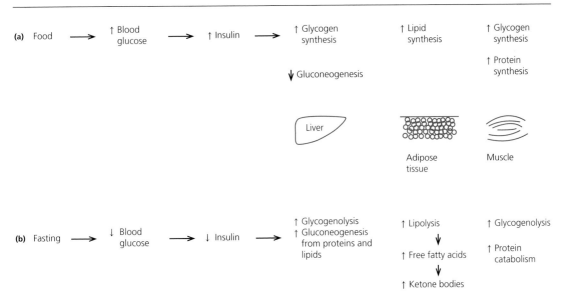

Figure 1.1 Glucose homeostasis: a comparison of (a) the fed state and (b) the fasting state.

- Dehydration
- Tachypnea; deep, sighing (Kussmaul) respiration
- Nausea, vomiting, and abdominal pain that may mimic an acute abdominal condition
- Drowsiness, confusion, progressive obtundation, and loss of consciousness.

Note that symptoms of systemic infection are infrequent; however, one must carefully look for an infection, especially if there is fever.

Examination

Patients with DKA typically are dehydrated. Clinical estimation of the degree of dehydration is imprecise and generally shows only fair to moderate agreement among examiners. The most useful signs for predicting 5% dehydration in young children are:
- prolonged capillary refill time (normal capillary refill is ≤1.5–2 seconds);
- abnormal skin turgor ('tenting' or inelastic skin).

Other useful signs to assess degree of dehydration include: dry mucous membranes, sunken eyes, absent tears, weak pulses, and cool extremities. More signs of dehydration tend to be associated with more severe dehydration; ≥10% dehydration is suggested by the presence of weak or impalpable peripheral pulses, hypotension, cool extremities, and oliguria.

Children diagnosed with diabetes should be immediately referred to a hospital for evaluation and management.

Differential diagnosis

The diagnosis of type 1 diabetes usually is obvious because the patient has classical symptoms (polyuria, polydipsia, and weight loss), random blood glucose is >11 mmol/L (200 mg/dL) and there is glucosuria with or without ketonuria. Diabetes should also be considered in the differential diagnosis of any child presenting with impaired consciousness and/or acidosis.

Tachypnea and hyperventilation in DKA may lead to the erroneous diagnosis of pneumonia or bronchiolitis. The lack of a cough or wheeze and the absence of abnormal findings on auscultation of the chest and a normal chest radiograph should raise the possibility of a metabolic acidosis such as DKA as the cause of tachypnea. Abdominal pain and tenderness in DKA may suggest a surgical emergency such as appendicitis or acute pancreatitis. Fluid, electrolytes, and insulin therapy will ameliorate the abdominal symptoms within hours. Diabetes should always be considered in children with secondary nocturnal enuresis and those with recurrent or persistent perineal candidiasis.

Acute illnesses such as severe sepsis or a prolonged convulsion may, occasionally, cause hyperglycaemia, glycosuria, and ketonuria. However, these biochemical abnormalities are almost always transient and are rarely associated with a history of previous polydipsia and polyuria. If in doubt, a fasting blood glucose measurement or OGTT (see Table 1.1) should be performed.

A doctor who either suspects or has made a definitive diagnosis of diabetes should immediately refer the child to a specialist for comprehensive assessment and initiation of treatment.

Investigations

At diagnosis, perform the following investigations:
- Plasma glucose concentration;
- Plasma BOHB concentration;
- Serum electrolytes, urea and creatinine concentrations (basic metabolic profile);
- Venous blood gas measurement;
- Complete blood count; note that leukocytosis and a raised C-reactive protein are common in DKA and do not necessarily indicate that an infection is present; an increased haematocrit reflects the degree of extracellular fluid (ECF) loss.
- A minority of children will have evidence of sepsis and need appropriate investigations (e.g. blood culture, chest radiograph, urine microscopy, and culture).
- HbA1c (glycated haemoglobin) is not necessary for initial management, but provides useful information about the duration and severity of antecedent hyperglycaemia.

The criteria for diagnosis of DKA are: plasma glucose ≥200 mg dL (11.1 mmol/L), venous pH < 7.30 or serum bicarbonate <15 mmol/L and 'moderate' or 'large' ketonuria, or serum BOHB ≥3 mmol/L (Wolfsdorf et al. 2018).

Initial management of newly diagnosed type 1 diabetes

Management of the child presenting without ketoacidosis

Hospitalization vs. Outpatient (home) treatment
The goals of initial management of the child with newly diagnosed diabetes mellitus are to restore the fluid and electrolyte balance, to stabilize the metabolic state with insulin, and to provide basic diabetes education and self-management training for the child (when age and developmentally appropriate) and caregivers (parents, grandparents, guardians, older siblings, daycare providers, and babysitters).

The diagnosis of diabetes in a child is a crisis for the family, who require considerable emotional support and time for adjustment and healing. Shocked, grieving, and overwhelmed parents require time to acquire basic ('survival') skills while they are coping with the emotional upheaval that typically follows the diagnosis of diabetes in a child. Even if they are not acutely ill, and depending on local resources and practices, children with newly diagnosed type 1 diabetes may be admitted to hospital to initiate insulin treatment and for diabetes education and self-management training. Outpatient or home-based management is preferred by some centres that have the requisite resources, in particular, the availability of travelling diabetes nurses who will need to visit at least daily in the first few days and maintain regular telephone contact, often outside normal working hours (Lowes and Gregory 2004). The size of the geographical area that needs to be covered is an important consideration. Outpatient or home-based management may have several advantages: the stress of a hospital stay is avoided, the outpatient setting or patient's home is a more natural learning environment for the child and family, and ambulatory treatment reduces the cost of care. Where adequate outpatient and/or home initial management of type 1 diabetes at diagnosis can be provided, studies have shown there is no disadvantage in terms of metabolic control nor increase in acute complications, hospitalizations, psychosocial or behavioural problems or total costs. The decision concerning whether a child with newly diagnosed diabetes should be admitted to hospital depends on several factors: most important are the severity of the child's metabolic derangements, the family's psychosocial circumstances, and the resources available at the treatment centre. Many paediatric diabetes centres offer ambulatory care and provide diabetes education and training in a day care unit for several days following diagnosis.

Hospital admission is necessary if intravenous (IV) therapy is required to correct dehydration, electrolyte imbalance, and ketoacidosis or if there are psychosocial challenges. Children who are ≤5% dehydrated, not nauseous or vomiting, who are not particularly unwell, and have a pH ≥7.30 usually respond well to subcutaneous insulin and oral rehydration.

Outpatient diabetes care

The diabetes team
Optimal care of children with type 1 diabetes is complex and time-consuming. Children with diabetes should be managed by a multidisciplinary diabetes team, which provides diabetes education and care in collaboration with the child's primary care physician. The team should consist of a paediatric endocrinologist or paediatrician with training in diabetes

management, a paediatric diabetes nurse educator (DNE) or diabetes nurse specialist (advanced practice nurse), a dietitian trained in paediatric diabetes nutrition, and a mental health professional (a clinical psychologist or medical social worker). The diabetes team should always be available by telephone to provide guidance and support to parents and patients and to respond to metabolic crises that require immediate intervention.

Initial diabetes education

Education is the foundation of diabetes care and is vital to ensure successful outcomes. Diabetes education provides the knowledge and skills needed to perform diabetes self-care and make the lifestyle changes required to successfully manage the disease. The diabetes education curriculum should be adapted to the individual child and family. Parents and children with newly diagnosed diabetes are usually anxious and overwhelmed and frequently cannot assimilate a large amount of abstract information. Therefore, the education programme should be staged. Initial educational goals should be limited to basic skills so that the child can be safely cared for at home and return to his or her daily routine as soon as possible. Initial diabetes education and self-management training should include: understanding what causes diabetes, how it is treated, how to measure and administer insulin, basic concepts of meal planning, self-monitoring of blood glucose (SMBG) and ketones, recognition, and treatment of hypoglycaemia, and how and when to contact a member of the diabetes team for advice.

Main topics for discussion following diagnosis

If several members of the diabetes team are involved in educating the newly diagnosed child and his or her family, good communication between team members to ensure consistency in the messaging and the specific information given is important. The following topics should be included in the curriculum and discussed with the child and family over a period of several weeks or months following diagnosis:

- Assessment of the family's pre-existing knowledge of diabetes.
- Current knowledge of the cause of diabetes.
- The consequences of having diabetes and its lifelong implications.
- The concept of the 'diabetes team' of professionals who will be involved in the child's care.
- The role of insulin in type 1 diabetes management.

- Practical details of insulin injections.
- When and how to monitor and interpret blood glucose concentrations.
- When and how to measure blood or urinary ketone concentrations.
- Advice about the crucial role of nutrition.
- The effect of exercise on carbohydrate and insulin requirements.
- The causes and consequences of hypoglycaemia and how to treat it.
- Management of diabetes during intercurrent illness ('sick days').
- The 'honeymoon period' of stable glycaemia and reduced insulin requirements following diagnosis.
- Long-term microvascular complications.
- Who to contact in an emergency (including phone numbers).
- Details of outpatient follow-up.
- The importance of always having identification (e.g. medical bracelet) indicating that the person has diabetes.
- Additional sources of information about diabetes.
- Availability of support groups.
- Health insurance issues, sources of and entitlement to financial assistance.
- Future developments.

Requirements on discharge from hospital

The child's primary care physician should be informed of the child's diagnosis, management plan, and discharge from hospital, and the diabetes nurse should communicate with the school nurse or daycare facility to ensure that details of the care plan are in place and understood. The equipment that a child will need on discharge is shown in Table 1.4.

Continuing diabetes education and long-term supervision of diabetes care

When the child is medically stable and parents (and other care providers) have mastered basic diabetes management skills, the child is discharged from the hospital or ambulatory treatment centre. In the first few weeks after diagnosis, frequent telephone contact provides emotional support and helps parents to interpret the results of blood glucose monitoring and, when necessary, insulin doses are adjusted to achieve blood glucose levels in a defined target range. Within a few weeks of diagnosis, many children enter a partial remission (the 'honeymoon' phase), evidenced by normal or near-normal blood glucose levels on a low

Table 1.4 Supplies required at time of discharge.

Lancing device and lancets

Blood glucose meter and test strips

Blood ketone meter and ketone strips or urine ketone test strips

Oral glucose tablets and gel

Glucagon emergency kit

Sharps container

Literature on diabetes management and how to obtain a Medic Alert bracelet/necklace

Pen insulin delivery system, disposable pre-filled pens, or syringes with needles for insulin injections

Insulin cartridges for non-disposable pen-delivery system or insulin vials

Rapid-acting and long- or intermediate-acting insulin (depending on insulin regimen)

Alcohol swabs

Needle clipper

dose (<0.25 U/kg/day) of insulin. By this time, most patients and parents are less anxious, have mastered basic diabetes management skills through repetition and experience, and are now more prepared to begin to learn the intricate details of intensive diabetes management. At this stage, the diabetes team should begin to provide patients and parents with the knowledge they will need to maintain optimal glycaemic control while coping with the effects of exercise, varying food intake, intercurrent illnesses, and the other challenges that normally occur in a child's daily life.

In addition to teaching facts and practical skills, education should promote desirable health beliefs and attitudes in the young person with a chronic incurable disease. For some children, this may be best accomplished in a non-traditional educational setting, such as a summer camp for children with diabetes. The educational curriculum must be concordant with the child's level of cognitive development and has to be adapted to the learning style and literacy and numeracy skills of the individual child and family. Parents, grandparents, older siblings, the school nurse, and other important people in the child's life are encouraged to participate in the diabetes education programme so they can actively share in the diabetes care and ensure that the child with diabetes is not excluded from normal childhood activities (sports, field trips, sleepovers, etc.).

In the first month after diagnosis, the patient and care providers are seen frequently by the diabetes team to review and consolidate the diabetes education and practical skills learned in the first few days and to extend the scope of diabetes self-management training. Thereafter, follow-up visits with members of the diabetes team should occur at least every three months. Regular clinic visits are necessary to ensure that the child's diabetes is being appropriately managed and the goals of therapy are being met. A focused history should obtain information about self-care behaviours, the child's daily routines, the frequency, severity, and circumstances surrounding hypoglycaemic events, details about insulin doses, and blood glucose monitoring data should be reviewed to identify patterns and trends. At each visit, height and weight are measured and plotted on a growth chart. The weight curve is especially helpful in assessing the adequacy of therapy. Significant weight loss usually indicates that the prescribed insulin dose is insufficient or the patient is not receiving all the prescribed doses of insulin. A complete physical examination should be performed at least once or twice each year focusing on blood pressure, stage of puberty, evidence of thyroid disease, examination of the injection sites for evidence of lipohypertrophy (from over-use of the site) or lipoatrophy, and mobility of the joints of the hands.

Each clinic visit provides an opportunity to reinforce the individual patient's blood glucose targets and HbA1c goal, and to increase the patient's and the family's understanding of diabetes management, the interplay of insulin, food, and exercise, and their impact on blood glucose levels. As the child's cognitive development progresses, the child should become more involved in diabetes management and increasingly assume *supervised* age-appropriate responsibility for daily self-care. Parents are encouraged to contact the diabetes team for advice if the pattern of blood glucose levels changes between routine visits, suggesting the need to adjust insulin doses or change the regimen. Eventually, when parents and patients have sufficient knowledge and experience to interpret blood glucose patterns and trends, they are encouraged to independently adjust insulin doses.

Psychosocial aspects of diabetes management

The diagnosis of diabetes in a child or adolescent hurls parents into a frightening and foreign world. They grieve the loss of their healthy child and have to cope with normal distress reactions, including shock, disbelief and denial, fear, anxiety, anger, and blame or guilt. During this emotionally intense time, parents are expected to rapidly acquire an understanding of the disease and manage the illness at home. Parents should receive the necessary support to begin coping with their emotional distress and not be overwhelmed by unrealistic expectations from a well-meaning diabetes treatment team.

Diabetes also presents family members with the task of being sensitive to the balance between the child's need for a sense of autonomy and mastery of self-care activities and the need for ongoing family support and involvement. The struggle to balance independence and dependence in relationships between the child and family members presents a long-term challenge and raises different issues for families at different stages of child and adolescent development. Focusing on normal developmental tasks at each stage of the child's growth and development provides the most effective structure to address this concern (Anderson et al. 2009).

A medical social worker or clinical psychologist should perform an initial psychosocial assessment of all newly diagnosed patients to identify families at high risk who need additional services. Thereafter, patients are referred to a mental health specialist when emotional, social, environmental, or financial concerns are suspected or identified that interfere with the ability to maintain acceptable diabetes control. Some of the more common problems in families who have a child with diabetes include parental guilt, resulting in poor adherence to the treatment regimen, difficulty coping with the child's frustration and rebellion against treatment, fear of hypoglycaemia, anxiety, depression, missed appointments, financial hardship, or loss of health insurance affecting the ability to attend scheduled clinic appointments and/or purchase supplies. Patients with poor glycaemic control and a history of frequent emergency department visits should be screened for depressed mood (Lawrence et al. 2006). Recurrent ketoacidosis is the most extreme indicator of psychosocial stress, and management of such patients must include a comprehensive psychosocial assessment.

Because childhood is characterized by cognitive and emotional immaturity, successful treatment of paediatric diabetes requires the continuous, active involvement of responsible adults. Moreover, diabetes treatment occurs within a family dynamic, and treatment-related conflicts are common, arising in part from a natural discord in goals between caretakers and the child. Each phase of childhood has unique characteristics that complicate treatment; for example, the normally erratic eating behaviour of toddlers and the unscheduled intense physical play of school-aged children that can hinge on unpredictable factors, such as the weather. Adolescence is characterized by multiple physiologic and psychosocial factors that make glycaemic control even more challenging. Diabetes treatment should be individually tailored to each child, based on age, family resources, cognitive ability, the schedule and activities of the child and family, and their goals and desires.

Rates of psychological ill health in youth with diabetes are high, and longitudinal data indicate that mental health issues in childhood are likely to persist into early adulthood and are prognostic of maladaptive lifestyle practices, long-term problems with diabetes control and earlier-than-expected onset of complications. For these reasons, mental health screening should be routinely performed in diabetes clinics. Screening for behavioural disturbance should begin in children at the time of diagnosis, with further assessment of parental mental health and family functioning for those children identified to be 'at risk'. Interventions can then be targeted based on the specific needs of individual children and families. Additional psychological support is often provided by diabetes nurses and other parents at local and national support groups.

Diabetes Control and Complications Trial (DCCT)

This clinical trial, completed in 1993, proved that near-normal glycaemia delays the onset and slows the progression of microvascular complications, and it set the current standards for treatment of type 1 diabetes. A total of 1441 subjects with diabetes aged 13–39 years were randomized either: (i) to continue with their conventional treatment; or (ii) to receive intensive therapy with increased support from the 'diabetes team' and insulin administered either by three or more injections daily or by a pump (The Diabetes Control and Complications Trial Research Group 1993). After a mean duration of 6.5 years, as compared with conventional therapy, intensive treatment resulted in a reduction in:

- mean HbA1c concentration of nearly 2% (22 mmol/mol);
- the risk of retinopathy by 76%;
- the occurrence of microalbuminuria by 39%;
- the occurrence of neuropathy by 60%.

For every 10% reduction in HbA1c (e.g. 8% vs. 7.2%), there was a 44% reduction in the risk of microvascular complications.

Intensive treatment using the insulin preparations available at the time (i.e. before the development of insulin analogues) was associated with a two-to-threefold increase in severe hypoglycaemia and a mean weight gain of 4.6 kg when compared with conventional treatment. This study clearly demonstrated that near-normal glycaemia (as measured by HbA1c) significantly reduced the risk of microvascular complications. In the 25 years since the results of this landmark study were announced, the challenge for clinicians has been to implement the principles of intensive diabetes therapy in children and adolescents in routine clinical practice.

Goals of therapy

The International Society for Pediatric and Adolescent Diabetes (ISPAD) recommends a target HbA1c of <7.5% (58 mmol/mol) for all age groups (DiMeglio et al. 2018). However, biochemical goals should be individualized, taking into account both medical and psychosocial considerations; i.e. each child should have individually determined targets with the goal of achieving an HbA1c value as close to normal as possible while avoiding frequent episodes of mild to moderate hypoglycaemia and severe hypoglycaemia. Less stringent treatment goals may be appropriate or more realistic for preschool-aged children, children with developmental handicaps, psychosocial challenges, lack of appropriate family support, children who have experienced severe hypoglycaemia, or those with hypoglycaemia unawareness.

Insulin therapy in type 1 diabetes

Initial insulin therapy

At the time of diagnosis, many children with type 1 diabetes are severely insulin-deficient and require insulin replacement to survive. The aim of insulin replacement therapy is to simulate normal plasma insulin patterns as closely as possible. Truly physiologic insulin replacement continues to be an elusive goal owing to: (i) delivery of insulin into the systemic circulation instead of the portal venous system, and (ii) the inability to mimic the first and second phases of normal insulin release in response to eating. Insulin pump therapy or multiple daily insulin (MDI) injections currently are the two methods that most closely mimic normal insulin secretion.

The *ideal* regimen for the newly diagnosed patient is a multiple dose, flexible basal-bolus regimen that provides basal insulin throughout the day and night and insulin boluses before meals and snacks. Rapid-acting insulin is injected approximately 15 minutes before eating; individual doses are adjusted meal-to-meal based on preprandial blood glucose values, anticipated meal macronutrient content, and physical activity. Practical considerations are vitally important when selecting an insulin regimen for a child with type 1 diabetes. Socio-economic circumstances, parental health literacy and numeracy, patient's age, supervision of care, ability and willingness to self-administer insulin several times each day, and difficulty maintaining long-term adherence, all conspire to make physiologic insulin replacement challenging. For these reasons, there is no universal insulin regimen that can be successfully used for *all* children with type 1 diabetes. The diabetes team must design an insulin regimen that meets the needs of the individual patient and is acceptable to the patient and family members(s) responsible for administering insulin to the child or supervising its administration.

The route of insulin administration initially is determined by the severity of the child's condition at presentation. Insulin is usually given intravenously for treatment of DKA; whereas insulin may be administered subcutaneously when children are metabolically stable without vomiting or significant dehydration and ketosis. Whenever appropriate, the newly diagnosed child should commence insulin replacement therapy with a flexible basal-bolus regimen. In some healthcare systems, it is now possible to start insulin pump therapy at the time of diagnosis regardless of the severity of presentation or age of the child.

Three major categories of insulin preparations, classified according to their time course of action, are available (Table 1.5) and various insulin replacement regimens consisting of a mixture of short- or rapid-acting insulin and intermediate- or long-acting insulin are used in children and adolescents, typically given at least two to four (or more) times daily.

Insulin analogues

Rapid-acting insulin analogues incorporate amino acid substitutions, which make them quickly dissociate into monomers following injection and are then rapidly absorbed. Compared with short-acting regular insulin, they produce lower postprandial glucose excursions.

Table 1.5 Types of insulin preparations and approximate insulin action profiles.

Insulin type	Onset of action (h)	Peak of action (h)	Effective duration of action (h)
Rapid-acting analogues			
Aspart, lispro, glulisine	0.25–0.5	1–3	3–5
Regular insulin	0.5–1	2–4	5–8
Intermediate-acting insulin			
Neutral Protamine Hagedorn (NPH), isophane	2–4	4–10	10–16
Long-acting analogues			
Detemir	2–4	None	12–20[a]
Glargine	2–4	None	20–24
Degludec	2–4	None	24–42
Premixed combinations			
50% NPH, 50% regular	0.5–1	dual	10–16
50% NPL, 50% lispro	0.25	dual	10–16
70% NPH, 30% regular	0.5–1	dual	10–16
70% PA, 30% aspart	0.25	dual	15–18
75% NPL, 25% lispro	0.25	dual	10–16

PA, protamine-crystallized insulin aspart suspension; NPL, neutral protamine lispro suspension. PA + soluble aspart and NPL + lispro are both stable pre-mixed combinations of intermediate- and rapid-acting insulins.

The human insulins and insulin analogues are available in vials, pre-filled disposable pen injectors, and cartridges for non-disposable pen injectors.

These data are approximations from studies in adult test subjects. The times of onset, peak, and effective duration of action vary within and between patients and are affected by numerous factors, including size of dose, site and depth of injection, dilution, exercise, temperature, regional blood flow, local tissue reactions.

[a] Dose-dependent; 12 hours for 0.2 U/kg; 20–24 hours for ≥0.4 U/kg.

The three long-acting insulin analogues are characterized by a relatively consistent and prolonged release of insulin without distinct peaks. Insulin glargine has a prolonged duration of action (22–24 hours) and can be injected at any time of day, but is usually given with dinner or at bedtime. The duration of action of insulin detemir is partly dependent on the dose – small doses may last only 12 hours; therefore, it usually has to be injected twice daily. Insulin degludec is an ultra-long-acting insulin with a flat, stable profile at steady state and a duration of action exceeding 24 hours and up to 42 hours. There is some evidence that both glargine and detemir lead to a decrease in the incidence of hypoglycaemia including nocturnal hypoglycaemia. Table 1.6 shows suggested starting total daily insulin dose (units per kg per day).

While clinical trials comparable to the Diabetes Control and Complications Trial (DCCT) have not been conducted in prepubertal children, it is logical to extrapolate that prepubertal children will also benefit from near-normal glycaemic control. Intensive treatment regimens (MDI injections or insulin pump) are

Table 1.6 Suggested starting total daily insulin dose (units per kg per day).

	No DKA at presentation	DKA at presentation
<6 years or HbA1c <7%	0.15–0.25	0.5–0.75
Prepuberty	0.25–0.5	0.75–1
Puberty	0.5–0.75	1–1.2
Postpuberty	0.25–0.5	0.75–1

the preferred form of therapy for all patients with type 1 diabetes. Insulin regimens based on one or two daily injections cannot achieve optimal glycaemic control in type 1 diabetes except during the remission ('honeymoon') period, and may incur a greater risk of hypoglycaemia. These regimens, including the use of pre-mixed combination insulins, should only be used when insurmountable barriers preclude the use of a multiple dose insulin regimen.

Split-mixed insulin regimens

When a *two-dose regimen* is used, the total daily dose (TDD) is typically divided as follows: two-thirds before breakfast and one-third is given in the evening. The relative proportion of rapid- or short-acting insulin to intermediate-acting insulin depends on the pre-meal blood glucose value and the carbohydrate content of meals. It is common to start by giving one-third of the pre-breakfast dose as rapid- or short-acting insulin and two-thirds as neutral protamine Hagedorn (NPH), and a similar ratio before dinner. For example, if the TDD for a 30-kg child is 0.75 unit kg (22.5 units): a mixed dose injected before breakfast would consist of 5 units of rapid-acting and 10 units NPH; the pre-dinner dose would be 2.5 units rapid-acting and 5 units NPH. Regular insulin should be injected at least 30 minutes before eating; rapid-acting insulin (lispro, aspart, glulisine) is given 15 minutes before eating.

The optimal ratio of rapid- or short-acting to inter-mediate- or long-acting insulin for each patient is determined empirically, guided by the results of frequent blood glucose monitoring. At least five daily blood glucose measurements are required to determine the effects of each component of the insulin regimen: before each meal, before the bedtime snack, and once overnight between midnight and 4 a.m. Parents are taught to look for patterns of hyperglycaemia or hypoglycaemia that indicate the need for a dose adjustment. Adjustments are made to individual components of the insulin regimen, usually in 5–10% increments or decrements, in response to patterns of consistently elevated (above the defined target range for several consecutive days) or unexplained low blood glucose levels, respectively. The insulin dose is adjusted until satisfactory blood glucose control is achieved, i.e. at least 50% of blood glucose values are in or close to the child's target range.

At the time of diagnosis, most children have some residual beta-cell function and within several days to a few weeks often enter a period of partial remission ('the honeymoon period'), during which normal or nearly normal glycaemia is achieved with a low dose of insulin. At this stage, the dose of insulin must be reduced to prevent hypoglycaemia, but should not be discontinued. As destruction of the remaining beta-cells occurs over time, the insulin requirement increases ('the intensification phase'), eventually reaching a full replacement dose. The average daily insulin dose in prepubertal children with long-standing diabetes is approximately 0.6–0.8 units/kg/day, and in adolescents 1–1.2 units/kg/day. Obese patients usually are insulin-resistant and require relatively higher TDDs, e.g. overweight or obese adolescents may require up to 1.5 units/kg/day.

Beyond the remission period it is seldom possible without a regimented lifestyle and rigid adherence to a meal plan to achieve near-normal glycaemia with two injections per day and without incurring a greater risk of hypoglycaemia, especially overnight. An important limitation of a two dose 'split-mixed' regimen is that the peak effect of the pre-dinner intermediate-acting insulin (isophane, NPH) tends to occur at the time of lowest insulin requirement (i.e. from midnight to 4 a.m.), increasing the risk of nocturnal hypoglycaemia (Figure 1.2). Thereafter, insulin action decreases from 4 a.m. to 8 a.m., when basal insulin requirements normally increase. Consequently, the tendency for blood glucose levels to rise before breakfast ('the dawn phenomenon') is compounded by the waning insulin effect before breakfast and/or by counter-regulatory hormones secreted in response to a fall in blood glucose levels during sleep, resulting in post-hypoglycaemic hyperglycaemia (the Somogyi phenomenon, see Section 1.7.7.2).

A *three-dose insulin regimen* with mixed short- or rapid- and intermediate-acting insulin before breakfast, only short- or rapid-acting insulin before dinner, and intermediate- or long-acting acting insulin at bedtime, may ameliorate these problems (Figure 1.2). The peak action of the morning dose of NPH occurring at midday may eliminate the need for a dose of rapid-acting insulin at lunchtime (provided lunch does not contain excessive carbohydrate), and this may be necessary in circumstances where nobody is available to administer a pre-lunch dose of rapid-acting insulin to a young child. Insulin regimens that employ intermediate-acting insulin demand consistency in the daily dietary regimen, both with respect to the amounts and timing of food consumed at each meal and snack, and the timing of insulin injections. Furthermore, owing to the time and duration of its peak action, NPH insulin given at bedtime is associated with increased frequency of nocturnal hypoglycaemia as compared to long-acting, 'peakless' basal insulin analogues.

Basal-bolus regimens and continuous subcutaneous insulin infusion (CSII)

Flexible basal-bolus insulin regimens utilize MDI (Figure 1.3) or continuous subcutaneous insulin infusion (CSII) with an insulin pump (Figure 1.3). Flexible regimens more closely simulate normal diurnal insulin profiles, overcome many of the

Split-Mixed Insulin regimen

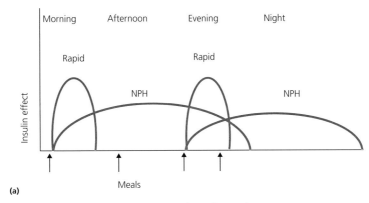

(a)

Split-Mixed Insulin Regimen

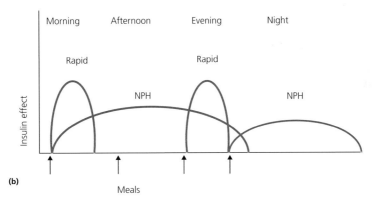

(b)

Figure 1.2 Schematic representations of commonly used insulin regimens. (a) Idealized insulin action profiles provided by a regimen consisting of twice-daily mixtures of rapid-acting insulin and intermediate-acting insulin (NPH) injected before breakfast and before dinner. A snack must be eaten at bedtime to reduce risk of nocturnal hypoglycaemia. (b) Idealized insulin action profiles provided by a regimen consisting of a mixture of rapid-acting insulin and intermediate-acting insulin (NPH) before breakfast, rapid-acting insulin before supper/dinner, and a second dose of NPH at bedtime, together with a snack to reduce risk of nocturnal hypoglycaemia.

limitations inherent in split-mixed regimens, and permit greater flexibility with respect to timing and content of meals, and adjustments for exercise. Doses of rapid-acting insulin are selected before each meal or snack, based on pre-meal glucose values, anticipated meal macronutrient content, and physical activity. In the 'basal-bolus' MDI regimen (shown in Figure 1.3), a peakless, long-acting insulin (insulin glargine, detemir, or degludec) is used to provide basal insulin (starting dose typically about 40–50% of the estimated TDD) together with short- or rapid-acting insulin injected 30 or 15 minutes, respectively, before each meal.

Insulin glargine is usually administered once daily in the evening with dinner or at bedtime or before breakfast. It should be injected at about the same time each day; short- or rapid-acting insulin is injected separately before each meal (and large snack), whenever it is eaten. Because it does not have the peak of activity characteristic of NPH, insulin glargine reduces the risk of nocturnal hypoglycaemia. Insulin detemir is an alternative long-acting, 'peakless' basal insulin with pharmacodynamics characteristics similar to those of glargine especially during the first 12 hours after administration. It has a shorter duration of action than glargine and usually has to be administered twice

Basal-Bolus Insulin Regimen

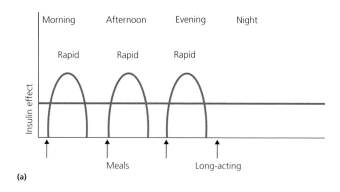

(a)

CSII (Pump) with Rapid-Acting Insulin Regimen

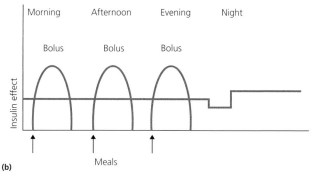

(b)

Figure 1.3 (a) Idealized insulin action provided by an insulin regimen consisting of four daily injections; rapid-acting insulin before each meal (denoted by arrows) and a separate single daily injection of a long-acting insulin analogue (glargine, detemir, or degludec), either at bedtime (as shown here) or at dinner or breakfast. (b) Idealized insulin effect provided by continuous subcutaneous insulin infusion via an insulin pump with rapid-acting insulin. In this figure, alternative basal rates are illustrated; insulin delivery is programmed to decrease from midnight to 3 a.m. to decrease risk of nocturnal hypoglycaemia and to increase from 3 a.m. until 8 a.m. to combat the dawn phenomenon. Arrows indicate times of insulin injection or boluses before breakfast, lunch, and the evening meal (supper or dinner).

daily in patients with severe insulin deficiency. Compared to NPH, studies in children and adolescents show a lower risk of hypoglycaemia and lower weight Z-score while its effect on HbA1c is equivalent. The most recently developed long-acting insulin formulation is ultralong-acting insulin degludec, which forms multihexamers resulting in a depot after injection into the subcutaneous tissue. The hexamers slowly dissociate to form monomers that are rapidly absorbed into the circulation. Degludec has a flat and stable pharmacokinetic profile; its major advantage is that it does not have to be injected at precisely the same time each day, which is an attractive feature especially for adolescents whose lifestyles make it difficult to adhere to an inflexible schedule.

Assuming the starting dose in a 60-kg adolescent is 0.75 unit per kg or 45 units per day, the initial dose of long-acting basal insulin might be 20 units (~45% of the TDD) and the insulin-to-carbohydrate ratio 1 unit of rapid-acting insulin per 10 g carbohydrate (calculated using the formula 450/TDD). The initial correction or insulin sensitivity factor is calculated using the formula 1800/TDD. In this example, it would be 1 unit of rapid-acting insulin to lower BG by 40 mg/dL (2.2 mmol/L) to a predetermined target; e.g. 120 mg/dL (11.1 mmol/L) during the day and 150 mg/dL (8.3 mmol/L) at bedtime and overnight. The actual prandial dose, administered ~15 minutes before the meal, is the sum of the individual doses required for carbohydrate coverage and the amount calculated to correct hyperglycaemia. The above simple formulae are useful to start insulin therapy; however, the optimal doses of rapid-acting insulin must be determined empirically guided by the results of frequent BG measurements, before and ~2 hours after a meal. At least five daily measurements are required to determine the effects of each component of the insulin regimen. The BG concentration should be measured before each meal, at bedtime, and once between midnight and 4 a.m. Patients and parents are taught to look for patterns of hyperglycaemia (>180 mg/dL or 10 mmol/L) or hypo-glycaemia (<70 mg/dL or 3.9 mmol/L) that indicate the need for a dose adjustment. Adjustments are made to individual components of the insulin regimen, usually in 5–10% increments or decrements, in response to patterns of consistently elevated (above the target range for several consecutive days) or unexplained low BG levels. The insulin dose is adjusted every 3–5 days until satisfactory BG control is achieved with at least 50% of BG values in the target range.

Practical aspects of insulin treatment

Insulin delivery systems

Insulin has an effective shelf life of at least two years if refrigerated at 4 °C and can be kept at room temperature for up to one month. However, in tropical climates or if kept in a car interior on a hot day, insulin degrades more rapidly. Insulin is administered by a pen delivery system or with a syringe and needle, or via an insulin pump. In general, vials of insulin are cheaper than insulin in disposable pens or pen cartridges. For children with needle phobia, spring-loaded automatic injection devices in which the needle is not visible may be helpful.

Insulin pens

Insulin may be administered using either a preloaded disposable pen or cartridges (different pens for rapid- and long-acting insulins) for a reusable pen device. Pen delivery systems are generally preferred by children as they are quicker and easier to use than syringes and needles, and lead to greater independence.

Syringes and needles

Insulin for injection may be drawn up from a vial and injected using an insulin syringe and needle. When mixing insulins, the rapid-acting clear insulin should be drawn up into the syringe before the intermediate-acting (NPH, isophane), which is a cloudy suspension, i.e. 'clear before cloudy insulin'. Before drawing up the dose into a syringe or injecting via a pen device, any preparation containing intermediate-acting insulin should be gently inverted several times to ensure that the insulin is uniformly suspended. Note that all insulin analogues are clear solutions; patients must be counselled to take special care not to confuse the rapid-acting with the long-acting analogue and accidentally (thinking it is the long-acting insulin) inject a large dose of rapid-acting insulin at bedtime.

Injections

The age at which children start to give their own injections is variable. Peer pressure, which may be experienced by a child attending a diabetes camp where children may see their contemporaries or even younger children administering injections, may motivate a child to learn to self-inject. Parents are strongly advised to supervise insulin injections when children wish to become more independent.

Appropriate injection sites are shown in Figure 1.4. The use of different injection sites and rotation of these sites should be encouraged to avoid the development of lipohypertrophy (Figure 1.5) which may be unsightly and lead to erratic absorption of insulin. If patients avoid injecting into these areas, lipohypertrophy will gradually resolve over a period of several months.

Injection technique

When using short (e.g. 4 or 5 mm) needles, the injection is given at a 90° angle without pinching the skin unless the patient is very thin. In those who find injections painful, distraction techniques can be used or the skin can be numbed with an ice pack before the injection.

Injecting small doses

In infants, the injection of doses as small as 0.5 to 1 unit can result in significant inaccuracies, with the dose actually delivered ranging from 0.89 to 1.23 units. In these circumstances, use of a pen-delivery system, which allows injections of insulin in increments of 0.5 units is recommended. If possible, infants should be managed using an insulin pump which permits accurate delivery of tiny amounts of insulin. Alternatively, insulin may have to be diluted to U10 concentration: 1 line on an insulin syringe corresponds to 0.1 unit of insulin.

Insulin preparations

In solution, human insulin forms hexamers (six-molecule units). The rate of absorption after subcutaneous injection is principally determined by how

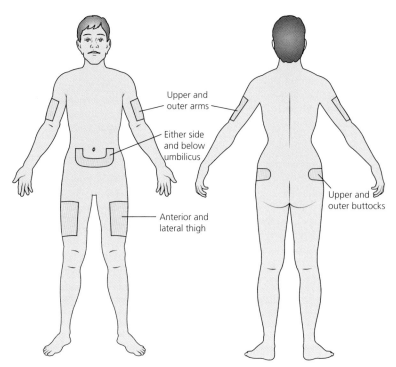

Figure 1.4 Insulin injection sites.

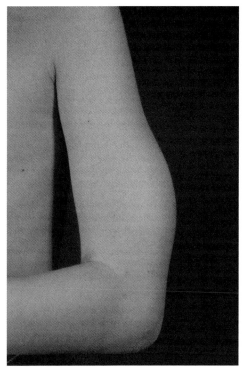

Figure 1.5 Lipohypertrophy on the arm.

quickly the hexamers dissociate into monomers (single molecules), which are absorbed across endothelial barriers. Children should be treated with human insulin analogues in a concentration of 100 units /ml (U100). Table 1.5 shows the most common insulin preparations and their durations of action.

Continuous subcutaneous insulin infusion (insulin pumps)

Despite the introduction of CSII (pump) therapy nearly 40 years ago, widespread adoption of this technology in paediatric diabetes practice has only occurred in the last 15 years. In 1996, less than 5% of patients who started pump therapy were < 20 years of age; over the intervening years there has been a worldwide steady increase in the number of children and adolescents using pump therapy. This may be attributable to recognition of the crucial importance of lowering HbA1c levels to prevent or delay vascular complications together with advances in pump technology. There is considerable worldwide variation in the frequency of pump use, e.g. use of insulin pumps is threefold greater in Germany, Austria, and the United States compared with England and Wales.

An insulin pump has several advantages over insulin injections, e.g. the ability to programme changes in basal insulin delivery to meet an anticipated increase or decrease in need. This feature can be advantageous in combating the dawn phenomenon (especially pronounced in adolescents) or preventing hypoglycaemia during or after strenuous exercise. In addition to programming various basal infusion rates over the course of the day and night, the use of dual wave and square wave bolus delivery significantly lowers postprandial blood glucose levels after meals with a high fat and protein content. Also, because the infusion set typically only has to be replaced every two or three days, the child is spared the discomfort of numerous daily injections. Registries that track outcomes of type 1 diabetes treatment and several single centre observational studies show that children who use a pump have significantly lower HbA1c levels and decreased glycaemic variability, decreased rates of severe hypoglycaemia, and improvements in diabetes-related quality of life, treatment satisfaction, and less fear of hypoglycaemia. A meta-analysis of randomized controlled clinical trials showed that CSII results in a small (~0.5%) improvement in HbA1c (Garvey and Wolfsdorf 2015). Even larger improvements in glycaemic control and hypoglycaemia reduction are possible with insulin pumps that incorporate continuous glucose monitoring (CGM), referred to as sensor augmented pump therapy (Slover et al. 2012).

Although an insulin pump is a complex and sophisticated medical device that requires extensive training in its proper use, with appropriate education and training and with support from parents and a school nurse, most children and adolescents can manage to successfully and safely use an insulin pump and benefit from its advantages. Because only short- or rapid-acting insulin is used with CSII, any interruption in insulin delivery rapidly leads to metabolic decompensation. To reduce this risk, patients must pay meticulous attention to insuring the integrity of the infusion system and must measure their blood glucose levels at least four times daily. A recent study showed a lower rate of DKA with pumps as compared to MDI therapy. Success requires motivation to achieve normal blood glucose levels, frequent blood glucose monitoring, accurate carbohydrate counting, good record-keeping, and frequent contact with the diabetes team. Patients must understand that to be successful CSII therapy requires more time, effort, and active involvement in diabetes care by patients and parents, and considerable education and support from the diabetes team. The individual who is unable to master an MDI regimen is not likely to be successful with CSII. Despite concerns that it might have adverse psychosocial consequences owing to the added burden of treatment, especially in adolescents, the opposite effect has been observed.

The insulin delivery system consists of a programmable pump (about the size of a cell phone) containing a reservoir filled with rapid-acting insulin, which is connected by a plastic infusion tube to a small plastic (or metal) cannula inserted subcutaneously - usually in the abdomen or posterior aspect of the upper arm, anterior thigh or buttocks (in toddlers and infants it is most often inserted in the buttocks) and fixed in place by adhesive tape. Depending on the specific device, changes in the insulin infusion rate as small as 0.025 units /hour can be made. The cannula is usually left in place for two to three days. If the cannula is not changed regularly or if the same site is used recurrently, there is a risk of developing lipohypertrophy or developing an infection at the site.

A 24-hour profile including measurements before each meal, two hours after the meal, at midnight, at 2.00–4.00 a.m. should be carried out at least every other week to enable any necessary dose changes to be made. The absence of a long-acting insulin depot means that if there is an interruption in insulin delivery, blood glucose levels will rise quickly and ketosis can develop in four to six hours. CSII therapy is considerably more expensive than MDI therapy.

Some patients prefer a tubeless disposable 'patch pump' (Figure 1.6), consisting of a micro pump, an insulin reservoir, and a cannula; the integrated device attaches directly to the skin. Insulin is delivered through a small subcutaneous catheter. Patch pumps are free of tubing and are waterproof, which makes them more discreet and allows greater freedom with

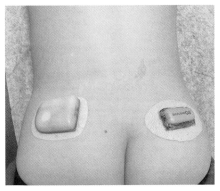

Figure 1.6 An Omnipod® patch pump is on the left buttock and a Dexcom G5® glucose sensor on the right buttock.

activities such as swimming. They are disposable and are lighter and smaller than conventional pumps. They usually need to be reapplied every two or three days. The pump is controlled by a remote device that has an integrated glucose meter and which communicates wirelessly with the patch pump.

CSII can also be used together with CGM sensors that measure glucose levels in the interstitial fluid every few minutes, referred to as sensor augmented pump therapy. The data can be transferred to the pump using Bluetooth technology so that if the blood glucose is below a certain value, for example, 4 mmol/L (72 mg/dL), the insulin pump sets off an alarm and suspends insulin delivery. Some insulin pumps can also be set to raise an alarm if the glucose level is falling rapidly and they will suspend insulin delivery if hypoglycaemia is anticipated to occur within the next 30 minutes ('predictive low glucose suspend'). Recently, interstitial glucose sensing and insulin delivery have been combined to produce a 'hybrid closed loop system', i.e. a version of an artificial pancreas that has been approved for use from 7 years. Such systems increase the number of BG values in the target range and decrease hypoglycaemia. Algorithms to cope with situations such as exercise are currently being devised and new technological innovations and device improvements have had a beneficial impact on the management of diabetes in children and adolescents. Use of an insulin pump permits a flexible lifestyle and eating patterns and is associated with a high degree of satisfaction in appropriately motivated patients.

Insulin regimens and glycaemic control

The technological innovations described above have provided patients with insulin preparations whose pharmacokinetic properties make it possible to crudely simulate physiologic insulin kinetics. It is now possible for children to safely achieve unprecedented levels of glycaemic control without excessive severe hypoglycaemia, and yet in most patients the goal of near-normalization of glycaemic control is not realized. Several recent studies have shown a persistent gap between target HbA1c ranges and the actual values patients attain. The successful implementation of intensive diabetes therapy remains a major challenge, and diabetes care providers should frankly discuss treatment options with the child and parents and explain the advantages and disadvantages of each in attempting to meet the overall goals of treatment. The most suitable regimen for a given child and family should be determined by mutual consent and should be the regimen they will most likely be able to afford

and adhere to. These considerations are particularly important in managing children living in economically and socially disadvantaged circumstances and when there is a shortage of food.

Potential problems with insulin therapy

The dawn phenomenon

The dawn phenomenon describes the rise in insulin requirements and blood glucose concentrations in the early morning, approximately 5.00–8.00 a.m. It is most pronounced during puberty and is thought to be caused primarily by the insulin resistance produced by nocturnal growth hormone secretion. This is a difficult problem to resolve in those using twice daily insulin regimens. Possible benefit may be obtained in such patients by dividing the evening injection so that rapid-acting insulin is given prior to the evening meal and intermediate-acting insulin before bedtime (see Figure 1.2a). Alternatively, in patients on a basal-bolus regimen, the pre-bedtime dose of intermediate-acting insulin or long-acting insulin analogue can be increased. When using an insulin pump, the overnight basal rate can be programmed to increase at 3 a.m. until 8 a.m.

The Somogyi phenomenon

This term refers to morning hyperglycaemia caused by the release of counter-regulatory hormones following the occurrence of nocturnal hypoglycaemia. However, when pronounced hyperglycaemia occurs after an episode of nocturnal hypoglycaemia, it usually is attributable to ingestion of an excessive amount of carbohydrate to treat the hypoglycaemia episode. Alternatively, when pre-breakfast hyperglycaemia occurs without preceding nocturnal hypoglycaemia, this usually is caused by inadequate or waning overnight insulinemia.

Insulin therapy in young children: special considerations

Caring for young children with diabetes is challenging for many reasons; one is the need to accurately and reproducibly measure and inject tiny doses of insulin supplied in a concentration of 100 units/ml (U100 insulin). To administer a dose of 1 unit requires the ability to accurately measure 10 μl (1/100 ml) of insulin. A dose change of 0.25 U translates into a volume difference of 2.5 μl in a 300 μl (3/10 cc or 30 unit) syringe. When parents attempt to measure insulin doses in increments of 0.25 U (e.g. 3.0, 3.25, 3.5 U) using a standard commercial 30 unit (300 μl) syringe, they consistently measure more than the prescribed amount. For these reasons, CSII can be a useful tool to provide U100 insulin in small doses to young children when there is appropriate caregiver education and diabetes team support. However, when injection regimens are used, to enhance accuracy and reproducibility of small doses, insulin should be diluted to U10 (10 units/ml) with the specific diluent available from the insulin manufacturers. Using U10 insulin, each line ('unit') on a syringe is actually 0.1 U of insulin.

Dietary management

Nutrition is a cornerstone of diabetes management and nutrition education and counselling are essential components of a comprehensive programme of diabetes self-management education for patients and their families. There is no 'diabetic diet' per se; rather, nutrition therapy should be individualized according to the family's and patient's usual eating habits and food preferences, religious or cultural considerations, and access to food. Combining blood glucose monitoring with intensive insulin therapy and mastery of carbohydrate counting enables children and adolescents to enjoy dietary flexibility while maintaining glycaemic control in the target range. The focus of dietary management differs between the two major types of diabetes. In type 1 diabetes, the primary goal is to match insulin delivery and carbohydrate consumption to achieve blood glucose levels in the target range. In contrast, children with type 2 diabetes are typically overweight or obese at presentation so that the emphasis is on weight loss, limiting calorie intake, and distributing meals evenly throughout the day.

Growth is an excellent indicator of the adequacy of energy intake, and should be regularly evaluated by plotting height and weight on a growth chart. If growth is not optimal, the diet should be reviewed and, in patients with type 1 diabetes, one should consider inadequate insulin delivery, hypo- or hyperthyroidism, coeliac disease, and adrenal insufficiency as possible causes. For overweight (BMI ≥85th percentile) and obese (BMI ≥95th percentile) youth with either type 1 diabetes or type 2 diabetes, energy consumption must be reduced to arrest weight gain. Table 1.7 shows a general approach to meal management for both type 1 diabetes and type 2 diabetes.

The numerous commercially available 'diabetic foods' are not recommended for children with diabetes, as such foods tend to be expensive and have no particular advantages over a healthy diet based on normal foods. Some 'diabetic foods' also contain the sweetener sorbitol that may lead to diarrhoea when consumed in large amounts. 'Diabetic foods' may also have a high calorie and fat content. Drinks containing sugar should be replaced with those containing artificial sweeteners.

Carbohydrate counting

Carbohydrate is the main nutrient in starches, fruits, milk, and sugar-containing foods and is the major determinant of postprandial blood glucose excursions. The most widely used method for youth with

Table 1.7 General approaches to meal management.

Type 1 diabetes	Split-mixed insulin regimen	• Three meals and two or three snacks daily • Meal times consistent from day-to-day • Meals and snacks spaced 2–3 hours apart • Consistent carbohydrate intake • Snack before bed to decrease risk of overnight hypoglycaemia • Continued education and assessment of readiness to change lifestyle to achieve a Heart Healthy diet
	Flexible basal-bolus or insulin pump therapy	• Carbohydrate content can vary • Must accurately count carbohydrate and match insulin dose using an insulin:carbohydrate ratio • Recommend eating three meals daily • Continued education and assessment of readiness to change lifestyle to achieve a Heart Healthy diet
Type 2 diabetes		• Meal plan to assist with evenly spaced carbohydrate intake and increased emphasis on reducing calories to promote weight loss

type 1 diabetes who use rapid-acting prandial insulin is an individualized insulin-to-carbohydrate ratio (e.g. 1 unit per x grams of carbohydrate). Carbohydrate counting allows flexibility in food choices and enables patients to include a wide variety of foods in their meal plan. An important limitation of carbohydrate counting is that it does not address carbohydrate quality, diet composition, or total caloric intake. Patients should be encouraged to learn about the glycaemic index (GI) of their favourite carbohydrate-containing foods ('fast' vs. 'slow' carbohydrates). Carbohydrates are absorbed slowly from low-GI foods, whereas high-GI foods lead to rapid carbohydrate absorption and a brisk increase in blood glucose levels. The amount of fat, protein, and fibre in food also influences the rate of carbohydrate absorption. For example, meals with a high fat content slow the rate of carbohydrate absorption.

An alternative method, employed by patients who use a fixed dose insulin regimen or for whom carbohydrate counting may be too difficult, is a prescribed carbohydrate meal plan that maintains day-to-day consistency in the carbohydrate content of meals and snacks.

Children and their parents are taught how to read the nutrition facts on food labels for total carbohydrate (grams) per serving. Periodically measuring and weighing foods is recommended to reinforce accurate portion sizes and carbohydrate amounts, which is essential for optimal insulin dosing and to minimize postprandial hyperglycaemia. Numerous nutrition 'apps' are available for smart phones and other digital devices.

Renewed attention has been given to the impact of fat and protein on postprandial glycaemic responses in youth with type 1 diabetes, and evidence suggests that additional insulin to account for protein and fat in a meal is superior to dosing insulin solely based on carbohydrate intake.

Fat

Diabetes is associated with a high risk of early subclinical and clinical cardiovascular disease (CVD), and children with type 1 diabetes are in the highest tier for cardiovascular risk. Saturated and *trans* fatty acids are the principal dietary determinants of plasma low-density lipoprotein (LDL)-cholesterol concentrations. To reduce the risk of CVD, consumption of saturated fat, *trans* fatty acids, and cholesterol must be limited while increasing intake of unsaturated fats and omega-3 fatty acids. Because both glycaemic control and cardioprotective nutrition improve the

lipid profile and reduce cardiac risk, patients should be advised to consume less red meat and high-fat dairy foods and eat more poultry, fish, and vegetable proteins, and drink low-fat milk. Children and adolescents with normal plasma lipid concentrations should derive less than 10% of their energy from saturated fats; the daily intake of cholesterol should be <300 mg per day, and consumption of *trans* fatty acids (principally formed by the hydrogenation of unsaturated fats and present in margarine, deep-frying fat, and some processed foods such as biscuits and cakes) should be minimal. In the overweight or obese child, total fat consumption should be reduced.

Nutrition education and formulation of the meal plan

Newly diagnosed children with type 1 diabetes usually present with weight loss; therefore, the initial meal plan includes an estimation of energy requirements to restore and then maintain an appropriate body weight and allow for normal growth and development. Energy requirements vary with age, height, weight, stage of puberty, and level of physical activity. Because the energy needs of growing children continuously change, the meal plan should be re-evaluated at least every six months in young children and annually in adolescents.

Dietary management begins at the time of diagnosis with an assessment by a registered dietitian (clinical nutritionist). The meal plan must take account of the child's school schedule, early or late lunches, physical education classes, after-school physical activity, and differences in a child's activities on weekdays compared with weekends and holidays. Young children typically have three meals and two or three snacks daily, depending on the interval of time between meals, age of the child, and level of physical activity. Although their daily energy intake is relatively constant over time, young children adjust their energy intake at successive meals. The highly variable food consumption from meal-to-meal typical of normal young children is especially challenging when the child has type 1 diabetes. The purpose of snacks is to prevent hypoglycaemia and hunger between meals. If the basal insulin component is adjusted appropriately, patients who use a basal-bolus insulin regimen or pump therapy may not require snacks.

The dietitian's role is to evaluate the patient's and family's knowledge and understanding of nutrition and to formulate an individualized meal plan. Nutrition education and counselling, like all aspects of diabetes education, should be an ongoing process with periodic review and revision of the meal plan and assessment of the child's and parents' levels of comprehension, ability to analyse and solve problems, and adherence to the nutrition goals. The patient should return to see the dietitian if glycaemic control is poor, growth is failing, weight gain is excessive, or if other problems arise related to dietary management.

The epidemic of obesity has not spared children with type 1 diabetes, and a recent report from the SEARCH study in the US showed a higher prevalence of overweight in youth with type 1 diabetes compared with similarly aged youth without diabetes (22% vs. 16%) (Liu et al. 2010).

Management of the child presenting with ketoacidosis

There is wide geographic variation in the frequency of DKA at presentation of diabetes; worldwide incidence rates range from approximately 15–80%. DKA is a presenting feature in 6–11% of patients with type 2 diabetes. In children with established diabetes, the risk of DKA is increased in those with chronic poor metabolic control and previous episodes of DKA, adolescent girls, children with psychiatric disorders, and those with psychosocial challenges. In patients who use a pump, interruption of insulin delivery for any reason can lead to DKA. Most DKA episodes are caused by insulin omission or treatment error, and the majority of the remainder are due to inadequate insulin treatment during an intercurrent illness.

The diagnostic criteria for the diagnosis of DKA include: hyperglycaemia (glucose>11 mmol/L [200 mg/dL]) with a venous pH < 7.30 or serum bicarbonate <15 mmol/L. Blood BOHB is typically ≥3.0 mmol/L and ketonuria is 'moderate or large'. DKA is classified by its severity: mild (venous pH < 7.30 or bicarbonate<15 mmol/)L, moderate (pH < 7.2 or bicarbonate<10 mmol/L) and severe (pH < 7.1 or bicarbonate <5 mmol/L). Partially treated children and children who have consumed little or no carbohydrate may have only modestly elevated blood glucose concentrations, referred to as 'euglycaemic ketoacidosis'.

The mortality rate from DKA is approximately 0.2%. Death is usually caused by cerebral oedema, but may also be caused by hypokalaemia-induced cardiac arrhythmia, sepsis, aspiration pneumonia, and numerous other rare complications.

Resuscitation

Acute management should follow the general guidelines for paediatric advanced life support (PALS). The protocol described below for the treatment of DKA is largely based on the guidelines published by the International Society of Pediatric and Adolescent Diabetes (Wolfsdorf et al. 2018).

- *Airway:* If the child is comatose, an airway should be inserted and if the level of consciousness is depressed or the child is vomiting, a nasogastric tube should be inserted, aspirated, and left to drain freely.
- *Breathing:* If there is evidence of hypoxia, give 100% oxygen and consider the need for intubation and ventilation. Airway and breathing problems are rare.
- *Circulation:* An IV cannula should be placed and blood samples (including a venous blood gas) obtained for investigations (see Section 1.5). In cases of circulatory impairment (suggested by the presence of prolonged capillary refill and tachycardia), give 10 ml/kg body weight of 0.9% saline intravenously as quickly as possible. The fluid bolus can be repeated (subsequent boluses can usually be given more slowly) until the circulation is restored.

If the child is too ill to weigh, for the purposes of calculating fluid requirements, weight can be estimated from a recent clinic weight or from a centile chart.

Antibiotics should be given if sepsis is thought likely after appropriate samples for culture have been taken.

Initial monitoring

Whenever possible, the child with DKA should be cared for in a high dependency or intensive care unit with experienced nursing staff, and with access to a clinical chemistry laboratory that can provide timely measurements of serum chemistries. In hospitals without a high dependency unit, high dependency care can still be given by providing a high level of nursing care, often on a one-to-one basis. Children with severe DKA – pH <7.1 or bicarbonate <5 mmol/L, compromised circulation, depressed level of consciousness, and those at increased risk for cerebral oedema (<5 years of age) should be treated in a paediatric intensive care unit or in a children's ward that specializes in diabetes and can provide comparable resources and supervision of care.

The following should be documented:
- Hourly vital signs.
- Weight should be measured twice a day.
- A strict fluid balance chart should be kept which includes measurement of urine volume and fluid losses from vomiting and diarrhoea.

- Hourly blood glucose measurements should be performed. Ideally, an additional cannula should be inserted for blood sampling to prevent recurrent, painful venipunctures or finger pricks, which may yield inaccurate blood glucose concentrations when peripheral circulation is poor.
- Venous or capillary blood ketone measurements 1–2 hourly, which measures the main ketone, BOHB, should be performed to quantify the suppression of ketogenesis.
- Venous blood gases, electrolyte and urea concentrations.
- A cardiac monitor should be used to monitor abnormal serum potassium concentrations.
- All patients with DKA should have at least hourly neurological observations and the Glasgow Coma Score should be recorded. The development of a severe headache or change in behaviour should be reported immediately to medical staff as this may be the first sign of cerebral oedema.
- If the patient is comatose or unable to void on demand (e.g. infants and very ill young children), the bladder should be catheterized.

Fluid therapy

The objectives of fluid and electrolyte replacement therapy are: (i) to restore circulating volume; (ii) to replace sodium, potassium, and the extracellular and intracellular water deficits; and (iii) to improve glomerular filtration and thereby enhance the clearance of glucose and ketones from the blood

Fluid requirements

Patients with DKA have a deficit in extracellular fluid (ECF) volume usually in the range 3–10%. Clinical estimates of the volume deficit are subjective and inaccurate. For fluid calculations, use 3–5% in mild DKA, 5–7% in moderate DKA, and 7–10% in cases of severe DKA. For patients with severe volume depletion but not in shock, volume expansion (resuscitation) should begin immediately with 0.9% saline to restore the peripheral circulation. The volume administered typically is 10–20 ml/kg over 1–2 hours, and may need to be repeated until perfusion is adequate. In the rare patient with DKA in shock, rapidly restore circulatory volume with isotonic saline in 20 ml/kg boluses infused as quickly as possible through a large bore cannula with reassessment after each bolus.

Subsequent fluid management (deficit replacement) can be accomplished with 0.45–0.9% saline or a balanced salt solution such as Ringer's lactate, Hartmann's solution, or Plasmalyte. Fluid therapy should begin with deficit replacement plus maintenance fluid requirements. All children will experience a decrease in vascular volume when plasma glucose concentrations fall during treatment. Therefore, it is essential to ensure that they receive sufficient fluid and salt to maintain adequate tissue perfusion.

Deficit replacement should be with a solution that has a tonicity equal to or greater than 0.45% saline (with added potassium chloride, phosphate or potassium acetate; see Section 1.9.5). The decision whether to use an isotonic or a hypotonic solution for deficit replacement should depend on clinical judgement based on the patient's hydration status, the serum sodium concentration, and the effective osmolality. In addition to providing the usual daily maintenance fluid requirement (see example in Table 1.9), replace the estimated fluid deficit at an even rate over 36–48 hours. Except for severely ill patients, oral intake typically begins within 24 hours. At this point, any remaining deficits are replenished by oral intake once DKA has resolved and patients are transitioned to subcutaneous insulin.

Clinical assessment of hydration status and calculated effective osmolality are valuable guides to fluid and electrolyte therapy. The aim is gradually to reduce serum effective osmolality to normal. There should be a concomitant increase in serum sodium concentration as the glucose concentration decreases (sodium should rise by 0.5 mmol/L for each 1 mmol/L decrease in glucose concentration).

Urinary losses should not routinely be added to the calculation of replacement fluid but this may be necessary in rare circumstances such as a patient with severe dehydration and extreme hyperglycaemia (i.e. mixed DKA and hyperglycaemic hyperosmolar state [HHS]).

The sodium content of the fluid should be increased if measured serum sodium concentration is low and does not rise appropriately as the plasma glucose concentration falls.

The fluid infused during initial resuscitation to restore the circulation should be taken into account when calculating fluid requirements and deducted from the total. Maintenance fluid requirements can be estimated using the Holliday-Segar method in Table 1.8 or the body surface area method, 1500 ml/m^2/24 hour (not suitable for use in children <10 kg). Using the Holliday-Segar method to determine the maintenance fluid requirement for an 8-year-old child weighing 25 kg yields 65 ml per hour or 1600 ml per day. This method is not suitable for neonates <14 days old and generally overestimates fluid needs in neonates.

The hourly infusion rate is calculated using the following formula:

Table 1.8 Maintenance fluid requirements in DKA.

Weight	Maintenance fluid requirements (ml per kg per hour)	Maintenance fluid requirements (ml per kg per day)
First 10 kg	4 ml/kg × 10 kg = 40 ml/hr	100 ml/kg × 10 kg = 1,000 ml/d
Second 10 kg	2 ml/kg × 10 kg = 20 ml/hr	50 ml/kg × 10 kg = 500 ml/d
Each additional 1 kg	1 ml/kg × 5 kg = 5 ml/hr	20 ml/kg × 5 kg = 100 ml/d

$$\text{hourly rate} = \frac{48\,\text{hour maintenance} + \text{defict} - \text{resuscitation fluid already given}}{48}$$

Table 1.9 Example of fluid volume calculation.

An eight-year-old boy weighing 25 kg who is estimated to be 8% dehydrated and who received 10 ml/kg 0.9% saline in the emergency department will need:

Daily maintenance = 1600 ml

Deficit = 25 kg × 8% = 2000 ml

Resuscitation fluid = 250 ml

Total requirements over
48 h = (2 × 1600) + (2000 − 250) = 4950 ml

Hourly rate = 4950/48 = 103 ml/h

An example of calculations to estimate fluid requirements for a child with DKA is shown in Table 1.9. It is important to double-check these calculations.

The serum sodium concentration is an unreliable measure of the degree of ECF contraction because glucose, largely restricted to the extracellular space, causes osmotic movement of water into the extracellular space, thereby causing dilutional hyponatremia. At presentation in DKA, the serum sodium concentration is usually low. A failure of measured serum sodium levels to rise or a further decline in serum sodium levels with therapy is an ominous sign of impending cerebral oedema.

Clinical assessment of hydration status and calculated effective osmolality (2× [plasma Na] + plasma glucose mmol/L) are valuable guides to fluid and electrolyte therapy. The aim is gradually to reduce serum effective osmolality to normal.

In the early stages of DKA, patients typically are extremely thirsty and request oral fluids. In severe dehydration with impaired consciousness, no fluids should be allowed by mouth. A nasogastric tube may be necessary in the case of gastric paresis, vomiting, or impaired consciousness to decrease the risk of aspiration pneumonia. Oral fluids should only be allowed after resolution of DKA. If substantial clinical improvement has occurred before the completion of the planned 48 hours of rehydration, oral intake can be permitted (provided the child is not vomiting) and the IV infusion rate reduced to take account of the oral intake.

Insulin therapy

Although rehydration alone frequently causes a marked decrease in blood glucose concentration, insulin therapy is essential to restore normal cellular metabolism, normalize blood glucose concentration, and suppress lipolysis and ketogenesis. Start the insulin infusion 1–2 hours after starting fluid replacement therapy, i.e. after the patient has received initial volume expansion. The recommended dose is 0.05–0.1 unit/kg/hour via intravenous infusion (dilute 50 units regular [soluble] insulin in 50 ml normal saline, 1 unit = 1 ml). An intravenous insulin bolus should *not* be used at the start of therapy; it is unnecessary and may increase the risk of cerebral oedema and exacerbate hypokalaemia.

The dose of insulin should usually remain at 0.05–0.1 unit/kg/hour until resolution of DKA (pH >7.30, bicarbonate >15 mmol/L, BOHB <1 mmol/L, and normal anion gap), which typically takes longer than normalization of blood glucose concentrations. If the patient is sensitive to insulin (e.g. some young children with DKA), the dose may be decreased provided that metabolic acidosis continues to resolve. For example, if a young child is receiving 0.05 unit/kg/hour, it may be necessary to reduce the insulin dose to 0.03 unit/kg/hour to prevent hypoglycaemia. During initial volume expansion, the plasma glucose concentration falls steeply. Thereafter, and after commencing insulin therapy, the plasma glucose concentration typically decreases at a rate of 2–5 mmol/L/hour (36–90 mg/dL/hour), depending on the timing and amount of intravenous glucose administration. To prevent an unduly rapid decrease in plasma glucose concentration and hypoglycaemia, 5% glucose should be added to the IV fluid when the plasma glucose falls to approximately 14–17 mmol/L (250–300 mg/dL), or sooner if the rate of fall is precipitous. It may be necessary to use 10% or even 12.5% dextrose to prevent hypoglycaemia while continuing to infuse the amount of insulin necessary to correct the metabolic acidosis. If blood glucose falls very rapidly >5 mmol/L/h (>90 mg/dL/h) after initial fluid expansion, consider adding glucose even before plasma glucose has decreased to 17 mmol/L (300 mg/dL).

In circumstances where continuous IV administration is not possible and in patients with uncomplicated DKA, hourly or two-hourly SC or IM administration of a short- or rapid-acting insulin analogue is safe and may be as effective as IV regular insulin infusion, but, if possible, should not be used in patients whose peripheral circulation is impaired. The initial dose SC is 0.3 unit/kg, followed one hour later by SC insulin lispro or aspart at 0.1 unit/kg every hour, or 0.15–0.20 units/kg every two hours. If blood glucose falls to <14 mmol/L (250 mg/dL) before DKA has resolved, reduce SC insulin lispro or aspart to 0.05 unit/kg per hour to keep blood glucose ≈11 mmol/L (200 mg/dL) until resolution of DKA.

Potassium

Potassium is mainly an intracellular ion and at presentation in DKA there is invariably a large depletion of total body potassium even though initial serum potassium concentrations may be normal or even high. Administration of insulin and the correction of acidosis drives potassium back into the cells, decreasing serum levels. The serum potassium concentration may decrease abruptly, predisposing the patient to a cardiac arrhythmia. Renal dysfunction reduces potassium excretion, contributing to hyperkalaemia. Early potassium therapy should be avoided if anuria is present as a result of acute tubular necrosis.

Replacement therapy is required regardless of the serum potassium concentration, except if renal failure is present. If the patient is hypokalaemic at presentation, start potassium replacement *at the time of* initial volume expansion and *before* starting insulin therapy. Otherwise, start replacing potassium *after* initial volume expansion and concurrent with starting insulin therapy. If the patient is hyperkalaemic, *defer* potassium replacement therapy until urine output is documented (may have to catheterize the bladder). If immediate serum potassium measurements are unavailable, an ECG may help to determine whether the child has hyper- or hypokalaemia. Prolongation of the PR interval, T wave flattening and inversion, ST depression, prominent U waves, apparent long QT interval (due to fusion of the T and U waves) indicate hypokalaemia. Tall, peaked, symmetrical, T waves and shortening of the QT interval are signs of hyperkalaemia.

The starting potassium concentration should be 40 mmol/L. Subsequent potassium replacement therapy should be based on serum potassium measurements with the goal of maintaining levels within the normal range. Potassium phosphate may be used together with potassium chloride or acetate, e.g. 20 mmol/L potassium chloride and 20 mmol/L potassium phosphate or 20 mmol/L potassium phosphate and 20 mmol/L potassium acetate. The maximum recommended rate of intravenous potassium replacement is 0.5 mmol/kg/hour. If hypokalaemia persists despite a maximum rate of potassium replacement, the rate of insulin infusion should be reduced.

Phosphate

Depletion of intracellular phosphate occurs as a result of osmotic diuresis. The fall in plasma phosphate levels is exacerbated by insulin therapy as phosphate re-enters cells. Clinically significant hypophosphataemia may occur if intravenous therapy without food intake is prolonged beyond 24 hours. Prospective studies have not shown a significant benefit from phosphate replacement and aggressive phosphate administration causes hypocalcaemia.

Acidosis and bicarbonate therapy

Acidosis is reversible by fluid and insulin replacement; insulin stops further ketoacid production and allows ketoacids to be metabolized, generating bicarbonate. Treatment of hypovolemia improves tissue perfusion and renal function, thereby increasing the excretion of organic acids. Clinical trials have shown no benefit from bicarbonate administration, which may cause paradoxical CNS acidosis and hypokalaemia. Nonetheless, bicarbonate administration may be beneficial in the rare patient with life-threatening hyperkalaemia and to improve cardiac contractility in patients who are severely acidotic (pH < 6.9) with circulatory failure despite adequate fluid replacement.

If bicarbonate is considered necessary, cautiously give 1–2 mmol/kg over 60 minutes.

Anticoagulant prophylaxis

There is a considerable risk of venous thrombosis in young and very sick children with DKA who have central venous catheters inserted and in patients with extreme hyperosmolarity. Prophylactic anticoagulation should be considered in such patients.

Introduction of oral fluids and transition to SC insulin injections

Oral fluids should be introduced only when substantial clinical improvement has occurred. Persistent ketonuria (urine ketone strips measure acetoacetate and acetone) characteristically occurs for several hours after serum BOHB levels have returned to normal; therefore, absence of ketonuria should *not* be used as an endpoint for determining resolution of DKA. When oral fluid is tolerated, IV fluid should be reduced accordingly so that the sum of IV and oral fluids does not exceed the calculated IV rate. When ketoacidosis has resolved and the change to SC insulin is planned, the most convenient time to change to SC insulin is just before a meal. To prevent rebound hyperglycaemia, the first SC injection should be given 15–30 minutes (with rapid-acting insulin) or 60 minutes (with regular insulin) before stopping the insulin infusion to allow sufficient time for the insulin to be absorbed. After transitioning to SC insulin, frequent blood glucose monitoring is required to avoid marked hyperglycaemia and hypoglycaemia.

Cerebral oedema

The mortality rate from DKA in children is approximately 0.15–0.30%. Cerebral injury is the major cause of mortality and morbidity accounting for 60–90% of all DKA deaths, and from 10% to 25% of survivors of cerebral oedema have significant residual morbidity.

The cause of cerebral oedema is controversial. Some have explained the pathogenesis as the result of rapid fluid administration with abrupt changes in serum osmolality. More recent investigations, however, have found that dehydration and cerebral hypoperfusion may be associated with DKA-related cerebral injury. This has led to the formulation of an alternative hypothesis; namely, that factors intrinsic to DKA and which could be worsened during treatment may be the cause of brain injury. It is noteworthy that the degree of oedema that develops during DKA correlates with the degree of dehydration and hyperventilation

at presentation, but not with factors related to initial osmolality or osmotic changes during treatment. Disruption of the blood–brain-barrier has been found in cases of fatal cerebral oedema associated with DKA, which further supports the view that cerebral oedema is not simply caused by a reduction in serum osmolality.

Demographic factors associated with an increased risk of cerebral oedema include: younger age (especially <5 years), new onset diabetes, longer duration of symptoms. These risk associations reflect the greater likelihood of severe DKA. Epidemiological studies have identified several risk factors at presentation or during treatment, including: greater hypocapnia (lower pCO_2) adjusted for degree of acidosis, increased serum urea nitrogen, more severe acidosis at presentation, administration of bicarbonate for correction of acidosis, a marked early decrease in serum effective osmolality, an attenuated rise in serum sodium concentration or an early fall in glucose-corrected sodium during therapy, greater volumes of fluid given in the first four hours, and administration of insulin within the first hour of fluid treatment.

Clinically significant cerebral oedema usually develops within the first 12 hours after treatment has started, but can occur before treatment has begun or, rarely, as late as 24–48 hours after the start of treatment. Symptoms and signs are variable. Onset of clinically overt cerebral oedema often follows an initial period of clinical and biochemical improvement; however, in some cases the patient's state of consciousness may decline from the time of admission.

Signs and symptoms of cerebral oedema include: onset of severe headache or worsening of a headache already present upon arrival, slowing of heart rate, change in neurological status (restlessness, irritability, confusion, increasing drowsiness, incontinence), specific neurological signs (e.g. pupillary abnormalities, cranial nerve palsies, papilloedema), rising blood pressure, decreased oxygen saturation, and respiratory impairment. Dramatic signs such as convulsions, papilloedema, and respiratory arrest are late signs associated with a grave prognosis.

A method of clinical diagnosis based on bedside evaluation of neurological state is shown in Table 1.10. One diagnostic criterion, two major criteria, or one major and two minor criteria have a sensitivity of 92% and a false positive rate of only 4%. Signs that occur before treatment should not be considered in the diagnosis of cerebral oedema.

A chart with the reference ranges for blood pressure and heart rate, which vary depending on height,

Table 1.10 Symptoms and signs of cerebral oedema.

Diagnostic criteria	Major criteria	Minor criteria
• Abnormal motor or verbal response to pain • Decorticate or decerebrate posture • Cranial nerve palsy (especially III, IV, and VI) • Abnormal neurogenic respiratory pattern (e.g. grunting, tachypnea, Cheyne-Stokes respiration, apneusis)	• Altered mentation/fluctuating level of consciousness • Sustained heart rate deceleration (decrease more than 20 beats per minute) not attributable to improved intravascular volume or sleep state • Age-inappropriate incontinence	• Vomiting • Headache • Lethargy or not easily arousable • Diastolic BP >90 mm Hg • Age < 5 years

weight, and gender, should be readily available at the bedside.

The appearance of diabetes insipidus, manifested by increased urine output with a concomitant marked increase in the serum sodium concentration, reflecting loss of free water in the urine, is a sign of cerebral herniation causing interruption of blood flow to the pituitary gland.

Treatment of cerebral oedema

Initiate treatment as soon as the condition is suspected.
• Give mannitol, 0.5–1 g/kg IV over 10–15 minutes.
• Hypertonic saline (3%), 5–10 ml/kg over 30 minutes, may be used as an alternative to mannitol.
• If mannitol has been used as first-line therapy and there is no initial response within 30 minutes, consider using hypertonic saline.
• Mannitol can be repeated after two hours.
• Hyperosmolar agents should be readily available at the bedside.
• Elevate the head of the bed to 30°.
• Transfer to pediatric intensive care unit.
• Reduce the rate of fluid administration by one-third.
• Intubation may be necessary for the patient with impending respiratory failure.
• *After* treatment for cerebral oedema has been started, cranial imaging may be considered, as with any critically ill patient with encephalopathy or acute focal neurologic deficit. The primary concern is whether the patient has a lesion requiring emergency neurosurgery (e.g. intracranial haemorrhage) or a lesion that may necessitate anticoagulation (e.g. cerebrovascular thrombosis).

Other uncommon or rare causes of morbidity and mortality in DKA include:
• Hypokalaemia
• Hypocalcaemia, hypomagnesemia
• Severe hypophosphatemia
• Hypoglycaemia
• Other central nervous system complications: dural sinus thrombosis, basilar artery thrombosis, intracranial haemorrhage, cerebral infarction
• Venous thrombosis
• Pulmonary embolism
• Sepsis
• Rhinocerebral or pulmonary mucormycosis
• Aspiration pneumonia
• Pulmonary oedema
• Adult respiratory distress syndrome (ARDS)
• Pneumothorax, pneumomediastinum, and subcutaneous emphysema
• Rhabdomyolysis
• Ischemic bowel necrosis
• Acute renal failure
• Acute pancreatitis
• Thrombocytopenia-associated multiple organ failure

The diabetes clinic

General principles

Children with diabetes should be seen in a designated diabetic clinic supervised by a paediatrician trained in the care of diabetes, paediatric endocrinologist or paediatric diabetologist. It has been recommended that there be a specialist diabetes nurse for every 100 children with diabetes. Age banding of the clinic may help bring families with similarly aged children together and facilitates group teaching of age-appropriate topics. The clinic should have the resources required to download data from blood glucose meters, insulin pumps, and CGM systems. It is highly advantageous to be able to perform point-of-care HbA1c measurements in the clinic so the results are available to the clinician during the consultation. The clinic should be equipped with a stadiometer for accurate auxology and should have suitable space for patient education and counselling. Educational literature (e.g. sick day guidelines), DVDs, information about diabetes camp and community resources, and other relevant information for children with diabetes should be available in the clinic.

The clinic visit

At each encounter in the diabetes clinic, the following issues should be addressed:

1 Documentation of general health and life events (e.g. changing school, participation in sports), recent hospital admissions or emergency department visits, insulin regimen, details of hypoglycaemic episodes and school absences.

2 Review of insulin regimen and blood glucose or CGM data.

3 Measurement of blood pressure, height and weight, and review of the growth chart.

4 Examination of injection or infusion sites and fingertips.

5 Measurement of HbA1c every three months.

6 If necessary, provision of advice on adjustments to the insulin regimen based on the results of glucose monitoring and physical activity.

An annual review of patients aged 10 years or older, who have had diabetes for ≥5 years should include:

7 a physical examination for microvascular and other complications of diabetes (Table 1.11);

8 assessment of puberty stage;

9 measurement of thyroid function tests and screening for coeliac disease (at suitable intervals);

10 measurement of cholesterol;

11 screening for microalbuminuria by measurement of the albumin:creatinine (ACR) ratio (ideally in a first morning urine sample);

12 referral to an ophthalmologist to screen for diabetic retinopathy or, if available, retinal photography in the clinic.

Given the multidisciplinary nature of a diabetes clinic, it is helpful to have a team meeting at the end of the clinic to share information about patients (especially those who are not achieving treatment goals) who have attended the clinic.

Monitoring and assessment of diabetes control

Self-monitoring of blood glucose (SMBG)

SMBG is the cornerstone of diabetes self-management and numerous studies show that frequency of SMBG correlates with glycaemic control. Routine SMBG is necessary to determine immediate insulin needs at meal times and to assess response to correcting hyperglycaemia with supplemental insulin or treatment of hypoglycaemia with glucose ingestion. Patients/parents should be encouraged to learn how to interpret patterns and trends of blood glucose data to assess the efficacy of therapy and to adjust individual components of their treatment regimen to achieve defined blood glucose goals. Most glucose meters have an electronic memory and data can be viewed on the device's screen or downloaded to a computer. In

Table 1.11 Points to note on clinical examination of patients with diabetes at annual review.

System	Points to note
Height	Growth failure
Weight	Poor or excessive weight gain
Puberty	Delayed puberty/menarche
Skin	Lipohypertrophy or lipoatrophy at injection sites, necrobiosis lipoidica
Mouth	Presence of caries or other signs of poor dental hygiene
Eyes	Presence of retinopathy/cataracts (through dilated pupils)
Feet	Signs of poor foot care (e.g. calluses from poorly-fitting shoes)
Hands	Finger-prick sites, limited joint mobility ('prayer sign')
Cardiovascular	Hypertension (if present, recheck at the end of the clinic visit)
Endocrine	Goitre, signs of hypothyroidism or hyperthyroidism; diffuse increased skin pigmentation suggestive of Addison's disease
Neurological	Impaired vibration or light touch (monofilament) sense; loss of ankle reflexes

recently diagnosed patients when insulin requirements are changing rapidly, it is valuable for patients/parents to manually record the results in a logbook and to examine the data for patterns and trends so that adjustments can be made when necessary.

For patients using intensive insulin regimens, SMBG should be performed before meals and snacks, occasionally two hours after meals, at bedtime, before, during, and after exercise, and after treatment of hypoglycaemia to ensure restoration of normoglycaemia. Blood glucose should be checked before driving and intermittently when driving for a prolonged period. To minimize the risk of nocturnal hypoglycaemia, blood glucose should be routinely measured at bedtime and between midnight and 4 a.m. once each week or every other week, and whenever the evening dose of insulin is adjusted. If HbA1c targets are not being met, patients should be encouraged to measure BG levels more frequently, including 90–120 minutes after meals. Children who are able independently to perform SMBG must be properly supervised because it is not unusual for children to fabricate data with potentially disastrous consequences.

Practical aspects of BG monitoring

- Children should be encouraged (but not coerced) to perform their own finger-prick BG measurements when they feel able to do so.
- Finger-pricks should be performed on the sides of the fingertips.
- Finger-pricking devices with variable depth settings can make lancing less painful.
- Forearm or thenar eminence blood glucose testing are accurate and acceptable alternatives to finger-prick testing.
- Blood glucose meters with electronic memory allow data to be downloaded to a computer or uploaded to 'the cloud' for review and discussion in clinic.
- Date-expired blood glucose testing strips should not be used as these may lead to inaccurate BG measurements.

Ketone testing

Urine or blood ketones should be measured during acute illness, whenever there is persistent hyperglycaemia (>250–300 mg/dL, 13.9–16.7 mmol/L), and when the patient experiences nausea, vomiting, or abdominal pain. When hyperglycaemia is prolonged in patients who use an insulin pump, ketone measurement provides an additional clue to the possibility of insulin infusion failure. Ketone measurement is a valuable guide to supplemental insulin therapy to prevent or reverse metabolic decompensation, and to determine when referral for urgent care is required (see Section 1.17 on 'sick day' management).

Urine ketone test strips detect acetoacetate (and acetone), and qualitative results are interpreted based on colour changes: 'trace', 'small', 'moderate', or 'large' ketones corresponding to 5, 15, 40, 80–160 mg/dL, respectively. The correlations between interquartile ranges of capillary blood BOHB and urine ketone values are:

0.1–0.9 mmol/L corresponds to + or 'small' urine ketones;

0.2–1.8 mmol/L corresponds to ++ or 'moderate' urine ketones;

1.4–5.2 mmol/L corresponds to +++ or 'large' urine ketones.

False negative readings may occur when the strips have been exposed to air or when the urine is highly acidic (e.g. after consumption of large doses of ascorbic acid). Urine ketone tests using nitroprusside-containing reagents can give false positive results in patients who take valproic acid or any sulfhydryl-containing drugs, including captopril.

Ketone meters for home use measure blood BOHB concentration, which, compared to urine ketone testing, offers the advantage of accurately assessing the biochemical response to treatment and is more efficacious in avoiding emergency room visits. Normally BOHB is <0.6 mmol/L; values >3 mmol/L may indicate impending or actual DKA. Blood ketone strips are, however, considerably more expensive than urine ketone strips; therefore, when expense is a consideration, a cost-effective approach is to reserve blood ketone measurements for young children who cannot reliably provide a urine sample on demand and when urine testing shows 'large' ketonuria.

Glycated haemoglobin or haemoglobin A1c

HbA1c is formed slowly and non-enzymatically when glucose attaches to haemoglobin. Because erythrocytes are freely permeable to glucose, HbA1c is formed throughout the lifespan of the erythrocyte, and its rate of formation is directly proportional to the ambient glucose concentration. HbA1c is a weighted average of blood glucose levels during the life of the erythrocytes (120 days). Therefore, glucose levels on days nearer to the test contribute substantially more to the HbA1c level than the levels in days further from the test.

Whereas blood glucose and ketone measurements provide valuable information for immediate day-to-day management of diabetes, HbA1c is a measure of average glycaemia over the preceding three months and is a biomarker of the risk for the development of diabetes complications. Laboratories should report their results adjusted to give comparable values to the assay used in the DCCT. The DCCT-aligned normal, non-diabetic range is 4–6% (20–42 mmol/mol).

HbA1c should be measured approximately every three months to determine whether a patient's metabolic control has reached or has been maintained within a target range. The HbA1c is primarily used to monitor the effectiveness of glycaemic therapy and as an indicator for when therapy needs to be modified (Table 1.12). HbA1c underestimates average glucose levels in conditions that shorten the average circulating erythrocyte lifespan, such as haemolysis, sickle cell disease, after blood transfusion, CF, and iron deficiency anaemia. When accurate HbA1c measurement is not possible, as in the above conditions, an alternative measure of chronic glycaemia such as fructosamine should be used. Fructosamine testing determines the fraction of total serum proteins that have undergone glycation. Since albumin is the most abundant protein in blood, fructosamine levels typically reflect albumin glycation. Albumin has a half-life of approximately 20 days; therefore, plasma fructosamine concentration reflects relatively recent (~2 weeks) glycaemia. Some tests specifically quantify glycation of albumin instead of all proteins.

Continuous glucose monitoring

Real-time CGM devices are minimally invasive and accurately measure glucose in the interstitial fluid with a subcutaneous glucose sensor and report a value every five minutes. Depending on the specific CGM system, finger-stick blood glucose values may be needed to calibrate the device. There is a lag of several minutes between plasma glucose and interstitial glucose concentrations; nonetheless, sensor glucose values provide detailed information about patterns and trends in the intervals between SMBG measurements, and especially after meals and during the night. The number of children with type 1 diabetes using CGM for routine diabetes care is rapidly increasing. The benefit of CGM on glycaemic control in type 1 diabetes is directly related to the duration and frequency of its use; near-daily use is associated with a significant reduction in HbA1c levels and less time spent in the hypoglycaemia range. Also, the number of daily finger-pricks can be reduced and parents and children experience less anxiety about nocturnal hypoglycaemia. In addition to cost, barriers to the use of CGM include insertion pain, annoying system alarms, contact dermatitis from the adhesive, and body image issues. For some patients, the hassles outweigh the benefits, which include glucose trend data (including the capability of remote monitoring), opportunities to promptly correct out-of-range glucose levels, and to detect actual or impending hypoglycaemia. As CGM technology improves and increasingly becomes integrated with insulin pumps, the acceptability of CGM devices for long-term use in youth with type 1 diabetes will undoubtedly continue to increase.

Table 1.12 Interpretation of glycated haemoglobin values.

HbA1c (%)[a]	IFCC-HbA1c mmol/mol	Comment
4–5.9	20–41	Within non-diabetic range
6–6.9	42–52	Optimal, ideal glycaemic control in absence of frequent or severe hypoglycaemia
7–7.5	53–59	Optimal, very good glycaemic control in absence of frequent or severe hypoglycaemia
7.6–8.9	60–74	Suboptimal, associated with increased risk of microvascular complications; action to improve control suggested
9–10.9	75–96	High risk, poor compliance; associated with high risk of microvascular complications; action required
≥11	≥97	High risk, poor compliance; insulin omission; associated with high risk of microvascular complications and DKA; action required

[a] DCCT standardized.

Exercise

Several cross-sectional studies of youth with type 1 diabetes show that physical fitness (measured by peak oxygen consumption [VO_2]) is inversely associated with HbA1c; lower peak VO_2 predicts higher HbA1c levels. Also, lack of physical activity (e.g. more time spent viewing television and computer screen time) is associated with poor glycaemic control. Although intervention/training studies in paediatric patients have not consistently shown a beneficial effect of regular physical activity on HbA1c levels, children with diabetes should, nonetheless, be encouraged to participate in sports and include regular exercise in their lives. Physical exercise has numerous benefits: it normalizes the child's life, enhances self-esteem, improves physical fitness, helps to control weight, and *may* improve glycaemic control. Regular exercise increases insulin sensitivity during and immediately after exercise, and again 7–11 hours later. Regular exercise also increases cardiovascular fitness and lean body mass, improves blood lipid profiles, and lowers blood pressure.

Physical exercise is complicated for the child with type 1 diabetes, especially by the need to prevent hypoglycaemia during and after exercise (Riddell et al. 2017). Children with type 1 diabetes are twice as likely to have nocturnal hypoglycaemia during the night after an exercise day as compared with a night after a sedentary day. Inability to spontaneously reduce insulin levels during exercise is the key factor that contributes to the increased risk of hypoglycaemia; however, with proper guidance and planning, exercise can be a safe and enjoyable experience.

In the child with poorly controlled diabetes, vigorous exercise can aggravate hyperglycaemia and ketoacid production; accordingly, a child with ketonuria should not exercise until satisfactory biochemical control has been restored. In type 1 diabetes increased levels of epinephrine and glucagon in response to acute strenuous anaerobic exercise may cause transient hyperglycaemia despite well-controlled diabetes. In contrast, sustained aerobic exercise acutely lowers the blood glucose concentration by variably increasing utilization of glucose depending on the intensity and duration of physical activity and the concurrent plasma insulin level. Hypoglycaemia can usually be prevented by a combination of anticipatory reduction in pre-exercise insulin dose or, with CSII, a temporary interruption or reduction of basal insulin infusion and/or supplemental carbohydrate containing snacks or drinks before, during, and after activity, depending on the intensity and duration of the physical activity and its timing. Nearly all forms of activity lasting more than 30 minutes require some adjustment to food and/or insulin. The optimal strategy depends on the child's insulin regimen and on the timing of exercise in relation to the child's meal plan. Several factors must be considered when selecting the content and size of the snack, including the current blood glucose level, the action profile of insulin most active during and after the period of anticipated exercise, the interval since the last meal, and the duration and intensity of physical activity. The appropriate adjustments for exercise are learned by trial and error; however, a useful initial guide is to provide 0.5–1 gram of carbohydrate per kg of body mass per hour of moderate to strenuous exercise. Prolonged strenuous exercise in the afternoon or evening should be followed by a 10–30% reduction in the pre-supper or bedtime dose of intermediate- or long-acting insulin, or an equivalent reduction in overnight basal insulin delivery in patients using CSII. In addition, to reduce the risk of nocturnal or early-morning hypoglycaemia caused by the lag effect of exercise and reduced counter-regulatory hormone responses during sleep, the bedtime snack should be larger than usual and contain a 'slow' carbohydrate, protein, and fat. Frequent blood glucose monitoring or CGM is essential for the active child with diabetes because it allows identification of trends in glycaemic responses. Records should include blood glucose levels, timing, duration, and intensity of exercise as well as the strategies used to maintain glucose concentrations in the target range.

Exercising the limb into which insulin has been injected accelerates the rate of insulin absorption. Therefore, if possible, the insulin injection preceding exercise should be given in a site (e.g. abdomen if running or cycling) least likely to be affected by exercise. Because physical training increases tissue sensitivity to insulin, when poorly conditioned youth commence participation in organized sports or dramatically increase their level of physical activity (e.g. at the start of summer camp), they should reduce the TDD of insulin by at least 20%, and further adjust the dose of insulin predominantly active during the period of sustained physical activity. The precise dose reduction is empirically determined by measuring blood glucose levels before and after exercise.

Diabetes in preschool-aged children

There are numerous unique features pertinent to the management of very young children with diabetes as shown in Table 1.13.

Table 1.13 Principles of managing diabetes in preschool-aged children.

- The target HbA1c is <7.5% (58 mmol/mol)
- Use an intensive insulin therapy regimen consisting of basal and preprandial meal-adjusted insulin together with frequent blood glucose monitoring.
- Insulin pump therapy is the preferred method of insulin administration; if unavailable, multiple daily injections should be used from the onset of diabetes.
- Preprandial administration of bolus insulin for correction of hyperglycaemia and for coverage of at least part of the meal is preferable to giving the entire dose during or after the meal.
- Introduce carbohydrate counting at onset of diabetes.
- It may be necessary to dilute insulin to be able to accurately administer the small doses required by young children.
- Use insulin syringes with ½ unit markings or insulin pens with ½ unit dosing increments.
- Continuous glucose monitoring is valuable to monitor glycaemia. If unavailable, frequent (up to 7–10) daily blood glucose measurements may be required to maintain optimal control.
- Injection, infusion and sensor insertion sites should be regularly rotated to reduce likelihood of lipohypertrophy, scarring, infection.
- Engage both fathers and mothers in diabetes care from the onset of diagnosis.
- Establish family-centred meal routines and restrict continuous snacking ('grazing') to ensure dietary quality and optimize glycaemic control.
- Provide diabetes education to staff at preschool and school to ensure safe and unrestricted participation in all school activities.
- Optimal glycaemic control with avoidance of extreme hyperglycaemia and hypoglycaemia enables the child to participate, concentrate, and learn.
- Monitoring growth, weight, and body mass index at each visit provides an indication of the adequacy of the child's nutrition and diabetes control.

Source: Modified from (Sundberg et al. 2017).

Diabetes in adolescence

Adolescence is the transitional phase of development between childhood and adulthood. It is a period of great physical and psychological change, including rapid physical growth and sexual maturation, ongoing identity formation, and increasingly powerful influences of social context and peer relationships. For patients with type 1 diabetes, adolescence presents special challenges related to diabetes self-care and glycaemic control, which often deteriorates during this period of life. This is attributable to physiologic increased insulin resistance during puberty as well as developmental and psychosocial factors that may decrease adherence to diabetes care tasks, including the shift in responsibility for care from parent to child, the impact of peer and romantic relationships, and increased risk-taking behaviours. For these reasons, the health care and emotional needs of adolescents differ substantially from those of younger children and adults. The overarching goal is to patiently and persistently educate, guide, support, and encourage the adolescent to maintain blood glucose levels as near to normal as possible, which reduces the risk of long-term complications, while avoiding hypoglycaemia

and DKA. Developing a trusting and motivating relationship between health care professionals and the adolescent patient and maintaining continuity of care provides the best opportunity to positively influence adolescent self-care.

The role of the family in adolescent diabetes

The family has a central role in the successful management of diabetes during adolescence and care should be family-centred from the time of diagnosis. Because the adolescent with diabetes is cognitively and emotionally immature, successful treatment requires the active involvement of responsible adults. At the same time, diabetes also requires family members to be sensitive to the balance between the youth's need for a sense of autonomy and mastery of self-care activities and the need for ongoing family involvement and support. The struggle to balance independence and dependence in relationships between the adolescent patient and family members presents a long-term challenge and raises different issues for families at different stages of child and adolescent development. Focusing on normal developmental tasks at each stage of the adolescent's growth and development provides the most effective framework for addressing these issues (Anderson and Schwartz 2014).

Family conflict around diabetes management is a strong predictor of poor adherence and poor glycaemic control; conversely, children living in supportive family environments with a high level of parent involvement generally have better adherence and glycaemic control. Counselling-based interventions to improve family communication and teamwork in diabetes care have been shown to improve treatment adherence and glycaemic control. Accordingly, the diabetes care team should encourage parents to foster family teamwork around diabetes management (e.g. schedule weekly brief family meetings to discuss 'the week in diabetes') and to view teamwork as a way to teach and empower their child to become a more active participant in his or her care. When communication between parents and the adolescent about diabetes is negative ('shaming and blaming'), involves sarcasm or yelling, or is dishonest (e.g. lying about blood glucose values), family teamwork is impossible to maintain.

Areas for intervention to improve adherence in adolescents with type 1 diabetes

Treatment adherence is closely associated with improved glycaemic control in adolescents with type 1 diabetes and efforts to support and enhance adherence to diabetes self-care tasks in adolescents are critically important. For example, use of a non-medically trained 'care ambassador' to deliver psychoeducational modules and facilitate clinic follow-up has been found to decrease HbA1c levels as well as diabetes-related emergency department visits and hospitalizations in adolescents with type 1 diabetes. Motivational interviewing techniques during routine clinic visits improve HbA1c as well as patient satisfaction. Mobile and internet health technologies are other promising avenues for engaging adolescents. For example, receiving a text-messaging support system ('Sweet Talk') to reinforce diabetes care goals improves diabetes self-efficacy and self-care adherence, and adolescents receiving internet-based education about both diabetes management and behavioural coping had lower HbA1c levels and higher quality of life and diabetes self-efficacy scores after 18 months.

Transition from pediatric to adult diabetes care

Adolescents will eventually need to transfer their care from paediatric to adult diabetes care providers. The developmental stage from the late teens through the twenties has been defined as 'emerging adulthood', a period of competing educational, social, work, and financial demands. As young adults with type 1 diabetes encounter these competing life priorities while simultaneously experiencing decreased parental support, adherence to self-care often declines and glycaemic control may deteriorate. Lack of effective transition from paediatric to adult diabetes care may contribute to fragmentation of health care and increase the risk for adverse outcomes.

The transition process entails numerous challenges, including suboptimal paediatric transition preparation, gaps in care, and increased post-transition hospitalizations. There is no evidence supporting an ideal transition age, and an individualized approach is recommended. A position statement of the American Diabetes Association, in collaboration with a number of professional societies, recommends that paediatric diabetes providers begin to prepare patients for transition to adult care during the early adolescent years and at least one year before actual transfer (Peters and Laffel 2011). Preparation should include a focus on diabetes self-management skills as well as coordination of transfer referrals, direct communication with the receiving adult providers, and a written care summary. Several organizations, including the National Diabetes Education Program and The Endocrine Society, have produced materials to support the transition process (http://www.Your DiabetesInfo.org/transitions; https://www.endocrine.org/education-and-practice-management/quality-improvement-resources/clinical-practice-resources/transition-of-care). In some health care systems, joint transition clinics staffed by both paediatric and adult physicians have been a successful care model for older adolescents and young adults.

Psychological and psychiatric problems

Depression

Major depressive disorders as well as subclinical depressive symptomatology are more common in adolescents with diabetes. A recent study in the US identified symptoms of depression in 13% of youth with type 1 and in 22% with type 2 diabetes, and subclinical depressive symptomatology is associated with poor clinical outcomes. Therefore, in addition to addressing family conflict related to type 1 diabetes and supporting adolescent adherence to diabetes self-management, adolescents with type 1 diabetes should be routinely screened for depression from the time of diagnosis. Interventions can then be targeted based on the specific needs of individual adolescents and families.

Eating disorders

Adolescent females with type 1 diabetes have a two-fold increased risk of developing an eating disorder compared to their peers without diabetes. Some adolescents manipulate insulin doses or dietary behaviours in order to lose weight. These behaviours should be suspected in adolescents, especially females, unable to achieve and maintain blood glucose targets or who have unexplained weight loss or deterioration of metabolic control. Efficient screening can be performed using a five-question SCOFF Questionnaire designed to clarify suspicion that an eating disorder might exist. Patients with identified eating disorders or deliberate misuse of insulin are at high risk for earlier onset and progression of microvascular complications and mortality, and should receive intensive multidisciplinary care that includes a mental health professional with expertise in eating disorders.

Miscellaneous problems

There is an increased incidence of polycystic ovary syndrome and menstrual irregularities in girls with both type 1 and type 2 diabetes. The menstrual cycle may also affect blood glucose control with rising values in the two to three days before the start of a period. In those in whom this occurs regularly, insulin dosage should be increased during this time.

Hypoglycaemia in youth with diabetes

Hypoglycaemia is the most common acute complication of treatment, and concern about hypoglycaemia is a central issue in treating people with type 1 diabetes. It is the most important barrier to the pursuit and maintenance of near-normal glycaemic control and patients, parents, and the diabetes team must continuously balance the risks of hypoglycaemia against those of long-term hyperglycaemia. Fear of hypoglycaemia is common in children with type 1 diabetes and their parents. An episode of severe hypoglycaemia undermines the confidence of the patient and parents, and fear of a recurrence may induce the patient or parents to change their diabetes management goals. Altered behaviours may include overeating and/or deliberate selection of lower doses of insulin to maintain higher blood glucose levels perceived as being safe, resulting in overall deterioration of glycaemic control over time. For some parents, concern about nocturnal hypoglycaemia may cause more anxiety than any other aspect of diabetes, including the fear of long-term complications.

The normal glucagon response to hypoglycaemia is lost early in the disease in parallel with loss of beta cells, and patients with type 1 diabetes must then depend on sympatho-adrenal responses to prevent or correct hypoglycaemia. Recurrent mild hypoglycaemia itself reduces epinephrine responses and symptomatic awareness of subsequent episodes of hypoglycaemia.

Symptoms and signs of hypoglycaemia

Patients with type 1 diabetes depend on the activation of the sympathetic nervous system and an increase in epinephrine secretion to detect a fall in blood glucose concentration. Symptoms and signs of hypoglycaemia are caused by the counter-regulatory response, which produces neurogenic (autonomic) symptoms, including sweating, trembling (shakiness), tingling, pallor, palpitations, nervousness, and anxiety, or are the result of neuroglycopenia (inadequate fuel for normal brain function), characterized by difficulty concentrating, blurred vision, confusion, odd behaviour, slurred speech, numbness, loss of coordination, drowsiness, seizures, coma, and death. Patients frequently report a combination of both neurogenic and neuroglycopenic symptoms. The most common signs and symptoms of hypoglycaemia in children are weakness, tremor, hunger, fatigue, drowsiness, sweating, headache, and pallor. In contrast to adolescents, autonomic symptoms are less common in children younger than 6 years old whose symptoms of hypoglycaemia are more often neuroglycopenic or nonspecific in nature. Behavioural changes (irritability, tantrums, erratic behaviour, inconsolable crying) are often the primary manifestation of hypoglycaemia in young children. In contrast to adults, who are usually able to distinguish between autonomic and neuroglycopenic symptoms, children and their parents report that symptoms tend to cluster.

The American Diabetes Association defines biochemical hypoglycaemia as blood glucose <70 mg/dL (3.9 mmol/L) (Seaquist et al. 2013). However, healthy 8- to 16-year-old children and adolescents and those with type 1 diabetes may begin to counter-regulate at a higher blood glucose level than adults. As a result, their hypoglycaemia symptoms may occur with blood glucose concentrations in the normal range. Hypoglycaemia in children is often classified in terms of its severity as mild, moderate, or severe, most episodes being mild. Cognitive impairment does not accompany mild hypoglycaemia and older children are able to recognize the symptoms and treat themselves. Mild symptoms abate within about 15 minutes after treatment with a rapidly absorbed carbohydrate. Moderate hypoglycaemia has both neuroglycopenic and autonomic symptoms, e.g. mood changes, irritability, decreased attentiveness, drowsiness, and behaviour change. Preschool age children, however, invariably require assistance with treatment because they are often confused and their judgement is impaired; also, weakness and lack of coordination may make self-treatment difficult or impossible. Moderate hypoglycaemia causes more protracted symptoms and may require a second treatment with oral carbohydrate. Severe hypoglycaemia is characterized by sufficient cognitive impairment that the assistance of another person is needed for treatment. Such events include episodes of unresponsiveness, unconsciousness, or seizures requiring emergency treatment with glucagon or intravenous glucose. This definition is not applicable to very young children, who, by definition, *always* require assistance for treatment of hypoglycaemia.

Children who have had diabetes for several years may describe a change in their symptoms over time. Autonomic symptoms tend to be less frequent and are more muted, and neuroglycopenic symptoms (e.g. drowsiness, difficulty concentrating, lack of coordination) are more common. Patients must learn to recognize the change in symptoms to prevent severe episodes. The blood glucose concentration at which symptoms occur varies among patients and the threshold may vary in the same individual in parallel with antecedent glycaemic control. Children with poorly controlled diabetes experience symptoms of hypoglycaemia at higher blood glucose concentrations than those with good glycaemic control.

Impact of hypoglycaemia on the child's brain

Owing to maturation of the central nervous system, the youngest children are at greater risk for cognitive deficits from hypoglycaemia. It is difficult, however, to dissect out the contributions of metabolic disturbances (hyperglycaemia and hypoglycaemia) and the psychosocial effects of chronic disease in a young child. Nonetheless, there is evidence linking hypoglycaemia (asymptomatic as well as severe hypoglycaemic events) to neuropsychological deficits. Preliminary findings suggest poorer memory skills, presumed but not proven to be the consequence of recurrent and severe hypoglycaemia. Exposure to severe hypoglycaemia has been associated with increased hippocampal volumes in children with type 1 diabetes, which may represent a pathological reaction to hypoglycaemia during brain development.

Even in the absence of typical symptoms, cognitive function deteriorates at low blood glucose levels. Moderate and severe hypoglycaemia is disabling, affects school performance, and makes driving a car or operating dangerous machinery hazardous. The utmost effort should be made to avoid such events. Repeated or prolonged severe hypoglycaemia can cause permanent central nervous system damage, especially in very young children. Fortunately, hypoglycaemia is a rare cause of death in children with type 1 diabetes.

Frequency of hypoglycaemia

The true frequency of mild (self-treated) symptomatic hypoglycaemia is almost impossible to ascertain accurately because mild episodes are quickly forgotten and are often not recorded. Increased use of CSII and the use of insulin analogues with multiple daily dose insulin regimens that more closely mimic physiologic insulin replacement, increased frequency of blood glucose monitoring, use of CGM, more widespread use of multidisciplinary diabetes care teams, and improvements in patient education have contributed to an overall reduction in risk of severe hypoglycaemia and lower HbA1c levels in recent years. In recent reports, rates of loss of consciousness or seizure are from 4 to 10 events per 100 patient-years.

Causes of hypoglycaemia in diabetes

Hypoglycaemia is the result of a mismatch between insulin, food, and physical activity and can be the result of therapeutic, biologic, and behavioural factors (see Table 1.14).

Nocturnal hypoglycaemia

An increase in plasma epinephrine concentrations is normally the main hormonal defence against hypoglycaemia in type 1 diabetes; however, sleep impairs counter-regulatory hormone responses to hypoglycaemia, both in normal subjects and in patients with

Table 1.14 Causes of hypoglycaemia in children and adolescents with diabetes mellitus.

Insulin errors (inadvertent or deliberate)
   Reversal of morning and evening dose
   Reversal of short- or rapid-acting insulin and
   intermediate- or long-acting insulin
   Improper timing of insulin administration in relation
   to food consumption
   Excessive insulin dosage
   Surreptitious insulin administration; suicide gesture
   or attempt

Erratic or altered insulin absorption
   Inadvertent intramuscular injection
   More rapid absorption from exercising limbs
   Unpredictable absorption from lipohypertrophy
   at injection sites
   More rapid absorption after sauna, hot bath,
   sunbathing

Diet
   Omission or reduced size of meals or snacks
   Delayed snacks or meals
   Variable meal composition: carbohydrate with/
   without protein and fat
   Eating disorders and disordered eating
   Gastroparesis
   Malabsorption, e.g. gluten enteropathy

Exercise
   Unplanned physical activity
   Prolonged duration and/or increased intensity of
   physical activity
   Strenuous exercise in the afternoon or evening
   Failure to reduce the dose of basal insulin to combat
   the 'lag effect' of exercise

Alcohol and/or drugs
   Impaired gluconeogenesis from excessive
   consumption of ethanol
   Impaired cognition from use of ethanol (may cause
   hypoglycaemia unawareness), marijuana, cocaine,
   other recreational drugs

Hypoglycaemia-associated autonomic failure
   Recurrent hypoglycaemia
   Hypoglycaemia unawareness
   Defective glucose counter-regulation

Miscellaneous uncommon causes of hypoglycaemia
   Adrenocortical insufficiency
   Hypothyroidism
   Growth hormone deficiency
   Renal failure
   Decreased insulin requirement in first trimester of
   pregnancy
   Insulin autoantibodies

diabetes, which explains the increased susceptibility to hypoglycaemia during sleep. Furthermore, asymptomatic nocturnal hypoglycaemia may impair counter-regulatory hormone responses. Thus, impaired defences against hypoglycaemia during sleep may contribute to the vicious cycle of hypoglycaemia, impaired counter-regulatory responses, and unawareness of hypoglycaemia (failure to experience autonomic warning symptoms before the onset of neuroglycopenia) either awake or asleep. Recurrent asymptomatic nocturnal hypoglycaemia is an important (but frequently undetected or overlooked) cause of hypoglycaemia unawareness, which, in turn, leads to more frequent and severe hypoglycaemia. Both children and adults studied either in hospital or at home with frequent intermittent or continuous blood glucose measurements during the night, show a high incidence of asymptomatic hypoglycaemia. For example, in the Juvenile Diabetes Research Foundation CGM randomized clinical trial, hypoglycaemic events (two consecutive CGM readings ≤60 mg/dL [3.3 mmol/L] in 20 minutes) occurred during 8.5% of nights (approximately twice per month) and lasted ≥2 hours on 23% of nights with hypoglycaemia. Hypoglycaemia during sleep may exceed four hours in duration, and up to half these episodes may be undetected because the subject does not wake from sleep. The incidence of hypoglycaemia on any given night is affected by numerous factors, including the insulin regimen, the timing and content of meals and snacks, and antecedent physical activity. Long after strenuous physical exercise has ended there is a sustained increase in insulin action on muscle and liver and blunting of the counter-regulatory response to hypoglycaemia. Low blood glucose concentrations in the early morning (before breakfast) are associated with a higher frequency of preceding nocturnal hypoglycaemia, and this knowledge is useful in counselling patients to modify the evening insulin regimen and bedtime snack to prevent more severe nocturnal hypoglycaemia.

Treatment of hypoglycaemia

The aim is to restore blood glucose to ≥100 mg/dL (5.6 mmol/L) as quickly as possible after the first symptom or sign is detected. Except in pre-school-aged children, most episodes of symptomatic hypoglycaemia are self-treated with a rapidly absorbed source of carbohydrate such as glucose tablets or gel, fruit juice, soft drinks, sweets, or crackers. Foods that contain fat together with carbohydrate should be discouraged because fat slows the absorption of carbohydrate from the gastrointestinal tract. Because glucose tablets raise blood glucose levels more rapidly than orange juice, and the dosage is easily calibrated, they should be the treatment of choice for children old enough to chew and safely swallow large tablets. The recommended dose of glucose is 0.3 grams per kg body weight (5–20 g depending on the child's body weight). The blood glucose concentration should be re-measured 15 minutes after treatment, and if the value does not exceed 70–80 mg/dL (3.9–4.4 mmol/L), treatment should be repeated. The glycaemic response to oral glucose usually lasts less than two hours; therefore, unless a scheduled meal or snack is due within an hour, the patient should be given either a snack or a meal containing carbohydrate and protein.

Hypoglycaemia is common when the child with diabetes is unable to consume or absorb oral carbohydrate because an intercurrent illness (e.g. gastroenteritis) causes nausea and vomiting or due to oppositional behaviour and food refusal in very young children. To maintain blood glucose concentrations in a safe range, parents may either seek emergency medical attention or attempt to force feed oral carbohydrate in an ill child, which often leads to more vomiting. 'Mini-dose' glucagon raises blood glucose by 60 – 90 mg/dL (3.3 – 5 mmol/L) within 30 minutes and its effect lasts approximately one hour. This is an effective method for managing most situations of impending hypoglycaemia at home. First dissolve 1 mg glucagon in 1 ml of diluent; then, using a U-100 insulin syringe children ≤2 years of age receive 2 'units' (20 μg) of glucagon SC, and children >2 years, receive 1 unit (10 μg) per year of age up to a maximum dose of 15 units (150 μg). Blood glucose should be measured every 30 minutes for one hour, and hourly thereafter until the crisis has resolved. If the blood glucose concentration does not increase within 30 minutes, repeat the treatment using double the initial dosage of glucagon.

Severe hypoglycaemia (unresponsiveness, unconsciousness, or seizures) requires emergency treatment with parenteral glucagon (IM or SC). The usual recommended dose is 0.5 mg if the child is <12 years and 1 mg if >12 years. The increase in blood glucose concentration is sustained for at least 30 minutes after glucagon administration. Therefore, it is unnecessary to repeat the dose or force the child to eat or drink for at least 30 minutes. In an emergency department or hospital, the preferred treatment is intravenous glucose (0.3 gram per kg). After bolus administration of glucose, the glycaemic response is transient; therefore, an intravenous glucose infusion should continue until the patient is able to swallow safely.

If severe hypoglycaemia was prolonged and the patient had a seizure, complete recovery of cognitive and neurologic function may take many hours despite restoration of normal blood glucose levels. Transient (Todd's) paralysis may occur; however, permanent hemiparesis and other neurologic sequelae are rare; however, the post-ictal period may be complicated by headache, lethargy, nausea, vomiting, and muscle ache.

Recurrent DKA and its prevention

Recurrent DKA is invariably the result of psychosocial problems and failure to inject insulin. Management of an episode of DKA is not complete until its cause has been identified and an attempt made to prevent recurrence.
- Infection is rarely the cause of DKA when the patient/family is properly educated in diabetes management and is receiving appropriate follow-up care by a diabetes team with a 24-hour telephone helpline.
- In most cases, the cause is either inadvertent or deliberate insulin omission.
- In insulin pump users, the most common cause of DKA is failure to take extra insulin with a pen or syringe when 'pump failure' (interrupted insulin delivery for any reason) occurs.
- Home measurement of blood BOHB concentrations, when compared to urine ketone testing, decreases diabetes-related hospital visits by permitting earlier identification, more accurate quantitation, and treatment of ketosis. Blood BOHB measurements may be especially valuable to prevent DKA in pump users because interrupted insulin delivery rapidly leads to ketosis.
- There usually is an important psychosocial reason for insulin omission such as:
  - an attempt to lose weight in an adolescent girl with an eating disorder;
  - teenage rebellion/rejection of diabetes;
  - a means of escaping an abusive home situation;
  - depression or other reason for inability of the patient to manage diabetes unassisted.
- A psychiatric social worker or clinical psychologist should be consulted to identify the psychosocial reason(s) contributing to development of DKA.
- Insulin omission can be prevented by comprehensive programmes that provide education, psychosocial evaluation, and treatment combined with adult supervision of insulin administration.
- Parents and patients should learn how to recognize and treat ketosis and impending DKA with additional rapid- or short-acting insulin and oral fluids.

- Families should have access to a 24-hour telephone helpline for emergency advice and treatment.
- When a responsible adult administers insulin, the frequency of recurrent DKA decreases dramatically.

The treatment of DKA is described earlier in this chapter (Section 1.9).

Management of diabetes during intercurrent illness ('Sick Day Rules')

An acute febrile illness often leads to a rise in blood glucose and ketone concentrations due to the effects of raised levels of stress hormones and increased insulin resistance. If not properly managed, progression to DKA may ensue. Conversely, diseases associated with diarrhoea and/or vomiting such as gastroenteritis may lead to hypoglycaemia. Families should have clear and concrete guidelines on the management of diabetes during intercurrent illness ('sick day rules'), see Table 1.15. Ketones should be measured whenever:

- the child has abdominal pain;
- there is nausea or vomiting;
- blood glucose is ≥300 mg/dL (16.7 mmol/L) on two consecutive measurements;
- blood glucose is ≥250 mg dL (13.9 mmol/L) upon waking up in the morning;
- the child is febrile.

The important principles for managing diabetes during intercurrent illness include:

- Do not omit or decrease the dose of long- or intermediate-acting insulin (see Table 1.15 for recommendations concerning doses of supplemental rapid-acting insulin).
- Regularly measure blood or urine ketone concentrations.
- Monitor blood glucose concentrations at least before each meal and before bedtime. More frequent monitoring, for example, hourly or every two hours, may be required.
- Consume carbohydrate regularly. If the child has a poor appetite, this may take the form of regular small snacks and/or sugar-containing drinks, rather than large meals.
- Drink plenty of water and/or reduced sugar fluids to counteract the potential dehydration that may be associated with glucosuria and a febrile illness.
- If hypoglycaemia occurs, particularly in association with gastroenteritis and mild ketosis, ensure that the child takes regular, frequent carbohydrate-containing snacks and/or sugary drinks. Oral rehydration solutions are sometimes necessary. Occasionally, glucose gel or mini dose glucagon (see Section 1.15 on hypoglycaemia) are required to treat hypoglycaemia and to help re-establish oral feeds. Vomiting may be treated with a single dose of an anti-emetic to try to improve carbohydrate intake.
- To treat the underlying illness, antibiotics may be required for some infections and antipyretics are also often required. Sugar-free medicines are preferable if available.
- If, despite these measures, the child has persistent vomiting and/or diarrhoea, significant hypoglycaemia, abdominal pain, drowsiness, tachypnoea, the blood glucose and/or ketone concentrations fail to

Table 1.15 Guidelines for managing sick days and correcting ketones.

Blood glucose (mg/dL mmol/L)		Urine ketones	Blood ketones (mmol/L)	Dose of rapid-acting insulin	Monitoring
≤180	≤10	≥Trace	≥0.6	Usual dose	Re-check glucose and ketones in two hours
181–300	10.1–16.7	≥Trace	≥0.6	Usual 'correction factor'[a]	Re-check glucose and ketones in two hours
>300	10.1–16.7	Small	0.6–0.9	Usual 'correction factor'[a]	Re-check glucose and ketones in two hours
>300	10.1–16.7	Moderate	1–1.5	15% of total daily dose or 0.15 units per kg	Re-check glucose and ketones in two hours
>300	10.1–16.7	Large	>1.5	20% of total daily dose or 0.2 unit per kg	Re-check glucose and ketones in two hours

Typical dosing guidelines are individualized based on age, weight, pubertal status, and duration of diabetes.
[a] 5–10% of total daily insulin dose or 0.05–0.1 unit per kg.

respond to changes in insulin treatment, or the parents remain concerned, then they should contact the diabetes nurse, doctor or hospital for further advice.

• In cases of severe gastroenteritis and in those with severe or persistent vomiting, IV fluids may be necessary (e.g. 5% dextrose/0.45% or 0.9% saline with 10 mmol of potassium per 500 ml). In such cases, it is often best to also administer IV insulin. Insulin infusion at a rate approximately equivalent to the child's basal insulin requirement may be used. For example, if the child's TDD of insulin is 0.8 units kg^{-1}, assume 50% (0.4 units kg^{-1}) is basal insulin. Divide this number by 24 to obtain an hourly dose of basal insulin for infusion. In this example, 0.4 divided by 24 = 0.017 unit per kg per hour (round down to 0.015 or up to 0.02 unit per kg per hour). Adjust the rate of insulin (and dextrose) infusion guided by hourly blood glucose measurements.

Management of diabetes when travelling

When travelling, the following principles are recommended for management of the diabetes (Pinsker et al. 2013):

• Patients who are planning to travel overseas should schedule a visit with their diabetes care provider at least 4–6 weeks before departure. Advanced planning will help prevent emergencies that may occur away from home.

• Travel with identification (diabetes identification card, Medic Alert necklace or bracelet), surplus insulin, glucose and ketone monitoring supplies (strips and lancets), spare batteries, syringes, pens, needles or infusion sets. Supplies should include glucose gel and glucagon. All diabetes-related medications and supplies should be taken as carry-on luggage and must NEVER be in checked baggage.

• A letter for the airlines, security and Customs should state the diagnosis and list all the diabetes supplies required.

• Appropriate health insurance must be arranged.

• Open insulin vials retain their potency at room temperature for at least one month. In hot climates, insulin should be stored either in a refrigerator or in thermal insulated bags or containers. Patients who use an insulin pump should change the insulin reservoir every one to two days.

• Suitable snacks (such as breakfast bars, granola bars, trail mix, cheese crackers, etc.) should be kept with the hand luggage in case the child does not like the food

on the plane or the meals contain inadequate carbohydrate or there are unexpected travel delays.

• Flying across time zones can cause confusion about how and when to adjust times of insulin administration and insulin dosage.

• Patients should obtain a travel itinerary showing departure and arrival times, duration of flights, and time differences between departure and arrival locations.

• Patients should obtain an individualized insulin dosage plan from their health care provider before departure. During the flight patients should leave their watches unadjusted so that they continue to correspond to the time at the point of departure. This makes it easier to determine the timing of their insulin injections and meals.

• With short flights or where the time zone between departure and arrival changes by less than four hours, no major changes to the insulin regimen are required.

• Travelling east shortens the day ('eastward = less insulin') and may necessitate a reduction in dose of long-acting insulin because insulin doses would, otherwise, be administered closer than normal and could cause hypoglycaemia.

• In contrast, travelling west means a longer day; insulin doses may need to be increased or an additional dose given to 'bridge the gap' ('westward = more insulin').

• Patients who use an insulin pump should continue to use their usual basal rates.

• A basal-bolus insulin regimen is the ideal injection regimen to cope with major time zone travel situations. Patients who are not using an insulin pump should be transferred to a basal-bolus regimen before travelling.

• With long-haul flights crossing time zones, on arrival at the destination, pump users must change the time in the pump to local time. Give usual pre-meal doses of rapid-acting insulin (using usual insulin:carbohydrate ratio and correction factor) before main meals on the airplane and revert to the usual regimen on arrival at the destination.

• Patients who have very tightly controlled blood glucose levels should be aware that changes in altitude can cause unintended insulin delivery from their pumps. During take-off, air pressure decreases and the pump can deliver additional insulin; the converse can occur during descent.

• Frequent blood glucose monitoring (at least every 4–6 hours) is essential for safety during flight and patients should maintain good hydration while in flight.

When on holiday, especially those involving more than usual physical activity, children with diabetes often require substantially less insulin (e.g. 20–30% reductions) than usual to avoid hypoglycaemia. At the start of the holiday, the child should be advised to monitor blood glucose concentrations regularly to guide changes in insulin doses.

Management of diabetes during surgery

The main goals of diabetes management during surgery are to avoid hypoglycaemia, marked hyperglycaemia, and DKA. When feasible, children with diabetes should not undergo elective surgery until they are metabolically stable and blood glucose control has been optimized (HbA1c approximately at or below 7.5%) in the weeks preceding elective surgery. If metabolic control is poor, surgery should be delayed if possible. Both the endocrinology and anaesthesiology services should participate in this assessment. Surgery should be performed in the morning with the patient first on the list whenever possible. In the case of an afternoon list, the patient should be first on the list. Children who present for emergency surgery (e.g. trauma or acute surgical conditions) require a multidisciplinary preoperative assessment with collaborative involvement of both the endocrinology and anaesthesiology services. Surgery often cannot be delayed even if metabolic control is poor, e.g. a child requiring emergency surgery who presents in DKA. The regimen for managing diabetes before, during, and after a surgical or diagnostic procedure should aim to maintain near-normoglycaemia, i.e. a blood glucose concentration in the range 100–200 mg/dL (5.6–11.1 mmol/L).

Evening prior to elective surgery
On the day before elective surgery, blood glucose should be measured before each meal and before bedtime. Blood or urine ketones should also be measured. In patients treated with glargine or detemir pre-bedtime, the usual dose should be administered.

Morning Operations
• No food from midnight.
• Clear fluids may be taken up to four hours pre-operatively.
• On the morning of surgery, no rapid- or short-acting acting insulin should be administered *unless* the blood glucose exceeds 250 mg/dL (13.9 mmol/L).

• Children using multiple daily injection regimens who are undergoing minor or brief procedures should receive their usual morning dose of long-acting insulin on the day of the procedure. Children who use NPH insulin should receive 50% of the usual morning dose.
• Children who require major surgery, especially procedures anticipated to last more than two hours, should have an IV insulin infusion as the preferred perioperative diabetes management plan.
• Patients who use an insulin pump should receive their usual basal rate of insulin until intravenous insulin and IV fluids are commenced.
• Measure blood glucose, serum urea, creatinine and electrolytes, and blood or urinary ketones before commencing surgery to ensure patient is metabolically stable and adequately hydrated.
• Start IV fluids, 5% dextrose/0.45% saline with 20 mmol of KCl/L, at a maintenance rate (for the first 10 kg body weight – 100 ml per kg per day, for each kg between 10 and 20 kg–50 ml per kg per day, and for each kg above 20 kg–20 ml per kg per day).
• Simultaneously start an insulin infusion using a syringe pump (1 unit of Regular insulin/ml) at a rate approximately equivalent to the child's basal insulin requirement. For example, if the child's TDD of insulin is 0.8 units per kg; assume 50% (0.4 units per kg) is basal insulin. Divide this number by 24 to obtain an initial hourly dose of basal insulin for infusion. In this example, 0.4 divided by 24 = 0.017 unit per kg per hour (round down to 0.015 or up to 0.02 unit per kg per hour). Adjust the insulin infusion rate hourly aiming for a blood glucose concentration of 100–200 mg/dL (5.6–11.1 mmol/L).
• Measure blood glucose hourly, or more frequently if necessary pre-, intra- and postoperatively.
• When blood glucose levels are stable in a satisfactory range, frequency of monitoring can be decreased to every two to four hours.
• Continue IV fluids and insulin until the patient tolerates oral fluids and snacks (this may not be until 24–48 hours after major surgery).
• Change to the usual subcutaneous insulin regimen before the first meal is eaten. The intravenous insulin infusion can be stopped 15 minutes after subcutaneous administration of a rapid-acting insulin analogue. Food should be given ~15 minutes after the insulin injection. In the case of children who use a pump, insulin delivery should be resumed 15 minutes before stopping the IV insulin, and a meal bolus dose using the pump can, likewise, be given ~15 minutes before commencing the meal.

• Following minor operations and procedures it usually is possible to discharge the patient after complete recovery from anaesthesia and consumption of oral fluids and a meal.

Afternoon Operations
• Patient can have breakfast with the usual dose of rapid-acting insulin. In patients who use an insulin pump, a bolus is given before breakfast and the usual basal rate can be continued until the IV fluids and insulin are commenced.
• Can have clear fluids up to four hours pre-operatively.
• Measure blood glucose, urea, creatinine and electrolytes, and blood or urine ketones pre-operatively.
• Start an infusion of regular insulin at midday and IV fluids and (see 'Morning operations').
• Then follow protocol for morning operations.

Emergency Surgery
• DKA may present with severe abdominal pain, which may be mistaken for a 'surgical abdomen'. Acute illness may also precipitate DKA.
• Keep patient nil by mouth.
• Obtain IV access.
• Check weight, blood glucose, complete blood count, serum urea, creatinine, electrolytes, venous blood gas, and blood or urine ketones pre-operatively.
• If ketoacidosis is present, follow the DKA protocol and, if possible, delay surgery until the circulating volume has been restored and any major electrolyte imbalances have been corrected.
• In the absence of ketoacidosis, start maintenance IV fluids and an insulin infusion as for elective surgery.

Minor procedures requiring fasting (e.g. endoscopy, grommets, sedated imaging)

For short procedures (with or without sedation or anaesthesia) where a rapid recovery is anticipated, a simplified protocol can be followed by the diabetes/anaesthesiology team. For example, for an early morning procedure between 8.00 and 9.00 a.m., basal insulin can be administered as usual, and breakfast and the pre-meal insulin bolus can be delayed until after completion of the procedure.

Long-term complications of diabetes

Monitoring for development of complications is an important component of comprehensive paediatric diabetes care. Complications are both microvascular (retinopathy, nephropathy, neuropathy) and macrovascular, causing coronary artery, cerebrovascular, and peripheral vascular disease and lead to ischemic heart disease, stroke, lower extremity gangrene, and amputation, respectively. Retinopathy causes visual impairment and blindness; nephropathy causes hypertension and renal failure; neuropathy causes pain, paresthesiae, muscle weakness, and autonomic dysfunction. Among teenagers and young adults who had been diagnosed with diabetes during childhood and adolescence, after a mean diabetes duration of 7.9 years approximately one in three with type 1 diabetes and almost three of four with type 2 diabetes have at least one complication (nephropathy, retinopathy, peripheral neuropathy, autonomic neuropathy) or co-morbidity (hypertension, arterial stiffness) (Dabelea et al. 2017). Clinically significant macrovascular complications affect older adults. Longer duration, older age, and puberty are risk factors for complications. The risk of complications is increased by genetic factors (i.e. a family history of complications), poor glycaemic control, and smoking in both type 1 and type 2 diabetes. Low socioeconomic status is the single strongest predictor of poor diabetes outcomes.

Diabetic retinopathy

Non-proliferative ('background') retinopathy is characterized by microaneurysms, retinal haemorrhages (blot, dot, and flame-shaped) (Figure 1.7), hard exudates (protein and lipid leakage), cotton wool spots (microinfarctions), intraretinal microvascular abnormalities and beading, dilatation, constriction and tortuosity of vessels. This stage is asymptomatic and does not impair vision. Risk factors for retinopathy include poor glycaemic control, longer duration of diabetes, hypertension, hyperlipidaemia, and smoking. Background diabetic retinopathy (BDR) may stabilize, regress with improved glycaemic control, or progress if poor control persists. BDR in childhood rarely progresses to proliferative retinopathy; nonetheless, all patients with retinopathy should be referred to an ophthalmologist.

Proliferative diabetic retinopathy (PDR) is characterized by neovascularization in the retina and/or vitreous posterior surface. The vessels may rupture or bleed into the vitreoretinal space and is vision-threatening. Advanced PDR can result in fibrosis and adhesions that can cause haemorrhage and retinal detachment. Diabetic macular oedema (DME) is characterized by decreased vascular competence and microaneurysm formation, which produces increased

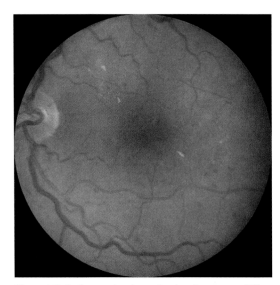

Figure 1.7 Background retinopathy showing scattered 'dots and blots' (microaneurysms and haemorrhages) and exudates. Source: Courtesy of Robert Cavicchi, CRA, FOPS, and Richard Calderon OD, FAOO, Beetham Eye Institute, Joslin Diabetes Center.

exudation and swelling in the central retina. DME is vision-threatening, but is very uncommon in children and adolescents with type 1 diabetes.

Cataracts may develop in patients with diabetes but are rare under the age of 20 years.

The most sensitive detection methods for retinopathy screening are bimicroscopic fundus slit lamp examination through dilated pupils by an ophthalmologist or optometrist and mydriatic seven-field stereoscopic retinal photography. Other commonly used screening methods include mydriatic and non-mydriatic two-field fundal photography, direct ophthalmoscopy, and indirect ophthalmoscopy.

Improvement in diabetes care has been associated with a marked reduction in diabetic retinopathy. For example, in one study, adolescents with a median diabetes duration of 8.6 years showed a decrease in retinopathy from 53% in 1990–1994 to 23% in 2000–2004, and then to 12% in 2005–2009. In a younger age group (11–17 years) with a shorter diabetes duration of only two to five years, the prevalence of mild BDR decreased from 16% in 1990–1994 to 7% in 2003–2006.

Once vision-threatening retinopathy (severe non-proliferative retinopathy and PDR) has been detected, treatment consists of panretinal photocoagulation (laser therapy consisting of multiple discrete outer retinal laser burns, sparing the central macula), which

reduces progression of visual loss by more than 50% in patients with PDR. Side-effects include decreased night and peripheral vision and changes in colour perception.

Because retinopathy can worsen rapidly when control is improved in patients with long-standing poor glycaemic control, frequent ophthalmologic monitoring is recommended both before and after initiating intensive diabetes treatment.

ISPAD recommends annual screening from age 10 years (or at onset of puberty if this is earlier), after a diabetes duration of two to five years. For patients with duration <10 years, minimal or no BDR, and well-controlled diabetes, screening by fundus photography may be performed biennially (Donaghue et al. 2018).

Diabetic nephropathy

Diabetic nephropathy is defined as persistent proteinuria >500 mg/24 h, albuminuria >300 mg/24 h, and is usually associated with hypertension and decreased glomerular filtration rate (Donaghue et al. 2018). End-stage renal failure requiring dialysis or kidney transplantation may occur many years later. The prevalence of microalbuminuria increases with duration of diabetes. Risk factors include poor glycaemic control, long-standing diabetes, cigarette smoking, hypertension, and a family history of diabetic nephropathy.

The first clinical sign of incipient nephropathy is a persistently elevated albumin excretion rate (AER), which can be determined by different methods:

- AER between 20 and 200 microgramme/minute
- AER between 30 and 300 mg/24 in 24-h or timed urine collections
- Albumin concentration 30–300 mg/L (early morning sample)
- Albumin:creatinine ratio (ACR) 2.5–25 mg/mmol or 30–300 mg/g in males and 3.5–25 mg/mmol in females (because of lower creatinine excretion).

Because timed urine collections can be difficult to obtain in children, the ACR is widely used to screen for nephropathy. First voided morning urine samples provide the most reliable measurements; however, in practice, it is usually most convenient to measure the ACR whenever the child is in clinic. If the value is abnormal, the measurement must be repeated on a first voided morning urine sample. Proteinuria may be caused by strenuous physical exercise, menstruation (do not obtain urine sample during menses), urinary tract infection, orthostatic proteinuria, and other types of nephritis. The latter should be excluded, especially in children with abnormal albumin excretion and a short duration of diabetes. Microalbuminuria is confirmed by finding two or all of three consecutive samples abnormal over a 3- to 6-month period. Microalbuminuria can regress, especially in adolescents; however, persistent microalbuminuria predicts progression to end-stage renal failure. In patients with microalbuminuria, attempts should be made to improve glycaemic control, ideally lowering the HbA1c to <7%, and this may lead to normoalbuminuria. Stopping smoking, strict blood pressure control, and exercise should also be advocated.

Angiotensin converting enzyme inhibitors (ACEI) or angiotensin receptor blockers (ARBs) should be used in patients with persistent microalbuminuria, even in the absence of hypertension, to prevent progression to proteinuria. ACEIs can have side effects such as cough and hyperkalaemia (serum electrolytes, urea, and creatinine concentrations should be measured five to seven days after starting treatment). ACEIs and ARBs are also associated with the potential risk of congenital malformations when used during pregnancy. Therefore, adolescent girls must be counselled about the risk and effective contraception recommended.

There is good evidence in adults with type 1 diabetes and microalbuminuria that ACEIs decrease ACR and, in some cases, lead to reversion to normoalbuminuria; as yet, there is no comparable evidence of long-term efficacy and safety in the paediatric population.

Early detection of diabetic nephropathy and timely treatment of hypertension have a pivotal role in the prevention of end-stage renal failure in young people and adults with diabetes. ISPAD recommends annual screening from age 10 years (or at onset of puberty if this is earlier) and after two to five years' diabetes duration (Donaghue et al. 2018).

Blood pressure (BP) should be measured at least annually. Hypertension is defined as average systolic BP and/or diastolic BP >95th percentile for gender, age, and height on more than three occasions. The BP target for adolescents is <130/80 mm Hg. Effective antihypertensive therapy in patients with nephropathy prolongs the time to end-stage renal disease. BP values between the 90th and 95th percentiles are defined as prehypertension. ACEIs are recommended for use in children and adolescents with hypertension.

Diabetic neuropathy

Diabetes insidiously and progressively damages diffusely all peripheral nerve fibres – motor, sensory, and autonomic. The earliest symptoms include numbness and paresthesiae of the feet or hands, decreased vibration sense and sensation to light touch (monofilament examination) and pinprick, and loss of ankle reflexes. Sensory loss in a stocking and glove distribution

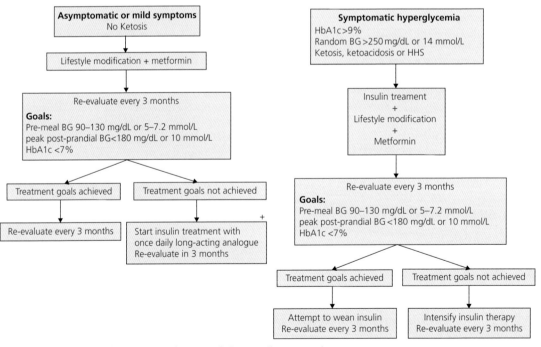

Figure 1.8 Recommended management for type 2 diabetes mellitus in youth.

typically precedes loss of motor function. Autonomic neuropathy can cause postural hypotension, gastroparesis, diarrhoea, bladder paresis, abnormal sweating, and impotence. Clinically significant neuropathy in adolescence is uncommon; however, prevalence rates of peripheral neuropathy varying from <10–27% have been reported.

Dyslipidaemia

The atherosclerotic process begins in childhood. Although CVD events are not expected to occur during childhood, youth with type 1 diabetes may have subclinical CVD within the first decade of diagnosis and are categorized as being in the highest tier for cardiovascular risk. Screening for dyslipidaemia should be performed soon after diagnosis (after glucose control has been established) in all children with type 1 diabetes ≥10 years of age. If LDL cholesterol is within the accepted risk level (<100 mg/dL or 2.6 mmol/L), lipid screening should be repeated every 3–5 years. If lipids are abnormal, annual monitoring is recommended. If the LDL cholesterol value is high (≥2.6 mmol/L, 100 mg/dL), interventions to improve metabolic control, dietary changes (reduced consumption of saturated fat), and increased physical exercise should be instituted. After the age of 10 years, if medical nutrition therapy and lifestyle changes fail to lower LDL cholesterol <160 mg/dL (4.1 mmol/L) or <130 mg/dL (3.4 mmol/L) in patients with one or more CVD risk factors, treatment with a statin should be considered. The goal of therapy is to lower LDL cholesterol to <100 mg/dL (2.6 mmol/L). Statins are potentially teratogenic; therefore, prevention of unplanned pregnancy is of paramount importance.

Premature mortality

Type 1 diabetes is associated with a substantially increased risk of premature death as compared with the general population. Among persons with diabetes younger than 30 years of age, excess mortality is largely attributable to DKA and hypoglycaemia. CVD is the main cause of death later in life. For patients who have very poor glycaemic control, the risk of death from any cause and from CVD is 8 to 10 times as high, respectively, as the general population risk. Several studies have shown an association between the level of glycaemic control (as measured by HbA1c) and all-cause mortality. Improving glycaemic control significantly reduces risk of microvascular complications and CVD.

Type 2 diabetes in children and adolescents

As early as 1916, a phenotypically distinct form of diabetes, now classified as type 2 diabetes mellitus, was recognized in childhood. Since the early 1990s, temporally coinciding with the worldwide increase in childhood obesity, an increase in the prevalence of type 2 diabetes has been reported from paediatric diabetes centres in North America and elsewhere in the world. In the US, type 2 diabetes now accounts for 22% of new cases of diabetes among youth. It is far more common in racial and ethnic minorities: 25% of diabetes cases in Hispanic, African-American and Asian/Pacific Islander patients have type 2 diabetes. Typical risk factors are shown in Table 1.16. In a recent report describing presentation of 503 youths with type 2 diabetes, 67% presented with symptoms of diabetes and confirming laboratory data, whereas 33% were identified by testing asymptomatic at-risk children.

The classic criteria (age at onset and weight) for distinguishing between the two major types of diabetes have become increasingly blurred. Owing to the current high prevalence of overweight and obesity in children and adolescents, many youths with type 1 diabetes are overweight or obese at diagnosis or become overweight within a few years after diagnosis. Both type 1 and type 2 diabetes often present during puberty, a period of life characterized by physiologic insulin resistance; however, type 2 diabetes can occur in severely obese prepubertal children. The increasing incidence of type 2 diabetes in youth now presents

Table 1.16 Risk factors for type 2 diabetes in youth.

- Overweight or obesity associated with insulin resistance
- Family history of type 2 diabetes in first- or second-degree relative
- Ethnicity: in North America, African-American, Hispanic, Pacific Islander, Native American, Canadian First Nation; children and adolescents from the Indian sub-continent living in Europe
- Maternal gestational diabetes
- Small size for gestational age (intrauterine growth restriction)
- Insulin resistance of puberty
- Acanthosis nigricans
- Polycystic ovary syndrome
- Lack of physical activity
- High calorie diet

clinicians with a diagnostic challenge when evaluating a paediatric patient with new-onset diabetes. Distinguishing between type 1 and type 2 diabetes cannot be based on ketone status, body weight, or insulin requirement. In contrast to type 2 diabetes in adults in whom ketonuria is unusual, a substantial fraction of adolescents with type 2 diabetes have ketonuria and between 5.6% and 11% have DKA at presentation, and 2% present with HHS. Furthermore, insulin requirements typically decrease after several weeks of treatment, which may resemble the remission or 'honeymoon' period of type 1 diabetes. Measuring pancreatic islet autoantibodies and a surrogate for insulin secretion (fasting C-peptide levels) in obese patients helps to distinguish between type 1 and type 2 diabetes. A fasting plasma C-peptide level > 0.85 ng/ml (0.28 nmol/L) suggests type 2 diabetes; however, plasma C-peptide levels obtained soon after diagnosis may be transiently low in type 2 diabetes owing to gluco- and lipotoxicity. Repeating the measurement after several weeks or months of therapy will sometimes demonstrate hyperinsulinaemia and insulin resistance, helping to establish a diagnosis of type 2 diabetes.

In summary, a binary classification is not always possible at the time of diagnosis. Patients may have clinical and biochemical features of both insulin deficiency and insulin resistance, i.e. characteristics of both major types of diabetes. Irrespective of the type of diabetes, the choice of initial therapy should be based on the metabolic state, as determined by clinical assessment. Subsequent therapy is then modified, if necessary, guided by the individual patient's response to treatment.

Treatment of type 2 diabetes

As for type 1 diabetes, a multidisciplinary diabetes team, including a physician, DNE, registered dietitian, and behavioural specialist (psychologist or social worker), is essential. In addition to blood glucose control, from the outset, treatment often must include management of comorbidities such as obesity, dyslipidaemia, hypertension, and microalbuminuria. Youth onset type 2 diabetes is an aggressive disease with a higher rate of complications than type 1 diabetes of comparable duration. Intensive intervention is required both for glycaemic control and to mitigate cardiovascular risk factors. An algorithm for managing type 2 diabetes in youth including HbA1c and glycaemic targets is shown in Figure 1.9. Treatment with metformin must not be started until ketosis/ketoacidosis has resolved and the patient is well hydrated.

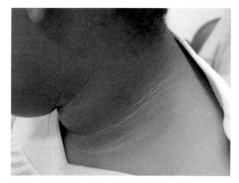

Figure 1.9 Acanthosis nigricans on the neck.

Nonpharmacologic therapy

Weight control and physical activity

Youths with type 2 diabetes are overweight or obese at presentation; the emphasis is on weight loss, limiting caloric intake, and distributing meals evenly throughout the day. Even modest weight reduction alone increases sensitivity to insulin and improves fasting and postprandial blood glucose levels. The aims of treatment are to lose weight, normalize fasting and postprandial blood glucose and haemoglobin A1c levels, identify and treat associated co-morbidities such as hypertension and dyslipidaemia, and to minimize the risk of acute and chronic complications associated with diabetes. Dietary management for patients with type 2 diabetes emphasizes healthy eating to optimize metabolic control while achieving sustained weight loss. Nutrition and lifestyle approaches to treatment should be given at least as much importance as drug therapy. A family-centred approach is essential in paediatric type 2 diabetes and patients and their families must prioritize lifestyle modifications such as eating a balanced diet, maintaining a healthy weight, and exercising regularly. Nutrition recommendations should be culturally appropriate and sensitive to family resources.

Patients and their family members should receive guidance on behaviour modification strategies to change their lifestyle, decrease their consumption of high-energy/high-fat foods, and incorporate daily aerobic physical activity into their lives. Regular physical activity facilitates weight loss, increases HDL cholesterol levels, lowers blood pressure, and improves metabolic control. Fasting serum insulin concentrations decrease and insulin sensitivity improves in obese children who lose weight and exercise regularly. To increase physical activity, the amount of time devoted to sedentary activities and 'screen time' (viewing television, playing video games, surfing the internet, etc.) must be strictly limited to less than two hours daily. Youths with type 2 diabetes should be encouraged to participate in aerobic exercise with a gradual increase in the frequency, intensity, and duration, aiming for at least 60 minutes daily of moderate/intense physical activity. Exercise tolerance is reduced in obese children; therefore, advice to increase physical activity should be realistic and individualized.

Pharmacologic therapy

Oral agents

Presentation with ketosis or ketoacidosis requires a period of insulin therapy until fasting and postprandial glycaemia have been restored to normal or near normal levels. Similarly, when the distinction between type 1 and type 2 diabetes is unclear, initial treatment should be with insulin. Recent clinical practice guidelines (Springer et al. 2013) recommend initiation of insulin therapy in patients with random blood glucose concentrations ≥250 mg/dL (13.9 mmol/L) or A1c >9% (75 mmol/mol).

Metformin

When insulin treatment is not required, current guidelines recommend a family-centred lifestyle modification programme plus initiation of metformin as first-line therapy for children and adolescents. Metformin is currently the only oral hypoglycaemic agent specifically approved for use in children with type 2 diabetes. Metformin is safe and often efficacious in paediatric patients with type 2 diabetes. Metformin suppresses basal hepatic glucose production and increases insulin-mediated glucose uptake in skeletal muscle, but does not affect insulin secretion or cause hypoglycaemia. It causes a mild reduction in triglyceride and LDL concentrations and its anorectic effect may contribute to modest weight loss. Its most common side-effects are nausea, vomiting, abdominal pain, and diarrhoea. Lactic acidosis is a rare, potentially fatal side-effect. Provided that it is not administered to patients with renal insufficiency (metformin is excreted unchanged in the urine) or poor tissue perfusion, the risk of lactic acidosis is extremely low. Metformin must be discontinued before radiographic studies with iodinated contrast agents, surgery under general anaesthesia, in patients with renal, liver, or heart disease, in patients with dehydration, and whenever tissue perfusion is poor. Because the absorption of vitamin B12 and/or folic acid may be compromised, patients are advised to take a daily multivitamin.

For children 10–16 years of age, the recommended starting dose of metformin is 500 mg once daily. The dose may be increased to 500 mg twice daily, and further increases may be made at weekly intervals in 500 mg increments to a maximum daily dose of 2000 mg. The acute, reversible gastrointestinal adverse effects of metformin may be minimized by administration with or after food, and by using lower dosages, increased slowly, as necessary. The extended release preparation should be initiated at a dose of 500 mg once daily, given with the evening meal. The maximum recommended dose of the extended-release product is 2000 mg per day. In overweight females with polycystic ovary syndrome, a condition that is often associated with type 2 diabetes, menstrual cycles and fertility may be restored to normal. Therefore, sexually active females should be counselled regarding the need for birth control.

Insulin secretagogues (Sulfonylureas and Meglitinides)

Although sulfonylureas have been used in adults for more than half a century, there is only limited evidence of their efficacy in children. A 24-week, randomized, single blind comparative study in type 2 diabetes paediatric patients showed that glimepiride was as safe and effective as metformin in terms of reduction of A1c and incidence of hypoglycaemia. The glimepiride-treated group, however, showed greater weight gain compared to patients treated with metformin.

Thiazolidinediones (TZDs)

Thiazolidinediones (TZDs) are insulin sensitizers that act on the nuclear receptor peroxisome proliferator-activated receptor gamma (PPARγ) and increase insulin sensitivity in muscle and adipose tissue. TZDs have favourable effects on lipid metabolism. Side effects include weight gain and fluid retention, which contraindicates their use in patients with heart failure. TZDs are not approved for use in children, and their use in adults is restricted due to concerns about risk of myocardial infarction with rosiglitazone, risk of bladder cancer with pioglitazone, and decreased bone density risk with both.

Insulin

Although many insulin regimens have been studied and successfully used in adults with type 2 diabetes, comparable data do not exist in paediatric type 2 diabetes. Metformin may be added after normalization of blood glucose, resolution of ketosis, and correction of dehydration.

Insulin therapy may be necessary in asymptomatic or mildly symptomatic patients who fail to achieve adequate glycaemic control (A1c <7%, 53 mmol/mol) after three months of lifestyle intervention and treatment with maximum doses of metformin. Long-acting insulin analogues (glargine, detemir, or insulin degludec) may be added to metformin at a starting dose of 0.2 units per kg per day at dinnertime or bedtime. Twice daily pre-mixed insulin regimens have been efficacious in adults with type 2 diabetes and a short trial with premixed insulin analogues was also beneficial in children. Basal-bolus therapy (once daily long-acting-insulin combined with short-acting insulin before meals) may be a suitable option in the motivated patient who is willing to perform carbohydrate counting.

Complications and comorbidities of type 2 diabetes

In youth with type 2 diabetes, complications may be present at the time of diagnosis or appear soon thereafter. A recent study showed that among youth with type 2 diabetes diagnosed before age 20 years, high rates of diabetic kidney disease, retinopathy, and neuropathy (20%, 9%, and 18%, respectively), occur after a mean duration of approximately eight years. Moreover, the risk of these complications is more than twofold higher than in those diagnosed with type 1 diabetes, after adjustment for age, disease duration, glycaemia, and obesity, emphasizing the need to begin monitoring youth with type 2 diabetes for development of complications from the time of diagnosis (Dabelea et al. 2017). Comorbidities associated with type 2 diabetes include: obesity, metabolic syndrome, hypertension, microalbuminuria, dyslipidaemia, non-alcoholic fatty liver disease (NAFLD), and acanthosis nigricans (Figure 1.9).

Hypertension

Strict control of blood pressure significantly reduces cardiovascular morbidity and mortality in adults, and similar effects would be expected in children. The aim is to reduce blood pressure to <90th percentile for age, height, and gender. If lifestyle intervention (weight control, regular exercise) is unsuccessful, pharmacological treatment should be initiated with an ACE inhibitor. If the highest recommended dose is ineffective or if the child experiences side effects, a second drug from a different class, such as an ARB, calcium channel blocker, cardioselective beta-blocker, and/or diuretic may be used.

Dyslipidaemia

Dyslipidaemia in childhood tracks into adulthood; therefore, it is reasonable to assume that untreated lipid disorders in children with diabetes increase the risk of CVD later in life. Initial therapy consists of weight control, exercise, optimization of glycaemic control, and discontinuation of tobacco use (if applicable), and a reduced fat diet. Specifically, total and saturated fat intake should be <30% and <10%, respectively of the total calories consumed. Some children with hyperlipidaemia will require lipid-lowering drug therapy; 3-hydroxy-3-methylglutaryl coenzyme A (HMG-CoA) reductase inhibitors (statins) are recommended as first-line pharmacologic treatment in children with hyperlipidaemia and are approved for use in children as young as 10 years old. Clinical trials in the paediatric age group have shown safety and efficacy similar to that observed in adult studies. The addition of lipid-lowering drugs is recommended when LDL cholesterol (LDL-C) levels are >190 mg/dL (4.9 mmol/L) and in patients with LDL-C > 160 mg/dL (4.1 mmol/L) and a family history of early CVD or other risk factors. Similarly, if after 6 to 12 months of medical nutrition therapy and lifestyle changes LDL-C levels remain >130 mg/dL (3.4 mmol/L), drug therapy is indicated. Lipid-lowering medications are not recommended in pre-menarcheal girls and boys younger than 8–10 years, unless there is a particularly high risk for atherosclerosis.

Miscellaneous practical matters

Driving

Patients with diabetes have a 1.23-fold increased relative risk of accidents compared with those without diabetes, which is the same order of risk as for those with epilepsy. If a teenager with diabetes wishes to drive, the following measures are required:

- The patient needs to inform the driving authorities who may request a medical form to be completed by the patient's physician. In the United Kingdom, assuming the patient has satisfactory health, is not affected by recurrent hypoglycaemia or hypoglycaemia unawareness and has visual acuity greater than 6/9, a licence for three years may be granted.
- Before driving, blood glucose concentrations should be checked, and a long journey should be broken by frequent rests and meals with blood glucose concentrations re-measured.

- If the patient feels hypoglycaemic, the car should be stopped, the engine turned off, the keys removed from the ignition and carbohydrate consumed.
- A supply of carbohydrate-containing snacks should always be kept in the car in case of unexpected delays.

School examinations

The stress of examinations can lead to impaired blood glucose control with adverse effects on academic performance. Glycaemic control should be optimized prior to sitting an examination.

Alcohol, smoking, and recreational drug use

Adolescents with diabetes risk their health by smoking cigarettes and using recreational drugs, and should be strongly discouraged from engaging in their use. Alcohol consumption has been associated with worse glycaemic control, increases the risk for severe hypoglycaemia as a result of impaired hypoglycaemia awareness and hormonal counter-regulatory responses, and hypoglycaemia may be confused with intoxication. Adolescents with type 1 diabetes must receive counselling about the effects of alcohol and be encouraged to abstain or at least consume alcohol in moderation. They should also receive education about blood glucose monitoring and how to prevent and treat hypoglycaemia, and must understand the considerable safety risks associated with driving.

Recreational drugs can lead to sympathetic over-activity (cocaine, amphetamines), hyponatraemia (ecstasy), and hunger (marijuana), leading to increased carbohydrate intake, and may precipitate ketoacidosis. As with alcohol, it may be difficult for the patient with diabetes and others to distinguish between the effect of drugs and hypoglycaemia. Drug addiction may lead to neglect of diabetes self-care with devastating adverse effects on glycaemic control.

The following guidelines are advised:
- The importance of avoiding drinking alcohol and driving must be stressed.
- Do not drink alcohol on an empty stomach or when blood glucose is low.
- Eat while drinking or shortly afterwards.
- If drinking in the evening, before bedtime check blood glucose to ensure it is between 100 and 140 mg/dL (5.6 and 7.8 mmol/L), and eat a snack if it is below this range.
- Do not omit food from your meal plan and replace it with alcohol.

- Avoid beers with low sugar content as these tend to contain higher alcohol concentrations and may lead to hypoglycaemia.
- Limit consumption of low-alcohol beers with increased sugar content.
- Consume dry or medium wines in preference to sweet wines.
- For mixed drinks, choose sugar-free mixers (diet soda, club soda, diet tonic water, water).
- Wear an I.D. that says 'I have diabetes.'

The adverse health effects of smoking are well recognized with respect to future cancer and CVD risk. Use of tobacco considerably increases the risk of onset and progression of nephropathy and macrovascular disease. Avoiding smoking is important to prevent both microvascular and macrovascular complications. A smoking history should be elicited at the initial and follow-up visits. Youth who do not smoke should be discouraged from ever starting and those who do smoke should receive help to quit.

Sexuality and Pre-conception counselling

Hyperglycaemia at conception and in the first weeks of pregnancy increases the risk of adverse maternal and foetal outcomes, including an increased risk of congenital malformations. Counselling about contraception and avoidance of unplanned pregnancy, therefore, is of utmost importance for adolescent females with diabetes.

Most sexually active teenagers with diabetes should be advised to use condoms to protect against sexually transmitted diseases together with a combined oral contraceptive pill. Adolescents with good glycaemic control and without microvascular complications can safely use a combined oral contraceptive pill containing ≤35 μg ethinylestradiol. Before prescribing the pill, hypertension and a family history of deep vein thrombosis should be excluded. Caution should also be exercised in patients with epilepsy and liver dysfunction.

Patients with microvascular disease or risk factors for coronary artery disease can safely use progesterone-only contraception. Further advice should be sought from a gynaecologist or family planning clinic.

Should a teenager with diabetes become pregnant, her medical care should be transferred to an adult physician and an obstetrician experienced in managing pregnant women with diabetes.

Endocrine and other disorders associated with diabetes

Thyroid disease

Autoimmune thyroid disease is the most common endocrinopathy associated with type 1 diabetes, occurring in 17–30% of patients. At the time of diagnosis of type 1 diabetes, approximately 25% of patients have thyroid autoantibodies; however, thyroid autoantibodies per se are poorly predictive of thyroid dysfunction (Triolo et al. 2011). Patients may develop hypothyroidism or, less commonly, hyperthyroidism (0.5%). Subclinical hypothyroidism may be associated with an increased risk of symptomatic hypoglycaemia and with reduced linear growth. Hyperthyroidism causes deterioration of metabolic control and increased insulin requirements. Asymptomatic individuals should be screened for thyroid dysfunction *after* metabolic control has been established (owing to frequent transient abnormalities of thyroid function at the time of diabetes diagnosis) by measuring thyroid stimulating hormone, and every one or two years thereafter. Further details of the investigation and treatment of thyroid disease can be found in Chapter 6.

Addison's disease

Adrenal autoantibodies occur in 1.6–2.3% of individuals with type 1 diabetes; only 1 in 200–300, however, progresses to develop clinical adrenocortical insufficiency. The risk increases to 1 in 30 in patients with two autoimmune processes (i.e. diabetes and thyroiditis). The development of adrenocortical insufficiency in type 1 diabetes is characterized by recurrent unexplained hypoglycaemia and decreasing insulin requirements. Other classical symptoms include fatigue, hyperpigmentation of the skin and mucous membranes, weight loss, abdominal pain or presentation with an adrenal crisis during an intercurrent illness.

The diagnosis of Addison's disease is confirmed by the presence of inappropriately low circulating serum cortisol and markedly increased plasma ACTH concentration in a person with adrenal autoantibodies (anti-21-hydroxylase). Further details of other relevant investigations and of treatment with glucocorticoids and mineralocorticoids can be found in Chapter 8. Adrenal insufficiency, hypothyroidism, and type 1 diabetes (Schmidt syndrome) are manifestations of polyendocrine syndrome type II, a rare autoimmune disorder.

Coeliac disease

Biopsy-confirmed coeliac disease affects from 1.9% to 7.7% of youth with type 1 diabetes <18 years, may be present before the onset of diabetes, and is often asymptomatic. Symptoms of coeliac disease may include diarrhoea, weight loss or poor weight gain, growth failure, abdominal pain or distension, chronic fatigue, anaemia, vitamin D deficiency, malnutrition due to malabsorption, a decrease in insulin requirements and intermittent unexplained hypoglycaemia, or erratic blood glucose concentrations. Approximately 75% of cases of coeliac disease are detected within the first five years after the diagnosis of type 1 diabetes; therefore, screening should be considered soon after the diagnosis of diabetes and repeated every two to five years thereafter. Screening entails measuring serum tissue transglutaminase or anti-endomysial antibodies (document normal total serum IgA levels), followed by small bowel biopsy in antibody positive children. Recent European guidelines suggest that biopsy may not be necessary in symptomatic children with extremely high antibody titres, provided that genetic or HLA testing is supportive, but asymptomatic children at increased risk should have a biopsy.

Treatment of coeliac disease is with a gluten-free diet. The combination of a gluten-free diet and the appropriate diet for a child with diabetes places a significant burden on individuals and families. The advice of a specialist dietitian is needed as compliance may be poor.

Necrobiosis lipoidica diabeticorum

This skin disorder is characterized by collagen degeneration with a granulomatous response, thickening of blood vessel walls, and fat deposition and affects 0.3–1.2% of people with diabetes. It is uncommon in children and more likely to be seen in adolescent females. The condition usually begins as red-brown or violaceous papules or nodules and slowly progresses to yellow-brown, atrophic telangiectatic plaques (Figure 1.10). Ulceration is common (usually occurring after trauma) and lesions may become infected. The lower legs, especially the shins and area above the medial malleoli, are most commonly affected; however, the scalp, face, trunk, genitals, or upper extremities can be affected. The aetiology is unknown. The development of necrobiosis lipoidica is not influenced by glycaemic control and there is no evidence that improving control of diabetes mellitus affects its course. The classic histologic finding is a

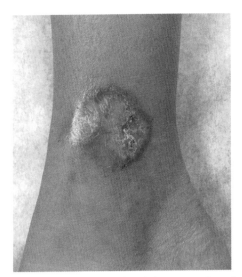

Figure 1.10 Necrobiosis lipoidica diabeticorum above the ankle.

palisaded and interstitial granulomatous dermatitis involving the dermis with extension into the subcutaneous tissue.

Numerous therapies have been used for necrobiosis lipoidica – with unsatisfactory results. Treatment should be directed by a dermatologist and focuses on managing signs and symptoms by inhibiting the inflammatory process and healing ulcerations. Non-ulcerated necrobiosis is often asymptomatic, may stabilize over time, and may not require treatment. The initial choice for non-ulcerated lesions is with a high potency topical corticosteroid applied under occlusion. If the response is unsatisfactory, the next treatment option is intra-lesional corticosteroid injections. Limited data suggest that other treatments may be useful for necrobiosis lipoidica; these include topical

tacrolimus, psoralen plus ultraviolet A (PUVA) photochemotherapy, systemic medications, and procedural therapies.

Unusual causes of diabetes in childhood

Monogenic diabetes or maturity onset diabetes of the young (MODY)

Maturity onset diabetes of the young (MODY) is a form of autosomal dominant diabetes mellitus that affects approximately 1–4% of people with diabetes in different populations and typically develops before the age of 25 years. Most patients have a family history of diabetes in two or more consecutive generations. It is characterized by β-cell dysfunction of variable severity depending on the specific gene mutation. Numerous different gene mutations have been shown to cause MODY; however, three genes (*GCK, HNF1A, HNF4A*) account for ~85% of MODY cases (Hattersley et al. 2018).

Biomarker tests help to identify appropriate candidates for genetic testing. Pancreatic islet autoantibodies are negative and patients with monogenic diabetes have significant residual endogenous insulin secretion (measured as stimulated serum or urinary C-peptide), in contrast to classical type 1 diabetes in which insulin secretion usually is minimal beyond the honeymoon period. An online probability calculator (http://www.diabetesgenes.org/content/mody-probability-calculator) can aid in the identification of these individuals.

Management of the most common subtypes (GCK, HNF1A, HNF4A MODY) differs from that of type 1 diabetes as shown in Table 1.17. Identification of the gene mutation in a child with MODY confirms

Table 1.17 Common subtypes of MODY and associated clinical features.

MODY subtype	Gene	Locus	Clinical features	Treatment
1	*HNF4A*	20q12-q31.1	Macrosomia, neonatal hypoglycaemia; renal Fanconi syndrome	Sulfonylurea
2	*GCK*	7p15-p13	Mild asymptomatic hyperglycaemia	No treatment; diet and exercise
3	*HNF1A*	12q24.2	Renal glucosuria	Sulfonylurea
5	*HNF1B*	17q12	Renal developmental abnormalities, genital tract malformations	Insulin

GCK glucokinase; HNF hepatocyte nuclear factor.

whether treatment is necessary, predicts the risk of future complications, and allows for specific genetic counselling.

Neonatal diabetes mellitus

Autoimmune type 1 diabetes is exceedingly rare before age of six months. Most patients diagnosed less than six months of age have a monogenic form of neonatal diabetes and should have genetic testing. In about half the cases, neonatal diabetes is transient and remits within a few weeks or months, but in at least 50–60% of cases diabetes recurs later in life, usually during puberty.

About two-thirds of cases of transient neonatal diabetes mellitus (TNDM) are caused by over-expression of paternally expressed imprinted genes on chromosome 6q24 (paternal uniparental disomy of 6q24 [UPD6], unbalanced paternal duplication of 6q24, or loss of maternal methylation). Most of the remaining cases are caused by activating mutations (prevent closure of the beta cell ATP-sensitive potassium [K_{ATP}] channel and impair insulin secretion in response to hyperglycaemia) in either of the genes (*KCNJ11* or *ABCC8*) encoding the two subunits Kir6.2 and SUR1, respectively, of the K_{ATP} channel. Patients with 6q24 abnormalities are born with severe intrauterine growth retardation (reflecting prenatal insulin deficiency) and usually develop severe non-ketotic hyperglycaemia during the first week of life. Initial treatment consists of rehydration and a continuous IV insulin infusion; thereafter, subcutaneous insulin is introduced and, when possible, patients are best managed by subcutaneous insulin infusion (pump) therapy. Insulin treatment of TNDM may be needed for a few days to 18 months.

The most common cause of permanent neonatal diabetes mellitus (PNDM) is an activating mutation of either *KCNJ11* or *ABCC8*. Heterozygous coding mutations in the *INS* (preproinsulin) gene are the second most common cause of PNDM after K_{ATP} channel mutations. *INS* mutations cause a misfolded proinsulin molecule that is trapped in the endoplasmic reticulum (ER) leading to ER stress and ß-cell apoptosis. There are no significant differences between TNDM and PNDM regarding the severity of intrauterine growth restriction or the age at diagnosis of diabetes. Patients with K_{ATP} channel activating mutations frequently present with DKA, and 20% of patients with *KCNJ11* mutations have associated neurological features, referred to as DEND (developmental delay, epilepsy, diabetes mellitus) syndrome. Approximately 90% of patients with activating mutations in the K_{ATP}

channel genes can be successfully switched from insulin to oral sulfonylureas (typical dose of glyburide/glibenclamide ~0.5 mg/kg day, but higher doses may be required).

Diabetes following pancreatectomy for persistent hyperinsulinemic hypoglycaemia of infancy

Infants with severe persistent hyperinsulinaemic hypoglycaemia caused by diffuse disease that is unresponsive to medical treatment often require near-total (95–98%) pancreatectomy to control hypoglycaemia (see Chapter 2 on Hypoglycaemia). A high proportion of these patients will eventually develop diabetes and require insulin treatment. The rate of progression to insulin dependence, however, varies from several months to 14 years or more after surgery.

Cystic fibrosis-related diabetes (CFRD)

Cystic fibrosis-related diabetes (CFRD) is the most common complication of CF in individuals of school age and older. The prevalence of CFRD increases with age from 2% in children ≤10 years of age to 40% in individuals 18–29 years. CFRD is caused by insulin deficiency resulting from slowly progressive destruction of pancreatic islets, and is a distinct form of diabetes mellitus different from either type 1 or type 2 diabetes. Insulin resistance caused by inflammatory cytokines and catecholamines plays a role in its pathogenesis, especially when there are acute exacerbations of pulmonary disease. Glucagon secretion is reduced and DKA is rare.

Development of CFRD is associated with deterioration of lung function and nutritional status, more frequent lung infections, and decreased survival. Insulin treatment can ameliorate these effects. Early diagnosis and treatment, therefore, are crucial to prevent morbidity. Annual screening with an OGTT at a time of baseline health is recommended beginning by age 10 years. In addition, fasting and postprandial blood glucose screening are suggested with acute pulmonary exacerbations. In patients receiving enteral tube feedings, blood glucose should be measured at the midpoint and immediately after a feed. HbA1c should not be used for screening because it is often normal despite hyperglycaemia and has low sensitivity for detecting CFRD.

Treatment consists of insulin therapy, which has beneficial effects on nutritional state, improves pulmonary function and survival, but adds substantially to the burden of CF treatment. The specific insulin regimen varies according to individual patient characteristics and preferences, responses, and dietary strategies. It should eliminate the catabolic state of CFRD, minimize postprandial hyperglycaemia while avoiding hypoglycaemia, and maintain HbA1c as low as possible. Although HbA1c is not recommended for screening, it is useful for monitoring glycaemic control. Patients with CF benefit from increased caloric intake, including calorie-rich beverages. Patients on insulin therapy should perform SMBG at least three times a day, and HbA1c should be measured every three months. The insulin regimen is adjusted to achieve targets and to ensure weight gain. Annual screening for microvascular complications should be performed, beginning five years after diagnosis.

Miscellaneous disorders

Diabetes is associated with numerous other disorders including Down syndrome, Turner syndrome, Klinefelter syndrome, Prader–Willi syndrome, Wolfram syndrome (diabetes insipidus, diabetes mellitus, optic atrophy, and deafness [DIDMOAD]), asparaginase and glucocorticoid treatment, thalassaemia, and the autoimmune polyendocrine syndromes.

Audit and benchmarking

Auditing and benchmarking against regional, national, or international standards is a valuable method to improve the quality of a diabetes service. A register of all patients is essential to allow auditing and benchmarking to take place. Several aspects of diabetes care can be audited including:

- the adequacy of management of newly diagnosed patients
- HbA1c concentrations;
- evidence of normal growth, weight gain, and puberty;
- frequency of follow-up in the clinic;
- frequency of DKA and severe hypoglycaemia in established patients;
- screening for co-morbidities;
- the incidence of complications;
- patient education;
- patients' satisfaction with the service.

Future developments

- Early diagnosis through genetic and immunological screening of high-risk children and, possibly, in the general population.

- Therapy to arrest progression of beta cell destruction and development of clinical diabetes.
- Immunomodulation in new onset diabetes to preserve or enhance residual insulin secretion.
- Non-invasive methods of accurate glucose monitoring.
- Closed loop insulin delivery systems ('artificial pancreas').
- More rapidly absorbed rapid-acting insulin analogues.
- Approval of medications (e.g. glucagon-like peptide analogues, DPP IV inhibitors, SGLT2, and combined SGLT1/2 inhibitors, etc.) currently used in adults, for treatment of type 2 diabetes in youth.
- The development of stem cell therapy to generate a potentially limitless source of genetically modified, artificially cultured pancreatic β-cells suitable for transplantation.

Controversial points

- Should a new patient with diabetes, but without DKA, be treated in hospital or in an ambulatory setting?
- What are the indications for starting insulin pump therapy?
- What effects do hyperglycaemia and hypoglycaemia have on brain development in preschool-aged children?
- How can the biochemical goals established after the DCCT be achieved in routine clinical practice?
- In adolescents, what is the role of ACE inhibitors in diabetic nephropathy and statins in those with dyslipidaemia?
- What is the role of psychological support and motivational interviewing in helping children and adolescents to improve their glycaemic control and well-being?
- What are the optimal fluid composition and rate of fluid administration to treat DKA?
- What causes cerebral oedema in DKA and how to prevent it?
- Should mannitol or hypertonic saline be used as first-line treatment for cerebral oedema?
- When should adolescents transition to adult care and how to design an effective paediatric to adult diabetes care transition programme?

Potential pitfalls

- Failure to realize that the blood glucose values in a patient's logbook are fictitious (may all be written in the same pen, may not be consistent with the HbA1c result).

- Recommending insulin doses in excess of 1.5 units/kg per day in a patient with a persistently high HbA1c when the most likely explanation is poor compliance and omission of injections or failure to bolus when using a pump.
- Failure to diagnose psychological/psychiatric problems, especially in adolescents, which may account for suboptimal or poor glycaemic control.
- Errors in fluid calculations during therapy of DKA.
- Stopping the insulin infusion during therapy for DKA when hypoglycaemia occurs.
- Inappropriately advising the omission of insulin because the child is ill and not eating, thus increasing the risk of DKA.
- Failure to identify early signs of retinopathy when using direct ophthalmoscopy.
- Losing track of patients, frequently adolescents, who repeatedly fail to attend clinic (more likely to occur if the clinic does not maintain a patient register).
- Failure to consider Addison's disease or coeliac disease as a possible cause for decreasing insulin requirements when the patient is beyond the 'honeymoon period'.
- Failure to distinguish between type 1 and type 2 diabetes, resulting in inappropriate therapy.
- Failure to diagnose MODY in a patient with a suggestive family history or in patients with de novo mutations.

Case histories

Case 1.1
A 14-year-old girl weighs 50 kg, has had recurrent severe hypoglycaemia with two episodes leading to a convulsion and hospital admission. She was diagnosed with type 1 diabetes at nine years of age and is using a basal-bolus insulin regimen with 18 units insulin glargine at 9 p.m. (~40% of the average TDD of 45 units or 0.9 units/kg per day) and pre-meal rapid-acting insulin aspart (1 unit per 10 g carbohydrate) three times daily. There have not been any recent changes in her diet or level of physical activity.

Questions and Answers
1 What investigations would you consider doing?

Measurement of HbA1c concentration to assess overall glycaemic control, thyroid function tests to exclude hypothyroidism, screening serologic tests (tissue transglutaminase and/or anti-endomysial antibody or deamidated gliadin titres) to exclude coeliac disease. Measurement of 21-hydroxylase (anti-adrenal autoantibody) titres, measurement of 8A.M. serum cortisol and plasma ACTH concentrations and consideration of a cosyntropin (Cortrosyn or Synacthen) stimulation test, if the latter are suspicious for adrenal insufficiency, to rule out Addison's disease.

2 If the results of these investigations are normal, what further explanations could account for her recurrent hypoglycaemia?

Self-administration of high doses of insulin. This adolescent girl was not coping with her diabetes and the recurrent hypoglycaemic episodes were 'a cry for help'. The episodes stopped following a referral and advice from the child psychiatry service.

Case 1.2
A 15-year-old boy has had type 1 diabetes for five years, frequently failed to attend diabetes clinic appointments and now presents with short stature and delayed puberty. He was receiving two insulin injections daily: 24 units in the morning before breakfast (mixed insulin with a ratio of short-to intermediate-acting insulin of 30:70) and 12 units in the evening; TDD 0.7 units/kg per day. His height had decreased from the 25th to the 2nd centile since diagnosis and his weight was on the 2nd centile. He had Tanner stage 2 pubic hair and the volume of his testes was 4 ml. His HbA1c concentration was 12.4%.

Questions and Answers
1 How would you investigate this patient?

Detailed dietary assessment and measurement of thyroid function tests and screening for coeliac disease.

2 How would you manage this patient?

The patient has delayed onset of puberty, which is likely to have contributed to his slow growth velocity. The dietary assessment revealed a low calorie intake and the results of his tests for hypothyroidism and coeliac disease were normal. There had been little change in his diet or insulin dosage since diagnosis. Poor glycaemic control because of an inadequate dosage of insulin and an inadequate dietary intake is the most likely cause for his delayed puberty and short stature. Therefore, he should be advised to increase his dietary intake and significantly increase his daily dosage of insulin (and consider switching to a multiple daily dose insulin regimen) in an effort to improve glycaemic control. If this proves successful, this is likely to stimulate further progression of puberty and the pubertal growth spurt.

Case 1.3

A 15-year-old white youth presented with a 6-week history of polyuria and polydipsia. His father was found to have non-insulin-dependent (type 2) diabetes at the age of 24 years, which was controlled by diet. His paternal grandfather had developed type 2 diabetes at 48 years of age, controlled by diet and an oral sulfonylurea. On examination, his body mass index was 22.4 kg/m², he was not dehydrated and appeared well. His blood glucose was 14 mmol/L (252 mg/dL). He had glycosuria but no ketonuria.

Questions and Answers

1 What is the likely diagnosis?

The most likely diagnosis is MODY. Because hyperglycaemia in MODY may be mild and asymptomatic, the age of diagnosis can be considerably later than the age of onset, which is the likely explanation for the late age of diagnosis in the father and grandfather.

2 How would you investigate this boy?

By screening of genes, mutations of which are known to cause MODY. This patient was found to have a mutation of the glucokinase gene (MODY2).

3 Why is it important to establish a precise diagnosis?

The patient can be reassured that he is extremely unlikely to experience complications from his MODY, and he and his family can be counselled about the autosomal dominant inheritance of MODY.

Case 1.4

A three-year-old girl presents for the first time with type 1 diabetes in DKA. She is severely dehydrated and acidotic with a venous pH of 7.08. She is resuscitated in accordance with the local DKA protocol and improves. However, 11 hours after admission she becomes irritable and more difficult to communicate with. She vomits once. The nurse looking after her notes that her heart rate has dropped from 120/min. to 88 min.

Questions and Answers

1 What is the most likely reason for this change in her condition?

The likeliest explanation is that she has developed the complication of cerebral oedema. This can be present at diagnosis but usually presents 4–12 hours after treatment has commenced. A headache (which in this girl may have been the cause of her irritability) and a decrease in the pulse rate of > 20/min (which cannot be explained by sleep or an improvement in the intravascular volume) are important features of cerebral oedema.

2 What immediate investigation should be done?

Measure blood glucose concentration to rule out hypoglycaemia as the cause of her altered behaviour. At a later stage, a CT scan *may* be required to rule out other intracerebral complications such as a thrombosis or a haemorrhage.

3 What should be the management?

A senior paediatrician and anaesthetist should be called urgently. Mannitol (0.5–1 gram per kg IV over 10–15 minutes) or hypertonic (3%) saline (2.5–5 ml per kg over 10–15 minutes) should be given immediately. The patient should be nursed in a 30° head-up position to help venous drainage. If not already in a paediatric intensive care unit, the child should be transferred there as soon as is safely possible. She is likely to require intubation and ventilation.

Case 1.5

A 14-year-old Asian girl presents with a six-week history of polyuria, polydipsia, and a 5-kg weight loss. Her grandfather had developed diabetes when he was in his fifties and takes tablets. On examination, she appears overweight and her BMI is 29 kg/m^2, which is between the 98th and 99.6 percentiles. She has pink stretch marks on her abdomen and acanthosis nigricans on the nape of her neck. Her blood glucose is 26 mmol/L (468 mg/dL). She is not acidotic but her urinalysis shows 3+ glucosuria and moderate ketonuria.

Questions and Answers

1 What is the likely diagnosis?

The most likely diagnosis is type 2 diabetes mellitus. She belongs to a high-risk ethnic group, has a family history, acanthosis nigricans, and her BMI centile places her in the obese category. Pink stretch marks can occur in anyone who is obese. The ketonuria is not unusual; occurs in many patients with paediatric type 2 diabetes. In some cases, especially in a patient such as this where there has been weight loss and ketonuria, it can be difficult to distinguish between type 1 and type 2 diabetes.

2 What investigations would help clarify the precise diagnosis?

Measuring pancreatic autoantibodies (islet cell, GAD, IA-2, insulin, ZnT8 antibodies) would help to clarify whether she is an obese girl with type 1 diabetes or has type 2 diabetes. Pancreatic autoantibodies would be negative in type 2 diabetes. Measuring C-peptide, which reflects the amount of insulin that the patient is producing, may also be useful. C-peptide measurement will be most informative after the patient has been treated for a few weeks and metabolic control has been established to minimize the impact of glucose toxicity on beta cell function. C-peptide levels would be normal or increased in type 2 diabetes but low in type 1 diabetes.

3 What treatment should be commenced?

Although this patient is likely to have type 2 diabetes, there is a possibility that she may have type 1. Some patients fall into a grey area between type 1 and type 2 diabetes, i.e. they have features of both types of diabetes. The results of the investigations listed in Answer 2 are likely to take several weeks. In view of this, the high blood glucose level and ketosis, it would be advisable to start this patient on a basal-bolus insulin regimen. Dietary treatment and an exercise regimen are also very important. When the ketosis has resolved, the patient is well hydrated, and the blood glucose has decreased to near normal levels, metformin should be gradually introduced with the aim of increasing the dose of metformin, decreasing the insulin dosages, and eventually, hopefully, treating the patient with metformin alone.

Significant Guidelines/Consensus Statements

American Diabetes Association (2018a). 2. Classification and diagnosis of diabetes: standards of medical care in diabetes – 2018. *Diabetes Care* 41 (Suppl. 1): S13–S27.
American Diabetes Association (2018b). 12. Children and adolescents: standards of medical care in diabetes – 2018. *Diabetes Care* 41 (Suppl. 1): S126–S136.
International Society for Pediatric and Adolescent Diabetes (ISPAD) Clinical practice consensus guidelines (2018). Website: www.ispad.org. Contains up-to-date consensus guidelines on virtually all aspects of pediatric diabetes (accessed 1 October 2018).
National Institute for Health and Care Excellence (NICE) (2015). Diabetes (type 1 and type 2) in children and young people: diagnosis and management. Guideline. NG18. Nice.org.uk/guidance/ng18 (accessed 1 October 2018).
American Diabetes Association (2018c) Standards of medical care in diabetes. http://care.diabetesjournals.org/content/41/Supplement_1 (accessed 1 October 2018).

References

American Diabetes Association (2018). 2. Classification and diagnosis of diabetes: standards of medical care in diabetes – 2018. *Diabetes Care* 41 (Suppl. 1): S13–S27.

Anderson, B. and Schwartz, D. (2014). Psychosocial and family issues in children with type 1 diabetes. In: *Therapy for Diabetes Mellitus and Related Disorders*, 6e (ed. G. Umpierrez), 134–155. Alexandria, VA: American Diabetes Association.

Anderson, B.J., Wolfsdorf, J.I., and Jacobson, A.M. (2009). Psychosocial and family issues in children with type 1 diabetes. In: *Therapy for Diabetes Mellitus and Related Disorders*, 5e (ed. H.E. Lebovitz), 97–104. Alexandria, VA: American Diabetes Association,.

Concannon, P., Rich, S.S., and Nepom, G.T. (2009). Genetics of type 1A diabetes. *New Engl. J. Med.* 360: 1646–1654.

Dabelea, D., Stafford, J.M., Mayer-Davis, E.J. et al. (2017). Association of type 1 diabetes vs type 2 diabetes diagnosed during childhood and adolescence with complications during teenage years and young adulthood. *JAMA* 317: 825–835.

Diabetes Control and Complications Trial Research Group (1993). The effect of intensive treatment of diabetes on the development and progression of long-term complications in insulin-dependent diabetes mellitus. *New Engl. J. Med.* 329: 977–986.

DiMeglio, L.A., Acerini, C.L., Codner, E. et al. (2018). ISPAD Clinical Practice Consensus Guidelines: Glycemic control targets and glucose monitoring for children, adolescents, and young adults with diabetes. *Pediatr Diabetes.* 19 Suppl 27: 105–14.

Donaghue, K.C., Marcovecchio, M.L., Wadwa, R.P. et al. (2018). ISPAD Clinical Practice Consensus Guidelines: Microvascular and macrovascular complications in children and adolescents. *Pediatr Diabetes.* 19 Suppl 27: 262–74.

Garvey, K. and Wolfsdorf, J.I. (2015). The impact of technology on current diabetes management. *Pediatr. Clin. N. Amer.* 62: 873–888.

Hattersley, A.T., Greeley, S.A.W., Polak, M. et al. (2018). ISPAD Clinical Practice Consensus Guidelines: the diagnosis and management of monogenic diabetes in children and adolescents. *Pediatr Diabetes.* 19 Suppl 27: 47–63.

Insel, R.A., Dunne, J.L., Atkinson, M.A. et al. (2015). Staging presymptomatic type 1 diabetes: a scientific statement of JDRF, the Endocrine Society, and the American Diabetes Association. *Diabetes Care* 38: 1964–1974.

Lawrence, J.M., Standiford, D.A., Loots, B. et al. (2006). Prevalence and correlates of depressed mood among youth with diabetes: the SEARCH for diabetes in youth study. *Pediatr.* 117: 1348–1358.

Liu, L.L., Lawrence, J.M., Davis, C. et al. (2010). Prevalence of overweight and obesity in youth with diabetes in USA: the SEARCH for diabetes in youth study. *Pediatr. Diabet.* 11: 4–11.

Lowes, L. and Gregory, J.W. (2004). Management of newly diagnosed diabetes: home or hospital? *Arch. Dis. Child.* 89: 934–937.

Morgan, E., Halliday, S.R., Campbell, G.R. et al. (2016). Vaccinations and childhood type 1 diabetes mellitus: a meta-analysis of observational studies. *Diabetologia* 59: 237–243.

Patterson, C., Guariguata, L., Dahlquist, G. et al. (2014). Diabetes in the young: a global view and worldwide estimates of numbers of children with type 1 diabetes. *Diabet. Res. Clin. Prac.* 103: 161–175.

Peters, A. and Laffel, L. (2011). Diabetes care for emerging adults: recommendations for transition from pediatric to adult diabetes care systems: a position statement of the American Diabetes Association, with representation by the American College of Osteopathic Family Physicians, the American Academy of Pediatrics, the American Association of Clinical Endocrinologists, the American Osteopathic Association, the Centers for Disease Control and Prevention, Children with Diabetes, the Endocrine Society, the International Society for Pediatric and Adolescent Diabetes, Juvenile Diabetes Research Foundation International, the National Diabetes Education Program, and the Pediatric Endocrine Society (formerly Lawson Wilkins Pediatric Endocrine Society). *Diabetes Care* 34: 2477–2485.

Pinsker, J.E., Becker, E., Mahnke, C.B. et al. (2013). Extensive clinical experience: a simple guide to basal insulin adjustments for long-distance travel. *J. Diabet. Metab. Disorders* 12 (59): https://doi.org/10.1186/2251-6581-12-59.

Pociot, F. and Lernmark, A. (2016). Genetic risk factors for type 1 diabetes. *Lancet* 387: 2331–2339.

Rewers, M.J. and Ludvigsson, J. (2016). Environmental risk factors for type 1 diabetes. *Lancet* 387: 2340–2348.

Riddell, M.C., Gallen, I.W., Smart, C.E. et al. (2017). Exercise management in type 1 diabetes: a consensus statement. *Lancet Diabet. Endocrinol.* 5: 377–390.

Seaquist, E.R., Anderson, J., Childs, B. et al. (2013). Hypoglycemia and diabetes: a report of a workgroup of the American Diabetes Association and the Endocrine Society. *Diabetes Care* 36: 1384–1395.

Skyler, J.S., Bakris, G.L., Bonifacio, E. et al. (2017). Differentiation of diabetes by pathophysiology, natural history, and prognosis. *Diabetes* 66: 241–255.

Slover, R.H., Welsh, J.B., Criego, A. et al. (2012). Effectiveness of sensor-augmented pump therapy in children and adolescents with type 1 diabetes in the STAR 3 study. *Pediatr. Diabet.* 13: 6–11.

Springer, S.C., Silverstein, J., Copeland, K. et al. (2013). Management of type 2 diabetes mellitus in children and adolescents. *Pediatr.* 131: e648–e664.

Sundberg, F., Barnard, K., Cato, A. et al. (2017). Managing diabetes in preschool children. *Pediatr. Diabet.* 18: 499–517.

Triolo, T.M., Armstrong, T.K., McFann, K. et al. (2011). Additional autoimmune disease found in 33% of patients at type 1 diabetes onset. *Diabetes Care* 34: 1211–1213.

Wolfsdorf, J.I., Glaser, N., Agus, M. et al. (2018). ISPAD Clinical Practice Consensus Guidelines: Diabetic ketoacidosis and the hyperglycemic hyperosmolarstate. *Pediatr Diabetes.* 19 Suppl 27: 155–77.

Ziegler, A.G., Rewers, M., Simell, O. et al. (2013). Seroconversion to multiple islet autoantibodies and risk of progression to diabetes in children. *JAMA* 309: 2473–2479.

Useful Information for Patients and Parents

American Diabetes Association (ADA) Website: www.diabetes.org (accessed 1 October 2018). Has a special section for children and adolescents.

Chase, H.P. and Maahs, D.M. (2012). *Understanding Diabetes: An Instruction Manual for Families on the Management of Diabetes*, 12e. http:/www.ucdenver.edu/academics/colleges/medicalschool/centers/BarbaraDavis/OnlineBooks/Pages/UnderstandingDiabetes.aspx (accessed 1 October 2018.

Children with Diabetes Website: www.childrenwithdiabetes.com. (accessed 1 October 2018). Contains educational materials, information on research, news and online support.

Diabetes UK Website: www.diabetes.org.uk (accessed 1 October 2018). Has a special section for children and adolescents.

European Society for Paediatric Endocrinology Website: http://www.eurospe.org/patient (accessed 1 October 2018). Information booklet on type 2 diabetes and obesity (available in English, French, Italian, Spanish, and Turkish).

Juvenile Diabetes Research Foundation International Website: www.jdrf.org (accessed 1 October 2018).

Advice on transition from paediatric to adult care

http://www.YourDiabetesInfo.org/transitions (accessed 1 October 2018). https://www.endocrine.org/education-and-practice-management/quality-improvement-resources/clinical-practice-resources/transition-of-care (accessed 1 October 2018).

2 Hypoglycaemia

Physiology

Glucose is the body's main fuel and the brain is the principal consumer of circulating glucose. The brain can neither synthesize glucose nor store more than a few minutes' supply as glycogen and depends on a continuous supply of glucose. Blood glucose concentrations are normally maintained within a relatively narrow range. Recurrent or persistent hypoglycaemia during the period of rapid brain growth and differentiation in infancy can cause permanent neurological sequelae, psychomotor retardation, and seizures. Prevention of hypoglycaemia and its prompt recognition, accurate diagnosis, and vigorous treatment are essential to prevent its devastating cerebral consequences.

Hypoglycaemia most often occurs in the newborn period and is the most common metabolic disorder of the newborn (see Table 2.1 showing neonates at increased risk for hypoglycaemia). The ratio of surface area to body mass of a full-term newborn baby is approximately three times that of an average adult, necessitating a high rate of energy expenditure to maintain body temperature. Also, the infant brain is large relative to its body mass (and hepatic glycogen stores) and its energy requirement is primarily derived from oxidation of circulating glucose. To meet the high demand for glucose, the rate of glucose production in newborn infants and young children (5–8 mg per kg per minute) is two to three times that of older children and adults (2.3 mg per kg per minute). As a consequence, until feeding is well established, maintenance of glucose homeostasis in the newborn period is more precarious than later in life. During infancy and childhood, hypoglycaemia most often occurs when night-time feeding is discontinued or when an intercurrent illness interrupts a child's normal feeding pattern, resulting in a period of relative starvation.

During prolonged fasting, infants and young children cannot sustain the high rate of glucose production. Compared to older children, adolescents, and adults, plasma glucose decreases and plasma ketone concentrations increase more rapidly.

In response to feeding, blood glucose concentrations increase, which stimulates insulin and inhibits glucagon secretion, to maintain plasma glucose concentrations below 7–9 mmol/L [126–162 mg/dL]. Insulin increases glucose uptake in skeletal muscle and adipose tissue by increasing GLUT4 expression, promotes hepatic and skeletal muscle glycogen synthesis, and inhibits glycogenolysis and gluconeogenesis. During fasting, plasma glucose concentrations decrease, insulin secretion is suppressed, and increased secretion of the counter-regulatory hormones glucagon, adrenaline (epinephrine), noradrenaline (norepinephrine), cortisol, and growth hormone (GH) prevent hypoglycaemia. The endocrine and metabolic responses involved in the transition from the fed to the fasted state are shown in Figure 2.1.

Practical Endocrinology and Diabetes in Children, Fourth Edition. Malcolm D.C. Donaldson, John W. Gregory, Guy Van Vliet, and Joseph I. Wolfsdorf.
© 2019 John Wiley & Sons Ltd. Published 2019 by John Wiley & Sons Ltd.

In healthy children, glycogen stores are largely depleted within approximately 12 hours of fasting. Thereafter, gluconeogenesis (from amino acids, glycerol, and lactate) is the sole source of glucose. Lipolysis is activated, increasing the supply of free fatty acids, an alternative energy source for most tissues, which reduces glucose consumption. The brain does not oxidize free fatty acids. However, water-soluble acetoacetate and ß-hydroxybutyrate (ketones), produced by hepatic ß-oxidation of fatty acids, readily cross the blood-brain barrier and become a major source of energy for the brain during prolonged fasting.

Table 2.1 Neonates at increased risk for hypoglycaemia and who require glucose screening.

Premature or postmature delivery
Foetal growth restriction (small for gestational age)
Maternal gestational diabetes; infant of a diabetic mother
Large for gestational age
Perinatal stress associated with transient neonatal hyperinsulinism
- Perinatal asphyxia/ischemia
- Caesarean delivery for foetal distress
- Maternal pre-eclampsia or eclampsia or hypertension
- Meconium aspiration syndrome, alloimmune haemolytic disease of the newborn, polycythemia, hypothermia
Maternal intrapartum treatment with glucose or with sulphonylureas
Abrupt interruption of an infusion with a high glucose concentration
Family history of a genetic form of hypoglycaemia
Congenital syndromes; e.g. Beckwith-Wiedemann or abnormal physical features (midline facial defects, micropenis, cryptorchidism) suggestive of hypopituitarism

Symptoms and signs of hypoglycaemia

During progressively severe hypoglycaemia, a hierarchy of physiological responses occurs, from sympathoadrenal activation to neuroglycopenia. Symptoms and signs are non-specific and reflect responses of the central nervous system to glucose deprivation (Table 2.2). Neurogenic (autonomic) symptoms result from the central nervous system-mediated sympathoadrenal discharge triggered by hypoglycaemia. Neuroglycopenic symptoms are caused by brain dysfunction from impaired energy metabolism, i.e. the direct result of brain glucose deprivation. Symptoms are particularly difficult to identify in newborns, who are at greatest risk of developing hypoglycaemia. Neonates with low blood glucose concentrations are frequently asymptomatic and hypoglycaemia is usually detected by routine screening of at-risk infants or as an incidental laboratory finding. With suspected hypoglycaemia, it is essential to accurately measure a confirmatory plasma or blood glucose concentration

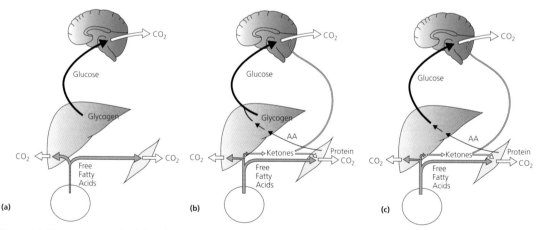

Figure 2.1 Transition from the fed to the fasting state. (a) Between meals: glucose is from hepatic glycogenolysis; free fatty acids from adipose tissue are an additional source of fuel for muscle. (b) Overnight fast: liver glycogen is depleted and gluconeogenesis becomes the principal source of glucose. Hepatic ketone production increases and rising plasma ketone body concentrations provide an alternative fuel for brain and muscle. (c) Prolonged starvation: fat-derived fuels are the predominant metabolic substrates. Brain utilization of ketones increases. Glucose is from gluconeogenesis. Source: *Pediatric Endocrinology*, ed. Fima Lifshitz, 5th edition, 2007.

Table 2.2 Symptoms and signs of hypoglycaemia in newborns.

Neurogenic (autonomic)	Neuroglycopenic
Jitteriness/tremors	Poor suck or feeding
Sweating	Weak or high-pitched cry
Irritability	Hypotonia
Tachypnoea	Change in level of consciousness (lethargy, coma)
Pallor	Seizures

and demonstrate that administration of glucose promptly relieves the symptoms and signs (Whipple's triad, see section 'Definition').

Additional signs of hypoglycaemia in newborns may include apnoea, bradycardia, cyanosis, and hypothermia. In older individuals, typical adrenergic symptoms include palpitations, tremor, and anxiety; cholinergic symptoms include sweating, hunger, and paresthesias. Typical signs include pallor, diaphoresis, tachycardia, and elevated systolic blood pressure.

Definition

The numerical definition of hypoglycaemia continues to be controversial, most especially in newborns, related to uncertainty regarding the definition of euglycaemia and the glucose threshold resulting in brain injury. In the absence of a consensus, several methods are employed to pragmatically define hypoglycaemia, including statistical, metabolic, neurophysiological, and neurodevelopmental (i.e. evidence that a particular blood glucose concentration is associated with long-term neurodevelopmental sequelae).

Clinical hypoglycaemia is defined as a plasma glucose concentration low enough to cause symptoms and/or signs of impaired brain function. This glucose concentration varies from one patient to another and depends on the availability of alternative fuels and previous blood glucose concentrations. Hypoglycaemia may be difficult to recognize, especially in neonates and young children in whom the symptoms and signs are not specific. Plasma glucose concentrations are also influenced by several factors, including when the sample is obtained relative to the last meal, the source of blood (arterial, capillary, or venous), and whether measurements are performed on whole blood, serum, or plasma (approximately 12–15% higher than whole blood). Furthermore,

a single low plasma glucose concentration, especially when measured on a point-of-care device (glucose meter), may be a measurement artefact. Confirmation of Whipple's triad is valuable in older children: (i) symptoms and/or signs consistent with hypoglycaemia; (ii) an accurately measured low plasma glucose concentration; and (iii) relief of symptoms and signs when plasma glucose concentration is restored to normal. Because reliance on Whipple's triad is not possible in infants and young children, recognition of hypoglycaemia may require confirmation by repeated measurements of plasma glucose concentration and, in certain circumstances, by performing a controlled fasting test.

In adults, the glycaemic threshold for a decrease in brain glucose metabolism is normally <54 mg/dL [3.0 mmol/L]. During acute insulin-induced hypoglycaemia, autonomic symptoms appear at a plasma glucose of approximately 60 mg/dL [3.3 mmol/L] and impaired brain function occurs at approximately 50 mg/dl [2.8 mmol/L]. In infants and children, functional changes in the central nervous system (brainstem and somatosensory evoked potentials) occur when the venous plasma glucose falls below 47 mg/dL [2.6 mmol/L]. These observations suggest that the physiologic threshold is a plasma glucose in the range 50–60 mg/dL [2.8–3.3 mmol/L]. For clinical care of children, a venous plasma glucose of ≥60 mg/dL [3.3 mmol/L] may be regarded as normoglycaemia and levels <50 mg/dL [2.8 mmol/L] as hypoglycaemia.

When considering management decisions, the above numerical definitions are useful; however, plasma glucose concentrations should also be evaluated in the context of the availability of other metabolic fuels (lactate and ketones). For example, a plasma glucose concentration <50 mg/dL [2.8 mmol/L] is not necessarily harmful if the blood ketone concentration is markedly elevated because infants and children can utilize ketones for cerebral metabolism. Note, however, that free fatty acid and ketone levels are suppressed by insulin, thus accounting for the increased risk of brain injury in infants with hyperinsulinaemic hypoglycaemia.

Aetiology

Hypoglycaemia occurs when the rate of blood glucose utilization exceeds the rate of glucose production and, beyond the newborn period, most commonly presents when an intercurrent illness is associated with reduced calorie consumption caused by anorexia (prolonged fasting), vomiting, and diarrhoea. Hypoglycaemia may also occur after a period of less protracted (e.g. overnight) fasting when blood glucose production is limited by an impaired counter-regulatory response resulting from cortisol and/or growth hormone deficiency, an inborn error of metabolism affecting glycogenolysis or gluconeogenesis, or when an increased rate of glucose utilization occurs together with decreased hepatic glucose production (hyperinsulinism, malaria, sepsis). The causes of hypoglycaemia in infants and children are shown in Table 2.3.

Table 2.3 The differential diagnosis of hypoglycaemia in children.

Accelerated starvation (idiopathic ketotic hypoglycaemia)
Hyperinsulinemic hypoglycaemia
- Congenital hyperinsulinism
- Dumping syndrome
- Beckwith-Wiedemann syndrome
- Exogenous insulin (diabetes, factitious hyperinsulinism)
- Insulinoma
- Insulin autoimmune syndrome
Hormone deficiency
- Primary adrenal insufficiency
- Secondary adrenal insufficiency (ACTH deficiency)
  - Withdrawal of exogenous glucocorticoids
  - Hypopituitarism
- Growth hormone deficiency
  - Hypopituitarism
  - Isolated growth hormone deficiency
- IGF-1 deficiency
Glycogenoses
- Glycogen storage diseases (types I, III, VI, IX)
- Glycogen synthase deficiency (GSD 0)
Glucose transporter defect
- Fanconi-Bickel syndrome
Disorders of gluconeogenesis
- Fructose-1,6-bisphosphatase deficiency
- Glucose-6-phosphatase deficiency (GSD I)
- Phosphoenolpyruvate carboxykinase deficiency
- Pyruvate carboxylase deficiency
Disorders of fatty acid oxidation
- Primary carnitine deficiency and carnitine cycle defects
- Disorders of ß-oxidation; e.g. medium chain acyl-CoA dehydrogenase deficiency
- Multiple acyl-CoA dehydrogenase deficiency
Disorders of ketogenesis
- HMG-CoA synthase and lyase deficiencies
Drugs (insulin, sulphonylureas, ß-blockers, aspirin, alcohol)
Infections (malaria, septicemia, gastroenteritis)
- Hereditary fructose intolerance and galactosemia
- Branched chain organic acidaemias and maple syrup urine disease
- Mitochondrial respiratory chain defects
- Severe liver disease

Preliminary examination and investigation

History and physical examination

When hypoglycaemia occurs in a *neonate*, the following details should be obtained:
- Pregnancy (duration, maternal health history, gestational or pre-existing diabetes, hypoglycaemia).
- Mode of delivery (breech delivery occurs more often in infants with hypopituitarism).
- Birth weight (may be increased in an infant whose mother had gestational diabetes or may be consistent with foetal growth restriction).
- Relationship between hypoglycaemia and feeding (hypoglycaemia despite adequate calorie intake is strongly suggestive of hyperinsulinism).

In the *older child*, clarify the following details:
- Feeding regimen and the maximum length of time that fasting has been tolerated without symptoms suggestive of hypoglycaemia.
- Symptoms suggestive of hypopituitarism (e.g. prolonged jaundice in the neonatal period).
- Use of oral or inhaled glucocorticoids.
- Consider the possibility of accidental ingestion or factitious symptoms following administration to the child of oral glucose-lowering medications or insulin.
- A careful family history: parental consanguinity or unexplained infant death may suggest an inborn error of metabolism; congenital hyperinsulinism may be inherited in an autosomal dominant or recessive fashion.
- Hypoglycaemic or other symptoms and signs, such as vomiting, diarrhoea, jaundice, hepatomegaly, or failure to thrive following consumption of lactose or foods containing fructose and sucrose, suggest galactosaemia or a disorder of fructose metabolism, respectively.

Individuals presenting with hypoglycaemia usually do not have abnormalities on clinical examination. Nonetheless, evaluation of growth (obtain all available growth records), weight gain, and a careful physical examination may identify abnormalities that will inform the cause of the child's hypoglycaemia. Table 2.4 lists the most common signs and associated disorders (see Figure 2.2).

Investigations

Although hypoglycaemia is a clinical emergency requiring prompt therapy, whenever possible, a blood sample (often referred to as the 'critical sample') for

Table 2.4 Clinical signs on examination.

Clinical sign	Possible diagnosis
Optic atrophy	Septo-optic dysplasia
Cranial midline defects	Growth hormone deficiency
Short stature or decreased height velocity	Growth hormone deficiency
Micropenis	Growth hormone deficiency
Diffusely increased skin or buccal pigmentation	Addison's disease
Hypotension	Addison's disease
Underweight or malnutrition	Accelerated starvation
Tall stature or increased height velocity	Hyperinsulinism
Excess weight	Hyperinsulinism
Abnormal ear lobe creases (Figure 2.2)	Beckwith–Wiedemann syndrome
Macroglossia	Beckwith–Wiedemann syndrome
Umbilical hernia	Beckwith–Wiedemann syndrome
Hemihypertrophy	Beckwith–Wiedemann syndrome
Hepatomegaly	Glycogen storage disorder

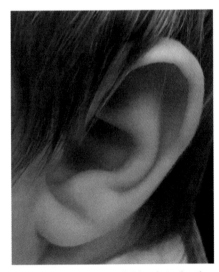

Figure 2.2 Ear lobe crease in a child with Beckwith–Wiedemann syndrome.

investigations should be drawn *before administering glucose*. Urine should be collected at the earliest opportunity and stored together with blood samples at −20 °C or below. The processing of these samples should be discussed with the laboratory to ensure proper storage of samples. The samples obtained at the time of hypoglycaemia may produce clear biochemical evidence of the cause of the hypoglycaemic episode and thus avoid having to subject the child to further costly and potentially hazardous investigations. Interpretation of the 'critical' blood and urine samples obtained at the time of presentation with hypoglycaemia (plasma glucose <50 mg/dL, <2.8 mmol/L), together with a careful physical examination, including assessment of the size of the liver, can frequently determine the specific aetiology of hypoglycaemia (Figure 2.3).

The preliminary investigation of hypoglycaemia is shown in Table 2.5. If blood and urine samples obtained at the time of initial hypoglycaemia do not elucidate its cause (or were not obtained), then additional investigations may be considered. These may include the measurement of intermediary metabolites before and after meals or a prolonged fast performed under controlled conditions, followed by the investigations listed in Table 2.5. Because a prolonged fast may result in severe hypoglycaemia and is potentially dangerous, fasting studies must be performed at a specialist centre. The length of the fast will be determined by the age of the child (Table 2.6). Children undergoing a fasting study should be closely supervised by staff who are experienced in dealing with hypoglycaemia. The timing of the latter stages of the fast when the child is most likely to become hypoglycaemic should be planned to coincide with a time of the day when appropriate staff are available to monitor the patient and assist in any required resuscitation. Intravenous (IV) glucose and

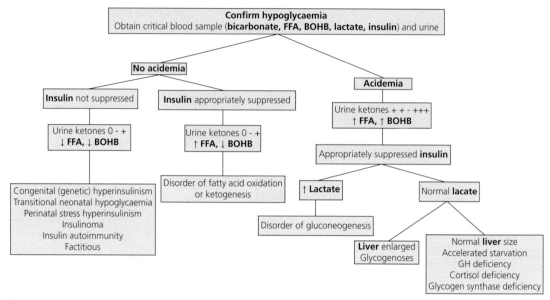

Figure 2.3 An algorithm for evaluation of hypoglycaemia. Urine ketones 0 to + indicates absent, trace or small ketonuria; ++ to +++ indicates moderate or large ketonuria; FFA, free fatty acids; BOHB, beta-hydroxybutyrate; serum insulin concentrations >100 µU ml^{-1} together with a low C-peptide level suggests factitious hypoglycaemia.

Table 2.5 Investigation of hypoglycaemia at time of presentation.

Sample	Investigation
Blood sample	Glucose
	Bicarbonate or venous pH
	Free fatty acids and β-hydroxybutyrate
	Lactate
	Insulin and C-peptide
	Cortisol and ACTH
	Growth hormone
	Liver function tests
	Ammonia
	Urea and electrolytes
	Alanine
	Acylcarnitines; total and free carnitine
Administer glucose	
Next urine sample	Ketones
	Glucose and reducing sugars
	Organic acid profile
	Glycine conjugates
	Carnitine derivatives
	Toxicology screen[a]

ACTH, adrenocorticotrophic hormone.
[a] Ethanol, salicylates, sulphonylureas.

Table 2.6 Length of fasts for children undergoing investigation of possible hypoglycaemia.

Age	Duration (hr)
<6 mo	8
6–8 mo	12
8–12 mo	16
1–2 yr	18
2–4 yr	20
4–7 yr	20
>7 yr	24

hydrocortisone should be available at the bedside. All symptoms should be carefully documented, sample times clearly recorded, and the patient must never be left unsupervised until the fast is complete and the patient is treated with glucose and/or food. Should hypoglycaemia occur during the planned fasting test, the treatment is described below (see section 'Treatment').

Investigations may fail to identify a specific cause of hypoglycaemia, which may occur in the context of a normal endocrine counter-regulatory response, associated with appropriately raised free fatty acids and ketones. Plasma lactate and pyruvate may be normal but alanine low, suggesting a reduced supply of gluconeogenic precursors. This disorder of unknown aetiology is known as 'accelerated starvation' or 'idiopathic ketotic hypoglycaemia'. It is more common in boys than girls and may be associated with a history of foetal growth restriction or a thin physique. Hypoglycaemia may occur after a day of unusually intense physical activity and/or decreased calorie consumption. Episodic hypoglycaemia usually resolves spontaneously by age 7–9 years. There are numerous causes of hypoglycaemia associated with hyperketonaemia (Figure 2.3). Therefore, accelerated starvation or idiopathic ketotic hypoglycaemia should only be diagnosed *after* other endocrine and metabolic causes of hypoglycaemia have been carefully excluded.

Treatment

Neonatal hypoglycaemia

The aim is to raise the blood glucose concentration, provide adequate fuel for the brain, and decrease the risk of brain injury. Owing to uncertainty regarding the definition of hypoglycaemia and appropriate thresholds for intervention, and a desire to promote breast-feeding and not separate infants from their mothers, the most common treatment for asymptomatic hypoglycaemia is to increase the frequency of feeding. Dextrose gel (200 mg/kg) massaged into the buccal mucosa before a feed is effective in raising blood glucose concentrations in hypoglycaemic late pre-term and term babies in the first 48 hours after birth. In conjunction with breast-feeding, dextrose gel is a non-invasive alternative to infant formula as a first-line treatment for neonatal hypoglycaemia. Babies who remain hypoglycaemic after initial treatment, or whose blood glucose concentrations are extremely low, are admitted to a newborn intensive care unit for treatment with intravenous dextrose (200 mg/kg of 10% dextrose as an IV bolus followed by a continuous infusion at a rate of 8 mg per kg per minute). For high-risk neonates without a suspected congenital hypoglycaemia disorder, the goal of treatment is to maintain plasma glucose >50 mg/dL [2.8 mmol/L] in infants <48 hours and >60 mg/dL [3.3 mmol/L] >48 hours from delivery.

Acute treatment at initial presentation in older children

Once the initial ('critical') blood samples have been obtained (see Table 2.5), the patient should be given IV dextrose (see section 'Emergency Management of Acute Hypoglycaemia'). The response to treatment should be monitored and the infusion rate adjusted to maintain blood glucose concentrations >4 mmol/L [72 mg/dL]. The use of intermittent boluses of glucose in concentrations greater than 25% should be avoided because of the risk of cerebral oedema.

If the patient remains unconscious despite normalization of the blood glucose concentrations, IV hydrocortisone should be administered empirically for possible undiagnosed adrenal insufficiency. If the patient does not respond to hydrocortisone, the possibility of an intracranial disorder or an inborn error of metabolism should be considered.

Emergency management of acute hypoglycaemia

1 Obtain initial diagnostic blood sample.
2 Give 0.2 grams glucose per kg body weight (2 ml/kg of 10% dextrose) intravenously over 4 to 6 minutes.
3 Start an infusion of IV 10% dextrose at an initial rate of 10 mg per kg body weight per minute (6 ml/kg/h) and adjust according to blood glucose response.
4 If patient remains unconscious, give 25 mg per metre^2 hydrocortisone intravenously.
5 Collect next urine sample for diagnostic investigations.

Hyperinsulinism

Medical treatment

Hyperinsulinism should be considered when glucose requirements to maintain normoglycaemia exceed 8–10 mg per kg body weight per minute (see Table 2.3 and diagnostic criteria in Box 2.1). Persistent hyperinsulinaemic hypoglycaemia, also referred to as congenital hyperinsulinism, is the most common cause of recurrent or persistent hypoglycaemia in infants. To date, mutations of 10 different genes involved in controlling insulin secretion have been described. Inactivating mutations in the genes *ABCC8* and *KCNJ11*, encoding SUR1 and Kir6.2, the two subunits of adenosine triphosphate (ATP)-sensitive (K_{ATP}) channels in the pancreatic beta cells, cause the most common and severe forms of congenital hyperinsulinism. Early recognition, accurate diagnosis, and immediate effective management to maintain normal blood glucose levels (at least 70 mg/dL, 4 mmol/L before feeds) are crucial. Delay in the diagnosis or ineffective management leads to hypoglycaemia-induced brain injury and adverse neurodevelopmental outcomes.

Infants with hyperinsulinism require frequent feeding; additional IV glucose is required when

---

> **Box 2.1 Diagnostic Criteria for Hyperinsulinaemic Hypoglycaemia**
>
> - Glucose infusion rate >8–10 mg per kg per minute
> - Plasma glucose ≤50 mg/dL [2.8 mmol/L]
> - Detectable serum insulin
> - C-peptide ≥ 0.5 ng/ml [0.17 nmol/L]
> - Serum beta-hydroxybutyrate <1.8 mmol/L
> - Serum free fatty acids <1.7 mmol/L
> - Glycaemic response to glucagon ≥ 30 mg/dL [1.7 mmol/L]
> - Serum IGFBP-1 ≤110 ng/ml
>
> Source: Adapted from Ferrara et al. (2016).

hypoglycaemia is recurrent or persistent despite enteral feeds. Glucose infusion rates may need to be increased up to 25 mg/kg/minute and such high concentrations of glucose must be administered through a central venous line. Many cases of neonatal hyperinsulinism (transient or stress-induced) will eventually resolve spontaneously; nonetheless, infants who require persistently elevated glucose infusion rates should receive vigorous and prompt treatment for hyperinsulinism.

The mainstay of medical therapy is diazoxide, which binds to the SUR1 subunit of the K_{ATP} channel. Diazoxide maintains the K_{ATP} channel in an open configuration, thereby preventing depolarization of the beta cell and insulin release. The majority of patients with biallelic *ABBC8* and *KCNJ11* mutations, as well as those with focal congenital hyperinsulinism (formed by focally hyperplastic islets), are unresponsive to diazoxide. Diazoxide is initiated at 5–25 mg/kg per day (subdivided 8–12 hourly), together with chlorothiazide (20 mg /kg per day, subdivided 12 hourly) to prevent fluid retention. Side effects of long-term diazoxide therapy include hypertrichosis, fluid retention, neutropenia, thrombocytopenia, and, rarely, pulmonary hypertension.

Somatostatin analogue (Octreotide) inhibits insulin release from beta cells through a different mechanism and is commonly used as a second-line medication. The starting dose of Octreotide is 5 mcg per kg per day by subcutaneous infusion, increasing every three to five days to a maximum dose of 30 mcg/kg/day. Once the effective dose has been determined, the subcutaneous infusion can be changed to an equivalent dose given as subcutaneous injections at 6-hourly intervals. Adverse effects include elevated levels of liver enzymes,

gastrointestinal side-effects (diarrhoea, abdominal discomfort), gallbladder pathology (sludge, gallstones), necrotizing enterocolitis, pituitary hormone suppression, and arrest of linear growth. Patients may develop tachyphylaxis to octreotide.

Sirolimus, a mechanistic target of rapamycin (mTOR) inhibitor, has been used to manage persistent hypoglycaemia in a small number of patients unresponsive to either diazoxide or octreotide. Its use should be restricted to specialist centres.

Surgical treatment

Surgery is the only alternative in patients who do not respond to medical therapy. Congenital hyperinsulinism occurs in two distinct histological forms: diffuse and focal. The diffuse form is inherited in an autosomal recessive (or, less frequently, dominant) manner, whereas the focal form is almost always sporadic. Surgical management differs for the two histological subtypes, therefore, it is essential to accurately distinguish between them. Focal lesions are identified by performing an [[18]Fluoro]-dihydroxyphenylalanine positron emission/computed tomography scan. Most cases are cured by resection of a focal lesion. Medically unresponsive diffuse disease requires near-total (95–98%) pancreatectomy, which is usually palliative, as the majority will continue to have abnormal glucose metabolism with recurrence of hypoglycaemia after surgery. Moreover, a near-total pancreatectomy is associated with a high risk of post-operative insulin-dependent diabetes mellitus and pancreatic exocrine insufficiency. If hypoglycaemia recurs post-operatively, medical therapy must be restarted. If this is unsuccessful, further pancreatic tissue should be removed, necessitating a total pancreatectomy.

Diabetes

See Chapter 1.

Hypopituitarism and adrenal insufficiency

Hypopituitarism in infancy may be associated with recurrent fasting hypoglycaemia resulting from cortisol or growth hormone deficiency. Hypoglycaemia should be prevented by the avoidance of prolonged periods of fasting and replacement of glucocorticoids (hydrocortisone 10–15 mg/m^2 per day) and growth hormone (0.17 mg per kg per week). At times of intercurrent illness, the dosage of oral hydrocortisone may need to be increased threefold, or the equivalent dosage of hydrocortisone may have to be given parenterally if the patient has vomiting or profuse diarrhoea. Management of hypoglycaemia during an adrenal crisis requires intramuscular or IV hydrocortisone (50–100 mg per metre^2 per day, administered at 6-hour intervals) together with intravenous glucose.

Inborn errors of metabolism

A detailed review of the treatment of inborn errors of metabolism is beyond the scope of this chapter. The principles of therapy are to prevent a catabolic state by frequent meals containing high carbohydrates and avoid prolonged periods of fasting. In common with children who suffer from accelerated starvation or idiopathic ketotic hypoglycaemia, the use of uncooked cornstarch (1–2g per kg body weight), which is digested slowly, can prolong the interval between feeds in patients with only short fasting tolerance. Uncooked cornstarch mixed with milk, a flavoured drink, or yoghurt at bedtime is useful to prevent nocturnal hypoglycaemia. For advice regarding the management of inborn errors of metabolism to prevent hypoglycaemia at times of intercurrent illness, the reader is referred to the review by Dixon and Leonard (1992).

Guidelines for follow-up

Careful neurodevelopmental surveillance of all children who have experienced severe hypoglycaemia in early life should be performed during childhood so that appropriate support can be provided where necessary. Individuals at risk of significant hypoglycaemia require continued follow-up so that their fasting tolerance can be re-evaluated as they grow. In general, the older the subject, the greater the fasting tolerance.

When to involve a specialist centre

The management of infants and children with severe and potentially life-threatening hypoglycaemia (e.g. persistent hyperinsulinemic hypoglycaemia of infancy, inborn errors of metabolism) requires urgent stabilization of blood glucose and, thereafter, referral to a specialist centre for rapid diagnosis and effective treatment. Such patients require a multidisciplinary team approach involving:
- paediatricians with expertise in endocrinology and metabolism;
- access to laboratories capable of performing the relevant endocrine and metabolic assays on small samples;
- paediatric surgical and intensive care expertise to ensure adequate venous access for the emergency administration of IV glucose, which may require the insertion of a central line.

Cases that should be discussed with a specialist centre are outlined below.
- persistent hyperinsulinemic hypoglycaemia of infancy;
- hypopituitarism;
- Addison's disease and other causes of adrenal insufficiency;
- recurrent hypoglycaemia of unknown aetiology;
- inborn errors of metabolism;
- those whose planned investigations may include a prolonged fast.

Patients who are identified as having hypoglycaemia secondary to an endocrine abnormality should be followed in a paediatric endocrinology clinic.

Transition

Many causes of hypoglycaemia such as accelerated starvation (idiopathic ketotic hypoglycaemia) or stress-induced hyperinsulinism in the newborn period are transient and resolve in early childhood or as a consequence of surgical intervention (e.g. excision of a focal lesion causing dysregulated insulin secretion). These individuals do not require follow-up into adult life. By contrast, children with hypoglycaemia that is secondary to disorders with life-long implications, such as hypopituitarism, adrenal insufficiency or an inborn error of metabolism, will need to be followed in adult life by physicians with expertise in the management of endocrine and metabolic disorders. Genetic counselling should be provided. Both males and females with activating glucokinase mutations should be informed that there is a 50% risk of transmission to their offspring, and affected newborns tend to be large-for-gestation age, reflecting the growth promoting effects of increased foetal insulin secretion.

Future developments

- Longitudinal studies are needed to describe the normal range of changes in blood glucose concentrations in breast-fed babies in current practice conditions.
- Randomized trials are needed to determine whether treatment of neonates at different blood glucose thresholds affects neurodevelopmental outcomes.

• New imaging techniques, such as functional brain spectroscopy, will allow *in vivo* neurological studies to assess the acute adverse effect of hypoglycaemia and evaluate mechanisms which may protect against these pathophysiological consequences.

• Despite the recent advances in understanding some of the causes of hyperinsulinemic hypoglycaemia, there are still a large number (approximately 50%) of patients in whom the genetic cause of hyperinsulinemic hypoglycaemia is not identified.

• What is the fundamental cause of stress-induced neonatal hyperinsulinemic hypoglycaemia?

• Research is required to develop novel therapies for children with the diffuse form of hyperinsulinemic hypoglycaemia.

• Diagnostic fasts are now performed less frequently and other diagnostic techniques, especially molecular genetics, have become more important.

• The role of continuous glucose monitoring in the management of high risk neonates and in the detection and management of hypoglycaemia in older children has yet to be defined.

Controversial points

• How to define hypoglycaemia in the newborn period?

• Should clinically significant hypoglycaemia be defined by different blood glucose concentrations at different ages?

• How extensively should a child with hypoglycaemia be investigated when initial tests fail to provide a diagnosis?

• What is the pathophysiological basis of 'accelerated starvation' or idiopathic ketotic hypoglycaemia?

Potential pitfalls

• Failure to obtain blood and urine samples for relevant investigations before treating a child to reverse hypoglycaemia.

• Failure to treat hypoglycaemia aggressively (e.g. with IV dextrose if necessary) to prevent further episodes.

• Failure to refer infants with severe, difficult-to-manage hypoglycaemia early enough to a specialist centre.

• During a planned fast for investigation into the cause of hypoglycaemia: inadequate skilled supervision, failure to extend the fast long enough to achieve hypoglycaemia, obtaining blood samples for measurement of hormones and intermediary metabolites before hypoglycaemia has occurred or failure to note time of blood samples on either the biochemistry request form or blood sample container.

• In children known to be at risk for hypoglycaemia, failure to make appropriate arrangements (e.g. planned use of IV dextrose and monitoring of blood glucose concentrations) to avoid hypoglycaemia while subjecting them to elective procedures requiring fasting.

• Failure to recognize the diagnostic significance of a high glucose requirement to avoid hypoglycaemia (suggesting hyperinsulinism) and the ineffective use of glucocorticoid treatment in these circumstances to prevent further episodes of hypoglycaemia.

Case histories

Case 2.1

A two-day-old boy presented with sleepiness, jitteriness, and hypoglycaemic convulsions. He required 20 mg glucose /kg body weight/min to prevent further episodes of hypoglycaemia. When IV glucose was temporarily discontinued, the following results were obtained from a blood sample drawn at the time of hypoglycaemia:

Plasma glucose 1.8 mmol/L [32 mg/dL]

Serum cortisol 141 nmol/L [5.1 µg/dL]

Serum GH 9.9 ng/ml

Serum insulin 72.4 mU/L

Serum C-peptide 4.0 pmol/ml(fasting reference range 0.14–1.39)

Serum non-esterified fatty acids 0.13 mmol/L (fasting reference range 0.1–0.6)

Serum 3-β-hydroxybutyrate 0.45 mmol/L (fasting reference range 0.03–0.3)

Questions and Answers

1 What do the above results demonstrate?

Hyperinsulinemic hypoglycaemia with an inadequate cortisol response. With a blood glucose of 1.8 mmol/L [32 mg/dL], serum concentrations of cortisol should be >550 nmol/L [>20 mg/dL], growth hormone >20 mU/L [>7 ng/ml] and insulin should be undetectable.

2 Are further investigations indicated?

A poor cortisol response in hyperinsulinaemic hypoglycaemia is common and usually does not indicate adrenal insufficiency in this circumstance (thought to be a response to recurrent hypoglycaemia). Nevertheless, a short Synacthen (Cosyntropin) stimulation test may be necessary to ensure that there is no associated adrenal disorder.

3 Is additional therapy indicated and, if so, what?

Given that glucose requirements are markedly elevated, this infant should be given a trial of diazoxide (and chlorothiazide) treatment. If this is unsuccessful, Octreotide should be tried next before surgery is considered.

Case 2.2

A nine-year-old boy presented to a hospital emergency department with a two-month history of recurrent abdominal pain, vomiting, and increasing lethargy. On examination, he appeared ill, dehydrated and hypotensive. An initial blood sample demonstrated the following:

Serum sodium 112 mmol/L
Serum potassium 7.9 mmol/L
Blood urea nitrogen 38.4 mg/dL [13.7 mmol/L]
Plasma glucose 2.6 mmol/L [47 mg/dL]
Serum cortisol 185 nmol/L [7 mcg/dL]

Questions and Answers

1 What additional investigations are necessary to confirm the diagnosis?

Measurement of plasma concentrations of 17-hydroxyprogesterone, adrenal autoantibodies, and urinary steroid metabolite analysis should distinguish the various causes of congenital adrenal hyperplasia from Addison's disease. Note that hyperkalaemia is not seen in central adrenal insufficiency. 17-hydroxyprogesterone, adrenal autoantibodies, and urinary steroid metabolite analysis should distinguish the various causes of congenital adrenal hyperplasia from Addison's disease.

2 What emergency treatment is required?

Ensure a patent airway and adequate respiratory support. Parenteral hydrocortisone (approximately 50-100 mg/m^2 per day, subdivided 6–8 hourly), IV glucose 200 mg/kg body weight given over four to six minutes and a bolus of 10–20 ml/kg body weight of IV saline (0.9%) should be given to restore the circulation.

Thereafter, an infusion of 0.9% saline with dextrose (5–10% as required) should be continued. When able to take medication orally, fludrocortisone should be started.

3 What further clinical sign may help to establish the diagnosis?

Diffusely increased skin pigmentation (without 'tan lines'), including the buccal mucosa, palmar creases, genitalia and areolae, is a consequence of increased melanin production in primary adrenal failure.

Case 2.3

An 18-month-old boy presented to a hospital emergency department in the morning with hypoglycaemia (confirmed laboratory plasma glucose of 1.7 mmol/l [31 mg/dL]) having refused his bottle of milk the night before and then having awoken vomiting. Most evenings when well, he consumes two biscuits and a bottle of milk before bed. On examination, he had a depressed level of consciousness. His height and weight were at the 5th centile; there were no other abnormal findings. An initial blood sample showed the following:

Serum sodium 134 mmol/L
Serum potassium 3.5 mmol/L
Blood urea nitrogen 5.4 mmol/L [15 mg/dL]
Serum cortisol 1,154 nmol/L [41.7 µg/dL]
Serum GH 8.1 ng/ml
Serum insulin and C-peptide undetectable

Questions and Answers

1 What additional investigations are necessary?

An inborn error of metabolism should be excluded by measurement of blood pH, liver function tests, ammonia, free fatty acids, β-hydroxybutyrate, lactate, amino acids, and urinary amino and organic acids.

2 What emergency treatment is required?

Ensure an airway and adequate respiratory support as required. IV glucose 200 mg/kg body weight should be given over four to six minutes and an infusion of 10% dextrose should be started at a rate of 6 ml/kg body weight per hour.

3 If no biochemical abnormalities of counter-regulation can be identified, what prognosis can the parents be offered?

If no other biochemical abnormalities are identified, the likely diagnosis is 'accelerated starvation'. The use of high calorie bedtime feeds or addition of uncooked cornstarch to a bedtime drink is likely to prevent further episodes. This predisposition to hypoglycaemia of unknown origin is likely to resolve by school age or shortly thereafter.

Case 2.4

A five-year-old boy was admitted for an elective 20-hour fast, 48 hours after discontinuation of diazoxide therapy. He had been diagnosed with persistent hyperinsulinaemic hypoglycaemia at one year of age, following investigations to elucidate the cause of a six-month history of convulsions. He had been clinically stable for four years on modest doses of diazoxide and chlorothiazide with no evidence suggestive of recurrent hypoglycaemia. He was asymptomatic during the fast with plasma glucose of 3.8 mmol/L after 15 hours and a blood sample at the end of the fast which demonstrated the following:

Plasma glucose 3.4 mmol/L [61 mg/dL]
Serum insulin <3 mU/L
Serum 3-β-hydroxybutyrate 0.41 mmol/L (fasting reference range 0.03–0.3)
Serum free fatty acids 0.87 mmol/L (fasting reference range 0.1–0.6)

Questions and Answers

1 What does this result demonstrate?

The result demonstrates an inadequate 3-β-hydroxybutyrate concentration (it should exceed 1.8 mmol/L) suggesting that he continues to have mild persistent hyperinsulinism.

2 What advice regarding management would you give?

The results suggest that further treatment with diazoxide and chlorothiazide is indicated. While he will probably tolerate overnight fasting without difficulty, his parents should be advised to monitor blood glucose concentrations at times of illness, particularly if he is 'off his food' as he may be at increased risk of hypoglycaemia in such circumstances. Deoxyribonucleic acid (DNA) should be analysed to search for a variant in one of the genes that may be mutated in persistent hyperinsulinaemic hypoglycaemia.

Case 2.5

A 35-month-old previously healthy girl presented to a local emergency department for evaluation of a non-febrile seizure. She was playing at her grandparents' house when she became lethargic and was noted to be sweating profusely. Within minutes, she lost consciousness and had a tonic-clonic seizure lasting about five minutes. Laboratory investigations obtained upon arrival in the emergency department:

Plasma glucose 28 mg/dL [1.6 mmol/L]
Serum sodium 136 mmol/L
Serum K 4.8 mmol/L
Serum total carbon dioxide 24 mmol/L
Blood urea nitrogen 3.6 mmol/L [4 mg/dL]
Serum AST 22, ALT 18 U/L, alkaline phosphatase 180 U/L
Plasma ammonia 50 mcg/dL [35.7 micromole/L] (reference range 20–65 mcg/dL)
Urinalysis showed no glucose or ketones.

Additional investigations obtained before administering IV glucose:

Serum cortisol 58 mcg/dL [770 nmol/L]
Serum insulin 14.6 uU/ml
Serum C-peptide 2.5 ng/ml (reference ranges: fasting 0.4–2.2; 2-hours mixed meal tolerance test 1.2–3.4)
Serum ß-hydroxybutyrate 0.1 mmol/L

Question and Answer

1 Which of the following is the most likely diagnosis and why?

1 Accidental ingestion of alcohol.
2 Accidental ingestion of sulphonylurea.
3 Deliberate injection of insulin lispro (factitious hypoglycaemia).
4 Hyperinsulinism hyperammonemia syndrome.

Elevated serum insulin concentration would not be expected to occur in a child with alcohol-induced hypoglycaemia. Both serum insulin and C-peptide concentrations are inappropriately elevated, suggesting endogenous insulin secretion. Although elevated, the serum insulin concentration is not extremely high (>100 µU/ml) as would be expected in factitious hypoglycaemia. The hyperinsulinism hyperammonaemia syndrome is characterized by asymptomatic twofold to threefold elevation of plasma ammonia concentrations. The cause of severe hypoglycaemia in this case was accidental ingestion of a long-acting sulphonylurea, which stimulates beta cells to secrete insulin.

Significant Guidelines

Kishnani, P.S., Austin, S.L., Arn, P. et al. (2010). Glycogen storage disease type III diagnosis and management guidelines. *Genet. Med.* 12 (7): 446–463.

Kishnani, P.S., Austin, S.L., Abdenur, J. et al. (2014). Diagnosis and management of glycogen storage disease type I: a practice guideline of the American College of Medical Genetics and Genomics. *Genet. Med.* 16 (11): e1.

References

Dixon MA, Leonard JV (1992) Intercurrent illness in inborn errors of intermediary metabolism. *Arch. Dis. Child.* 67(11)1387–1391.

Ferrara, C., Patel, P., Becker, S. et al. (2016). Biomarkers of insulin for the diagnosis of hyperinsulinemic hypoglycemia in infants and children. *J. Pediatr.* 168: 212–219.

Further Reading

Arya, V.B., Mohammed, Z., Blankenstein, O. et al. (2014). Hyperinsulinaemic hypoglycaemia. *Horm. Metab. Res.* 46 (3): 157–170.

Brown LM, Corrado MM, van der Ende RM, et al. (2015) Evaluation of glycogen storage disease as a cause of ketotic hypoglycemia in children. *J. Inherit. Metab. Dis.* 38(3), 489–493.

Cornblath, M., Hawdon, J.M., Williams, A.F. et al. (2000). Controversies regarding definition of neonatal hypoglycemia: suggested operational thresholds. *Pediatrics* 105 (5): 1141–1145.

De Leon, D.D. and Stanley, C.A. (2017). Congenital hypoglycemia disorders: new aspects of etiology, diagnosis, treatment and outcomes: highlights of the Proceedings of the Congenital Hypoglycemia Disorders Symposium, Philadelphia, April 2016. *Pediatr. Diab.* 18 (1): 3–9.

Ghosh, A., Banerjee, I., and Morris, A.A. (2015). Recognition, assessment and management of hypoglycaemia in childhood. *Arch. Dis. Child.* 101 (6): 575–580.

Guemes M, Rahman SA, Hussain K (2015) What is a normal blood glucose? *Arch. Dis. Child.* 101(6), 569–574.

Harding, J.E., Harris, D.L., Hegarty, J.E. et al. (2017). An emerging evidence base for the management of neonatal hypoglycaemia. *Early Hum. Dev.* 104: 51–56.

Harris, D.L., Weston, P.J., and Harding, J.E. (2012). Incidence of neonatal hypoglycemia in babies identified as at risk. *J. Pediatr.* 161 (5): 787–791.

Harris, D.L., Weston, P.J., Signal, M. et al. (2013). Dextrose gel for neonatal hypoglycaemia (the sugar babies study): a randomised, double-blind, placebo-controlled trial. *Lancet* 382 (9910): 2077–2083.

Lord, K., Dzata, E., Snider, K.E. et al. (2013). Clinical presentation and management of children with diffuse and focal hyperinsulinism: a review of 223 cases. *J. Clin. Endocrinol. Metab.* 98 (11): E1786–E1789.

Morris, A., Thekekara, A., Wilks, Z. et al. (1996). Evaluation of fasts for investigating hypoglycaemia or suspected metabolic disease. *Arch. Dis. Child.* 75: 115–119.

Stanley, C.A., Rozance, P.J., Thornton, P.S. et al. (2015). Re-evaluating "transitional neonatal hypoglycaemia": mechanism and implications for management. *J. Pediatr.* 166 (6): 1520–1525.

Thornton, P.S., Stanley, C.A., De Leon, D.D. et al. (2015). Recommendations from the Pediatric Endocrine Society for evaluation and management of persistent hypoglycemia in neonates, infants, and children. *J. Pediatr.* 167 (2): 238–245.

van Veen, M.R., van Hasselt, P.M., de Sain-van der Velden, M.G. et al. (2011). Metabolic profiles in children during fasting. *Pediatr.* 127 (4): E1021–E1027.

Useful Information for Patients and Parents

Congenital Hyperinsulinism International (CHI) is an organization founded by parents of children with hyperinsulinism and is supported by an international Scientific Advisory Group comprising leading specialists in congenital hyperinsulinism. CHI is dedicated to improving the lives of children, adults, and families living with congenital hyperinsulinism by providing education information and support to those living with the disease. Information is available at www.congenitalhi.org (accessed 3 October 2018).

The Association for Glycogen Storage Disease is an organization for parents of and individuals with glycogen storage disease to communicate, share their successes and concerns, share useful findings, provide support, create an awareness of this condition for the public, and to stimulate research in the various forms of glycogen storage diseases. The website (www.agsdus.org) (accessed 3 October 2018) provides basic information about the glycogen storage diseases. The information is intended to be useful to people affected by one of the glycogen storage diseases, their families, and other interested parties.

3 Short Stature

Introduction

The term 'auxology' (Greek root, αὐξάνειν, *auxanein*, to grow) is used to describe the study of human growth using repeated measurements of the same individual over successive time periods. It was Professor James Mourilyan Tanner (1920–2010), who in the 1970s established auxology as a scientific discipline and introduced its routine use as an essential part of clinical growth assessment.

Definitions of short stature, failure to thrive, and growth failure

Short stature can be defined both in terms of auxology and perception. In auxological terms, short stature refers to *height* which is less than two standard deviations below the mean for the population concerned; this corresponds to height below the 2nd or 3rd centile, depending on which growth charts are used. In terms of perception, short stature can be defined as small size sufficient to cause physical, psychological, or social concerns in the child and family. Short stature should be distinguished from *failure to thrive* or weight faltering, a term usually applied to infants and pre-school children which denotes failure to gain weight at an

appropriate rate so that the child looks thin; and *growth failure* – failure to maintain a *height velocity* which is appropriate for both age and maturity.

In most patients, short stature is a variation of normal physiology rather than a pathological process. The challenge to the paediatrician is to identify the relatively few children with pathology without subjecting essentially normal children to unnecessary investigation.

Physiology of growth

Normal linear growth

Human linear growth can be divided into three phases – infancy, childhood. and puberty as described by Karlberg (Karlberg 1989 – see Figure 3.1). These are not distinct entities, for the process of growth is a continuum. However, during these periods of development distinct features of growth can be recognized, corresponding with different regulatory mechanisms.

Infantile phase

This can be regarded as a continuation of the foetal growth curve, beginning at conception. The infantile curve is rapid but decelerating, with a mean of 25 cm of growth in the first 12 months of life, and 12.5 cm

Practical Endocrinology and Diabetes in Children, Fourth Edition. Malcolm D.C. Donaldson, John W. Gregory, Guy Van Vliet, and Joseph I. Wolfsdorf.
© 2019 John Wiley & Sons Ltd. Published 2019 by John Wiley & Sons Ltd.

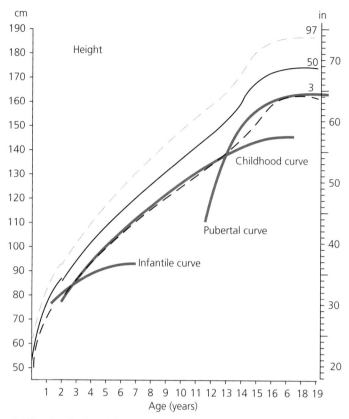

Figure 3.1 The infancy, childhood and pubertal (ICP) concept of Karlberg showing the three growth curves. Source: After Karlberg (1989).

during the second year. The major regulating influences on growth in infancy are nutritional and thyroidal status. Intrauterine growth restriction (IUGR) results in impairment of the infantile growth curve.

Childhood

The childhood growth pattern starts from approximately six months of age and predominates from the age of three years. During childhood, nutrition becomes less important and hormonal influences, particularly the effects of the growth hormone (GH)–insulin-like growth factor (IGF) axis and thyroid hormones – become the principal regulating mechanisms for linear growth. Impairment of the childhood growth curve will result from GH or thyroxine (T4) deficiency.

Puberty

During puberty, the pattern of human growth changes dramatically, but differs in important ways between females and males, as described by Tanner (Tanner 1986 – Figure 3.2).

In females, the adolescent growth spurt starts approximately two years earlier than in males. Its onset coincides with breast development, the first sign of puberty. Peak height velocity (PHV) occurs on average at approximately 12 years of age and menarche (the onset of menstruation) follows PHV by a variable interval, being close to PHV in early developers and more distant in late developers. Consequently, menarche occurs when height velocity is falling and is followed by approximately two years of gradually diminishing growth rate. A further difference between females and males is the amplitude of PHV which, in females reaches, on average, approximately 8 cm per year compared with 10 cm per year in males.

In males, the adolescent growth spurt begins when puberty is already well established and coincides with a testicular volume of 10–12 ml. PHV is reached at an average age of approximately 14 years (15 ml testicular volume). The average difference in adult height between males and females is 12.5–14 cm, (roughly 5 in.) according to UK standards, being accounted for by two additional years of prepubertal growth, a

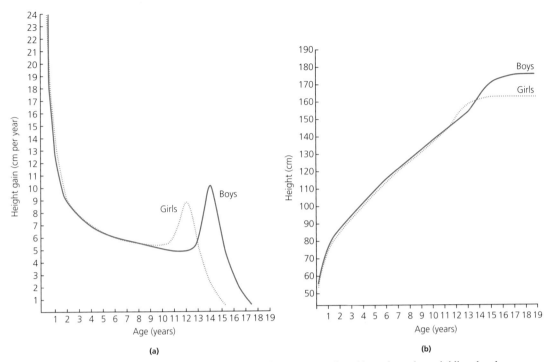

Figure 3.2 (a) Height velocity and (b) typical individual height curves in girls and boys throughout childhood and adolescence. Source: (a) from Tanner (1986).

greater amplitude of the adolescent growth spurt, and greater prepubertal height in males.

Absence of the pubertal acceleration, with prolongation of the childhood curve, will be seen with delayed puberty. Lack of a pubertal growth spurt despite normal pubertal development is seen in isolated GH deficiency, indicating that both sex steroids and GH are required for a peak to occur.

Endocrine control of growth

GH secretion

GH is the major endocrine regulator of postnatal linear growth. GH is a single-chain polypeptide consisting of 191 amino acids, which circulates in the blood bound to growth hormone binding protein (GHBP) that results from cleavage and shedding of the extracellular part of the GH receptor. The predominant form (75%) of GH exists as a 22 kDa protein with 5–10% of pituitary GH release represented by a smaller 20 kDa form that lacks amino acids in positions 32–46. GH is secreted by somatotroph cells of the anterior pituitary gland under the dual regulation of two hypothalamic peptides: growth hormone-releasing

hormone (GHRH), which is stimulatory, and somatostatin, which is inhibitory to GH release. These two peptides are, in turn, influenced by central neurotransmitters. Ghrelin, secreted from the gut, is a third GH secretagogue. GH is secreted in an episodic or pulsatile manner, reflecting the interaction of GHRH and somatostatin. Secretion of GH, mostly via its hypothalamic control, is influenced by a wide variety of environmental, genetic, and physiological factors including nutrition, sleep, exercise, and stress.

The growth hormone-insulin-like growth factor (GH-IGF) axis

Figure 3.3 shows the GH-IGF axis. The insulin-like growth factors (IGF-I, IGF-II) are related peptides, so named because of their close structural relationship with proinsulin and their weak insulin-like metabolic effects. GH is believed to have little *direct* effect on linear growth. IGF-1 is directly responsible for linear growth, particularly during the childhood and pubertal phases.

IGF-1 is primarily secreted by the liver into the circulation and exerts an *endocrine* effect on target tissues, including bone. IGF-1 is also synthesized by bone, the cells exerting an influence on adjacent

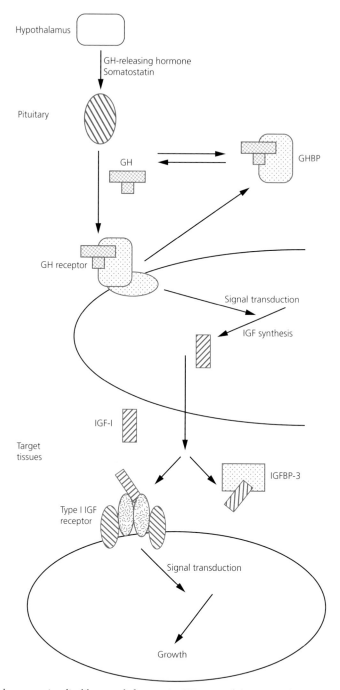

Figure 3.3 The growth hormone–insulin-like growth factor axis. GH = growth hormone, GHBP = growth hormone binding protein, IGF = insulin-like growth factor, IGFBP = IGF binding protein.

cells – the *paracrine* effect – as well as on the cells which secrete it – the *autocrine* effect. The relative contribution of endocrine versus paracrine IGF-1 on bone remains unclear (Crane and Cao 2014).

IGF-I is a single-chain polypeptide of 70 amino acids which is encoded from a complex gene on chromosome 12. IGF-I synthesis occurs after binding of GH to its receptor in the liver and other target organs.

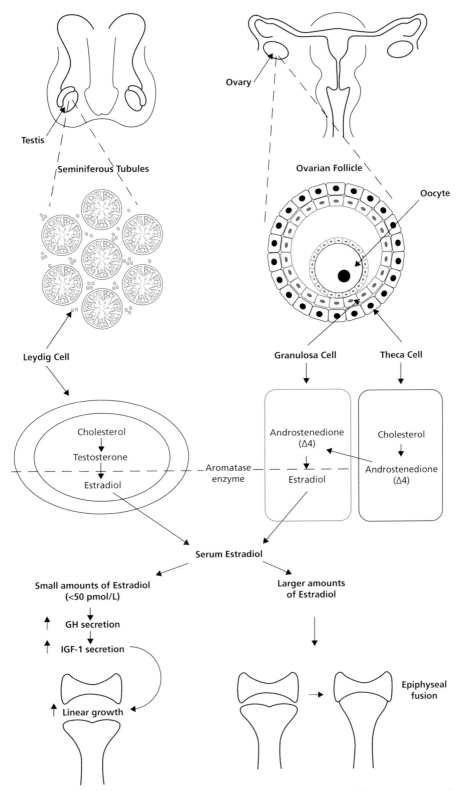

Figure 3.4 Schematic representation of effect of estradiol on growth. Estradiol is aromatized from testosterone in boys and androstenedione in girls. Serum estradiol levels of 15–30 pmol/L in girls and boys are associated with enhanced growth velocity (Albin et al. 2012; Ankarberg-Lindgren and Norjavaara 2008) via an effect on the growth hormone axis. Larger amounts of estradiol result in growth deceleration and epiphyseal fusion via an effect on the growth plate.

The concentration of IGF-I in the circulation is closely related to physiological secretion of GH, although this relationship may be disturbed in pathological states. IGF-I interacts specifically with soluble proteins called insulin-like growth factor-binding proteins (IGFBPs). The principal carrier protein for IGF-I is IGFBP-3, the systemic levels of which depend on GH status. When IGFBP-3 has an IGF molecule bound to it, it can then associate with another GH-dependent glycoprotein, 'acid-labile subunit' (ALS), to form a ternary complex.

Unlike insulin, most IGF-I circulates in an inactive or bound form. The IGFBPs extend the half-life of the IGF peptides, transport them to target cells and modulate their interaction with their respective receptors. IGF-I binds to the type 1 IGF receptor in target tissues, such as the growth plate at the ends of long bones.

Growth at puberty: the effect of sex hormones on the GH-IGF axis and growth plate

Estradiol is the key hormone influencing the GH-IGF axis at puberty in both sexes (Figure 3.4). The enzyme *aromatase* is responsible for estradiol synthesis from *testosterone* in the *Leydig* cell of the *testis*; and from *androstenedione* in the *granulosa* cell of the *ovary*.

The effect of serum estradiol on growth is paradoxical and relates to the level of secretion. Small to moderate levels of serum estradiol accelerate growth by stimulating the hypothalamus to enhance GHRH secretion, resulting in an increase in the amplitude of GH secretion, especially at night (Rose et al. 1991), and increased GH secretion raises IGF-1 levels. Larger amounts of estradiol inhibit growth through action on the growth plate, accelerating epiphyseal fusion. Thus, estradiol is indirectly responsible for the pubertal growth spurt and directly responsible for the cessation of linear growth in both sexes.

Clinical assessment of growth

See Appendix 1 for Growth Charts.

Techniques of measurement

Accurate measurement is essential for growth assessment and an important clinical skill. Errors may be the result of unreliable equipment and faulty measurement technique. To optimize the accuracy of measurement, a single trained measurer – or, at the most

two – should measure children in a single clinic. The following techniques enable reliable data to be collected from the most commonly used measurements.

Weight

Ideally, babies and infants up to the age of two years should be weighed nude, using specialized digital baby/toddler scales. Nappies should always be removed. If the infant is especially fractious and will not lie or sit still enough for a reading to be taken it is acceptable to weigh the parent and child together and then the parent separately and calculate the child's weight by subtraction. For children over two years, weight should be taken with the subject wearing the minimum of clothing on standing or sitting scales. Where possible, automated equipment should be used and follow national guidelines Measurements should be given in metric units.

Measurement of standing height

The cost of equipment for measuring height varies considerably. The stadiometer is recommended for use with children from the age of two years and should be calibrated daily using a metal rod of known length. The subject stands with heels (without shoes and socks), buttocks and shoulder blades against the backplate and the measurer ensures that the imaginary line from the centre of the external auditory meatus to the lower border of the eye socket (the Frankfurt plane) is horizontal. The measurer then applies upward pressure on the mastoid processes and the reading is taken at maximum extension without the heels losing contact with the baseboard.

Measurement of supine length in children from birth to two years of age

Neonates and toddlers are notoriously difficult to measure accurately. The supine table and neonatometer, both consisting of a flat surface with a fixed headboard and moving baseplate, are two devices developed to reduce error in measuring babies and children too young to stand up (Figure 3.5). Two people are necessary to obtain a reliable measurement. The assistant holds the child's head in firm contact with the headboard, so that the Frankfurt plane is vertical; with neonates, it is also advisable to use the forefingers to pin the shoulders down. At the same time, the legs of the (by now almost always crying) child are straightened and when the measurer is satisfied that the head is still in contact with the headboard, the measurement can be taken.

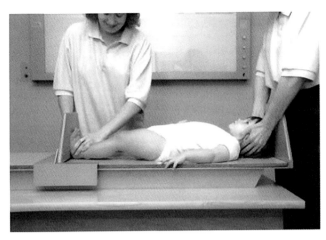

Figure 3.5 Measurement of supine length.

Sitting height

Technically more difficult to measure than standing height, sitting height is required to derive subischial leg length and thus assess body proportion. A sitting height table is required and the subject sits on the table with the back of the knees resting on the edge, with the feet supported on a variable height step so that the upper surface of the thighs is horizontal. The subject is then asked to sit up straight. The headboard is placed on the subject's head, upward pressure is then applied to the mastoid process and the measurement is taken.

Upper arm circumference

Upper arm circumference is not used in routine clinical practice in the developed world but is related to body mass index (Brito et al. 2016) and hence a valuable tool in screening for malnutrition when measurement of height and weight is impractical. The site for measurement is mid-way between the acromion and the olecranon process.

Head circumference

Head circumference is an important measurement of normal growth and should be routine in children under the age of two years. The tape is slipped over the head and passed around the occipital prominence to measure maximal head circumference. Accurate positioning of the tape is vital to ensure reliability and the average of three measurements should be taken.

Reliability

There will always be a degree of intra-observer error, however competent the operator. With good technique, an error of 0.2–0.3 cm for height measurement by a single observer is achievable (Voss et al. 1990).

Decimal age

Expression of age as a decimal makes calculations, particularly height velocity, much simpler. The Table of Decimals of Year, which normally accompanies clinical growth charts, shows what decimal fraction of a year has elapsed by each day. For example, on 2 July 2009 the year has passed 0.501 of the way to 2010 and that date can be expressed as 2009.501.

To calculate the decimal age of a child seen at the clinic on 9 May 2018 and born on 26 August 2008, the decimal birthday (108.649) is subtracted from the decimal clinic appointment (118.351) to give a decimal age of 9.702 years.

Calculation of height velocity

Height velocity should be calculated using measurement intervals of 6–12 months (minimum/maximum 4/14 months), dividing the difference in height (cm) by the difference in interval (years). For example, a child born on 28 March 2002, measuring 132.6 cm on 3 February 2011 and 138.2 cm on 4 January 2012 will have decimal ages at the times of 8.854 and 9.772 so that the height velocity is:

$$\frac{138.2 - 132.6}{9.772 - 8.854} = \frac{5.6}{0.918} = 6.1 \, \text{cm/year}$$

An idea of height velocity can also be obtained by examining the growth curve constructed from a series of accurate measurements. A height curve which crosses the centile bands downwards or upwards indicates a change in height velocity from the norm which requires an explanation.

Parental height and target range

Parents should be measured whenever possible. Reported parental heights are notoriously inaccurate, especially in fathers (Cizmecioglu et al. 2005). The mean height difference in men and women from the United Kingdom is 13 cm (Tanner et al. 1970). When a boy is seen in the clinic, the father's height is plotted directly on the right-hand side of a growth chart for boys (see Figure 3.6). The mother's height is then plotted after adding 13 cm to her height. The mid-parental height (MPH) centile is the mid-point between the father's height and the mother's corrected height. The target range is calculated as the MPH ± two standard deviations = 8.5 cm (6.5–10 cm depending on population data) and represents the 95% confidence limits.

When a girl is seen in the clinic, the mother's height is plotted directly, the father's height is plotted after subtracting 13 cm. The MPH and target range are then calculated as for boys.

With normal parents and healthy children, the children's final heights will be normally distributed around the MPH, with only a 5% probability of falling outside the target range.

Pubertal staging

Staging of pubertal development using the criteria of Tanner and the Prader orchidometer in boys is important in the clinical assessment of *all* patients, irrespective of age. Details of the criteria for pubertal staging are given in Chapter 5.

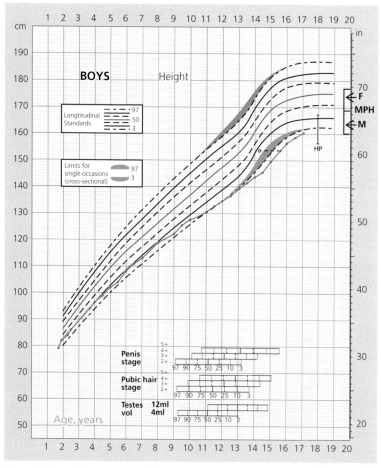

Figure 3.6 Growth chart of a boy with constitutional delay in growth and adolescence associated with mild asthma. The father measures 174 cm and his height is plotted directly on the growth chart (F). The mother measures 151 cm and 13 cm are added to her height to correct for the sex difference = 164 cm and this corrected height (M) is plotted. The mid-parental height (MPH) is 174 + 164/2 = 169 cm with target range ±8.5 cm = 160.5–177.5. Mean (2SD) height prediction (HP) according to the Tanner Whitehouse RUS TW2 system is 162.5 (5) cm.

Height and height velocity standard deviation score

Height for chronological age and bone age can be expressed as standard deviation scores (SDSs) according to the following formula:

$$\text{Height SDS} = \frac{\text{child's height} - \text{mean height for age}}{\text{SD for height at that age}}$$

Height velocity SDS can be calculated according to the following formula:

$$\frac{\text{Child's height velocity} - \text{mean height velocity (for the mid age over which height velocity was measured)}}{\text{One SD for height velocity at that age}}$$

The SDS for height and height velocity at different ages can be obtained by consulting the original publications from which local growth standards have been derived or by downloading software such as Professor Tim Cole's LMS system, based on UK 1990 data which is available as a free download: http://www.healthforallchildren. com/shop-base/shop/software/lmsgrowth. Using SDS to express height and height velocity values enables data on groups of children of both sexes and different ages to be pooled and compared statistically. It is also more informative to express extremely short or tall stature as SDS rather than < or ≪ 0.4th centile, > or ≫ 99.6th centile, etc. When SDS values are calculated for patients in puberty, adjustments must be made for the pubertal stage of the child and the age at which PHV occurred.

Body mass index

The relationship between weight and height of an individual can be expressed as body mass index (BMI) which is calculated as body weight (in kilogrammes)/height^2\(metres). This method has been criticized for assessment of obesity in children because the average values for BMI vary considerably with age. Normal standards for BMI are available for British children using UK 1990 data (Freeman et al. 1995) or since 2009 the UK-World Health Organization data (see Chapter 11 and Appendix 1 for more information)

Assessment of skeletal maturity

Several methods have been developed to assess the skeletal maturity or 'bone age' of growing children using an X-ray of the left wrist. The two most commonly used methods are the 'atlas method' (e.g.

Greulich and Pyle) and the 'bone-specific scoring system' (e.g. Tanner–Whitehouse). Figure 3.6 shows how bone age is represented on the growth chart as an open circle using height at the time of measurement and bone age as coordinates, and linking bone and chronological age with a broken line.

The Greulich and Pyle method

An atlas of standard or typical X-rays of the left hand and wrist of normal girls and boys at specific ages throughout childhood and adolescence is used. The overall standard that most closely resembles the film in question is chosen and this becomes the bone age. Critics of this method claim that a single radiograph may yield bone ages that are several years apart when assessed by different observers. The standards, which are derived from North American children, are also relatively advanced (six to nine months) compared with European children. However, this method is the most widely used throughout the world, with relatively little specialized training being required.

The Tanner–Whitehouse method

In this method, criteria have been established for set stages in skeletal maturation. The most commonly used system is the TW2 method, which also incorporates a methodology for predicting adult height (see Figure 3.6). The system is a bone-by-bone, stage-by-stage method and the assessor assigns a score to each bone according to written criteria. The composite score is translated into the bone age. This system is generally considered by connoisseurs in the field as being superior to the atlas method as subjectivity is almost eliminated. However, specific training of the assessor is required and use of this method outside the United Kingdom is relatively limited. In 2001, this system of bone age assessment was updated to TW3 to reflect the secular trend towards more rapid physical maturation seen in many countries.

Automated bone age assessment

In recent years automated systems for bone age assessment have been introduced in clinical practice, with evidence to show comparable accuracy with single-observer assessment and the advantage of saving labour (Lee et al. 2017). Since 2012, bone age in Glasgow has been calculated using an automated system (http://www.bonexpert.com).

Growth charts

Growths charts are compiled using cross-sectional and/ or longitudinal data. Cross-sectional charts are based on single measurements of large numbers of individuals, covering the whole age range. Longitudinal charts are based on regular, serial measurements of a smaller number of individuals. Three main types of growth charts are currently available in the United Kingdom. The UK 90 charts published by the Child Growth Foundation in 1990 are cross-sectional and were compiled using contemporary UK data. They incorporate a novel nine-centile format with each centile 'band' being 2/3 SDS apart. The resultant growth curves are similar to the conventional 3rd–97th centiles, with additional curves −2.67 SD (0.4th centile) and + 2.67 SD (99.6th centile) about the mean to give more useful cut-offs for stature screening. The Buckler-Tanner charts (1995) are a revised version of the former Tanner-Whitehouse charts and incorporate both cross-sectional (in the childhood curve) and longitudinal (in the pubertal curve) data, making them particularly useful for the interpretation of serial measurements.

In 2010, UK–WHO growth charts for the age range birth to four years were introduced. These charts are based on the World Health Organization (WHO) international child growth standards which describe the optimal growth of healthy breast-fed children from six countries. In 2012, the Royal College of Paediatrics and Child Health (RCPCH) among other organizations recommended use of the 2–18 year WHO growth charts (www.rcpch.ac.uk/resources/ uk-world-health-organisation-growth-charts-2-18-years).

In the USA, many of the major centres use growth charts incorporated into electronic medical record systems. The National Center for Health Statistics (NCHS) Centers for Disease Control and Prevention (CDC) growth charts and the WHO growth charts are widely used. NCHS recommends the WHO growth charts for children aged 0–2 years and the NCHS (CDC) charts for children aged 2 years and older (https://www.cdc.gov/growthchart /).

In Canada, the Canadian Pediatric Endocrine Group (CPEG) officially endorsed the 2014 revision to the WHO Growth Charts for Canada, with a preference for the use of the Set 2 charts (https://www.cpeg-gcep.net/content/who-growth-charts-canada).

For clinical use we find that the split format of the WHO charts is not ideal for monitoring, and demonstrating to families, the growth status and height trajectory of patients with problems such as constitutional delay, growth hormone deficiency and congenital adrenal hyperplasia. The UK editors prefer the Child Growth Foundation (CGF) and Buckler-Tanner charts for children aged two years or more with endocrine and growth problems while the North American editors often use the Tanner and Davies longitudinal growth charts (Tanner and Davies 1985), especially for children with short stature and delayed onset of puberty. There is agreement that the WHO charts are indicated for children aged 0–2 years.

Appendix 1 therefore reproduces the WHO 0–4 year and CDC 2–20 year height and weight charts; the Tanner and Davies 2–19 year height velocity charts; and the UK-WHO body mass index (BMI) 2–20 year charts for girls and boys. In addition, Appendix 2 shows disease-specific growth charts for Turner, Down and Noonan syndromes, and achondroplasia.

Clinical assessment of short stature

Much of this is within the scope of all healthcare professionals who deal with children, including family practitioners, school nurses, and health visitors. With a combination of meticulous auxology, thorough history, and focused examination, a sensible diagnosis and management plan can be achieved.

Auxology

The following should be carried out *before* the child/ adolescent and family enter the consulting room:

- *Measurement:* The heights of patient and *both* parents should be obtained and the patient weighed.
- *Calculation:* Decimal age, MPH and target range; and height velocity (when previous height data are available).
- *Plotting:* Patient and parental height data are plotted onto an appropriate growth chart as shown in Figure 3.6.

History

- *Presenting complaint.* Establish who is worried about what (e.g. parents but not child concerned about small size).
- *History of presenting complaint* (three sections). Growth history (supplemented by previous measurements if available); general health, including energy levels and activities; and degree of psychological upset in the child/adolescent.
- *Past medical history.* Birth weight and length, gestation and mode of delivery; history of atopy (an important factor in constitutional delay); relevant medical events (e.g. orchidopexy for cryptorchidism).

- *Family history*. Name, age, and health of each family member; parental and sibling heights/height status; consanguinity; size during childhood and pubertal history in father and mother (including age at menarche in the latter).
- *Social and educational history*. Name of school; school year (whether age-appropriate or not); school attendance, academic status (including need for extra help), relationship with peers (teasing and bullying) and authority figures; sport and leisure activities.
- *System review* (where appropriate).

Examination (with child standing initially)

- General appearance and nutrition
- Body proportions
- Dysmorphic features
- Systemic examination, including heart and blood pressure measurements
- Fundi
- Pubertal status

Clinical diagnosis

The most likely diagnosis and differential diagnosis should be formulated *before* any investigations are contemplated.

Investigation of short stature

This is unnecessary in most short children, for example, those with normal familial short stature and/or constitutional delay in growth and adolescence. Clinical features suggesting that investigation of short stature is indicated are given in Table 3.1. Investigation should always be seriously considered in a child whose height centile falls below the parental target range centiles.

Laboratory investigations for short stature

Once the decision has been made to perform laboratory investigations on the child with short stature, the doctor must proceed as a general paediatrician and not as a paediatric endocrinologist. If the approach is too specialized, disorders such as anaemia, malabsorption, renal disease, Crohn disease, or even Turner syndrome can easily be missed. Baseline investigations for short stature are shown in Table 3.2. Note that no investigations of GH status other than IGF-1 are included at this stage.

Table 3.1 Clinical features suggesting that investigations for short stature are indicated.

Marked short stature (Ht SDS < −2.5)
Height centile below parental target range centiles
Abnormal/inappropriate height velocity for stage of maturity
History suspicious for chronic disease
History of neonatal hypoglycaemia and prolonged jaundice (suggestive of hypopituitarism)
Dysmorphic features suggestive of underlying syndrome (e.g. Turner and Noonan syndromes)
Pubertal delay
Extreme parental concern

Table 3.2 Baseline investigations for short stature.

X-ray of left wrist and hand for skeletal maturity ('bone age')
Full blood count, ESR
Creatinine, urea, electrolytes
Calcium, phosphate, liver function tests
Ferritin, tissue transglutaminase (TTG) (for coeliac disease)
Karyotype
T4, TSH
IGF-I, cortisol, prolactin
Skeletal survey if dysplasia suspected

The decision to investigate GH secretion is made only after the above investigations have been performed and documented to be normal. At the second and third consultations additional auxological information, particularly on height velocity, will be available. Further investigation of the child can now be considered. Indications and procedures for investigation of possible GH insufficiency are covered in section on the diagnosis of GH deficiency, which discusses this disorder in detail.

Differential diagnosis of short stature

Short stature may result from a combination of factors (composite short stature) rather than a single cause. For example, a child might be short due in part to IUGR but may also have short parents, poorly controlled asthma, and psychosocial difficulties. A suggested classification of the major aetiological

Table 3.3 Classification of short stature.

Normal short stature
- Familial/genetic
- Constitutional delay

Short stature following smallness for gestational age (SGA)
Dysmorphic syndromes
- SGA a constant feature (e.g. Russell Silver and Foetal Alcohol Spectrum disorder)
- SGA not a constant feature (e.g. Turner and Noonan syndromes)

Skeletal dysplasias (e.g. hypochondroplasia)
Chronic disease (e.g. coeliac disease, Crohn disease, cystic fibrosis)

Psychosocial deprivation
Endocrine disorders
- GH insufficiency
- Thyroid deficiency
- Cortisol excess
Other
- Idiopathic short stature

categories is shown in Table 3.3. This classification separates idiopathic short stature (ISS) from normal familial short stature. There is some overlap between categories; some dysmorphic children are small-for-gestational age (e.g. foetal alcohol syndrome), while skeletal dysplasia is a component of other syndromes (e.g. Turner syndrome).

Normal short stature

Familial/Genetic short stature

This is the most common cause for referral of a child with short stature. Essentially, the child is perfectly healthy but has inherited short stature genes from one or both parents or, occasionally, a more distant relative. There is no endocrine abnormality and the bone age is usually not delayed, unless there is also a component of growth delay.

NB: Do not assume that familial short stature is always normal. If one of the parents is markedly short, a dominantly inherited growth disorder, such as a skeletal dysplasia, neurofibromatosis, or GH deficiency, should be considered.

Constitutional growth delay

The diagnosis of constitutional growth delay (see Figure 3.6) is suggested when the child is healthy but looks young for his/her age, has evidence of late maturation in terms of bone age and pubertal delay, and often the history that one parent or second degree relative (e.g. an uncle) was short during childhood with subsequent delay in puberty. A history of atopic asthma, often mild, is common. The condition is seen more often in boys and typically there is a component of genetic short stature since it is the shorter children who tend to show slow maturation.

Frequently, the slow maturation starts in early childhood and the delay of physical development accumulates. Consequently, an 11-year-old boy could well have the physical maturity, bone age, height, and appearance of an 8-year-old. The short stature in this situation is then compounded by the delay in pubertal development. Typically, final adult height is within but in the lower half of the parental target range (see Figure 3.6).

Short stature related to smallness-for-gestational age and intrauterine growth restriction

Smallness-for-gestational age (SGA) is linked with, but distinct from, intra-uterine growth restriction (IUGR) (see Figure 3.7). SGA is defined according to weight and varies with the paediatric discipline involved. Neonatologists define SGA as birth weight below the 9th or 10th centile for gestational age, recognizing that this population is at risk of postnatal hypoglycaemia, and should be targeted for early feeding and capillary glucose monitoring. Endocrinologists define SGA in auxological terms – birth weight below the 2nd or 3rd centile (i.e. more than 2 SD below the mean). Using the latter definition of SGA will include many small normal babies. Short stature at birth can only be reliably identified if birth length is measured accurately, and is only roughly correlated with birth weight (Sardar et al. 2015).

IUGR means intrauterine growth failure. Affected infants are usually but not always light/short at birth (see Figure 3.7). The diagnosis of IUGR is *secure* if serial antenatal ultrasound has demonstrated growth failure; and in defined syndromes such as Russell-Silver; *likely* in the context of severe SGA; and can be *inferred* in SGA or non-SGA infants with birth weight < 25th centile and a combination of postnatal feeding difficulties and impaired infantile growth curve.

If weight, length, and head circumference are proportionate at birth, the SGA is termed *symmetrical* and reflects either a small/normal baby or IUGR related to early growth failure. *Asymmetrical* SGA, when weight is reduced but with preservation of head and linear growth, occurs because of late deprivation of nutrients usually related to placental insufficiency and is the foetal equivalent of failure to thrive. Babies with asymmetrical SGA are more

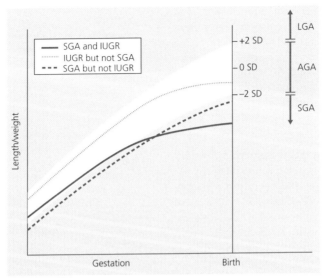

Figure 3.7 Intrauterine growth chart showing three patterns of intrauterine growth. The solid line shows impaired foetal growth with birth length/weight below the – 2 standard deviation (SD) curve, i.e. both small for gestational age (SGA) and intrauterine growth restriction (IUGR). The broken dashed line shows normal growth below but parallel to the – 2 SD curve, i.e. SGA but no IUGR. The dotted line represents impaired foetal growth but birth weight/length is appropriate-for-gestational age (AGA), i.e. IUGR but no SGA.

likely to show postnatal catch-up growth. The overall catch-up rate within two years of birth in SGA subjects is 87% (Albertsson-Wikland and Karlberg 1994).

SGA also can be classified according to the cause:
- *foetal*: genetic syndromes, intrauterine infection, exposure to irradiation, smoking, alcohol;
- *placental*: impaired placental function, especially during 3rd trimester;
- *maternal*: chronic illness such as renal disease and hypertension.

Dysmorphic syndromes

Dysmorphic syndromes can be defined as conditions arising from a specific event – chromosomal, genetic, environmental – during foetal life and resulting in a variable constellation of features (Jones 1997). These include:
- unusual phenotype (especially face, hands, body proportions);
- growth problems – usually short but sometimes tall stature;
- developmental delay/learning disability;
- congenital anomalies (especially cardiac, renal, and gastrointestinal);
- gonadal problems.

Diagnosis is important not only to provide a cause for the short stature but also to identify associated problems (e.g. ovarian failure in Turner syndrome) and giving the patient and family a prognosis.

The paediatrician seeing children with short stature needs to become experienced in recognizing clinical patterns suggestive of a dysmorphic process, and being aware of the heterogeneity of each syndrome. Professor James Tanner taught that identification of dysmorphic features is easier with the patient standing opposite the seated doctor. Every patient in Professor Tanner's clinic was photographed, which also accentuated unusual features. The involvement of a clinical genetic colleague is invaluable, particularly in assessing the many patients with dysmorphism who do not fit into an obvious diagnostic category.

A detailed account of all the relatively common recognizable dysmorphic syndromes is beyond the scope of this chapter; however, a selection of six syndromes which may present undiagnosed to the growth clinic are briefly described here.

Russell-silver syndrome

Birth weight is usually <2nd centile and almost invariably <9th centile, feeding difficulties are the rule, and nocturnal sweating (suggestive of hypoglycaemia) is common. On examination, affected individuals are short and thin, some showing asymmetry with hand, foot, arm, or leg shorter on one side. Head is relatively large, often with expanded vault, and facies are characteristically triangular with down-sloping eyes. Intelligence is normal. The condition results from maternal and/or paternal iso- and heterodisomy causing abnormal methylation in imprinted genes. Causes include, but are not confined to, hypomethylation at 11p15.5 and to maternal disomy of chromosome 7 (Dias et al. 2012). Hypomethylation at 11p15.5 has been shown to affect postnatal mRNA expression of IGF-2.

Foetal alcohol spectrum disorder (FASD)

Birth weight is invariably reduced, and there is postnatal short stature associated with poor concentration, behaviour and learning difficulties. Facies are variable but may show smooth philtrum, short palpebral fissures, and malar hypoplasia. Head circumference is reduced. A history of maternal alcohol ingestion is crucial to making the diagnosis but is not always evident at initial presentation. Hence, SGA/IUGR children with developmental delay and poor concentration should be followed up so that foetal alcohol spectrum disorder (FASD) can be recognized.

Turner syndrome

Turner syndrome (see Table 3.4 and Figure 3.8) occurs in about 1 in 2500 liveborn girls. There is loss or abnormality of the second X chromosome in at least one major cell line in a phenotypic female. The principal features are outlined in Table 3.4 and include dysmorphic traits (see Figure 3.8), short stature (an almost constant sign) and ovarian dysgenesis (in about 90%). Associated features include congenital heart disease (15%), middle ear disease which can be very troublesome (65%), hypertension and aortic root dilatation, renal anomalies (common but rarely problematic), a predisposition to autoimmunity, specific learning difficulties (particularly with mathematics), and a degree of social vulnerability.

Genetic aspects

Partial inactivation of the second X chromosome in all the body's cells from early foetal life partly explains the remarkably mild phenotype of Turner syndrome. However 30% of the short arm genes of the second X chromosome are not inactivated, and these include the *Short Stature Homeobox* (*SHOX*) gene. Loss of this and other genes results in skeletal dysplasia with short stature. Loss of genes controlling lymphogenesis, ovarian function, and skin naevi result in lymphoedema, accelerated atresia of oocytes, and

Table 3.4 Principal features of Turner syndrome.

Features attributable to skeletal dysplasia
- Short stature (with disproportion affecting lower extremities)
- Short 4th/5th metacarpals
- Cubitus valgus
- High palate
- Micrognathia; dental overcrowding
- Broad chest

Ovarian dysgenesis

Chronic middle ear disease

Lymphoedema-related
- Hyperconvex nails ± nail-fold oedema
- Neck webbing
- Lymphoedema hands/feet/limbs

CNS-related
- Sleeping difficulties and hyperactivity
- Specific learning difficulties: number work, visuo-spatial tasks
- Social vulnerability and isolation

Systemic malformations and problems
- Cardiac abnormalities (aortic coarctation, bicuspid/stenotic aortic valve, aortic root dilatation/dissection, anomalous venous drainage, essential hypertension)
- Renal abnormalities (horseshoe, duplex, elongated and posteriorly rotated kidneys)

Immune and inflammatory disease (e.g. Hashimoto's thyroiditis, coeliac and inflammatory bowel disease)

Miscellaneous – naevi, ptosis, epicanthic folds, oblique palpebral fissures, low set/rotated ears, low hairline

increased naevi (particularly on the face), respectively. The second chromosome may be completely lost (45,X), undergo duplication of the long arm (q) with concomitant loss of the short arm (p) to form an isochromosome (isoXq), undergo ring formation (rX), or deletion in the short or long arm (Xp⁻ or Xq⁻). Complete 45,X monosomy accounts for 40–60% of the karyotypes on peripheral blood lymphocytes, while most of the remaining karyotypes show a mosaic pattern; for example, 45,X/46,XX, 45,X/46,X,iXq, 45,X/46,XY, 45,X/46,X,rX. There is little specific phenotype/genotype correlation for most karyotypes but phenotype is milder in the 45,X/46,XX and 45,X/47,XXX variants.

Growth (see Appendix 2)

All three components of Karlberg's ICP model are impaired in Turner syndrome, with a degree of IUGR (usually mild) in almost all cases; subnormal growth during infancy and childhood with 15 cm loss in

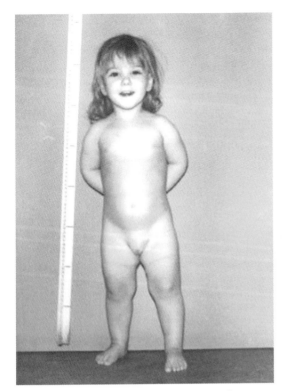

Figure 3.8 Three-year-old child with Turner syndrome showing 'shield' chest and relatively short legs.

height compared with normal girls between the ages of 3 and 12 years; and impaired pubertal growth spurt even with oestrogen therapy, related to the underlying skeletal dysplasia. Adult height in European populations ranges from 142 to 147 cm (Ranke 1998). There is a positive correlation between adult height and parental height.

Diagnosis and follow-up

Because of the subtlety and variable incidence of many of these features, Turner syndrome is easily missed. The diagnostic key is short, or borderline short, stature in a girl whose height is inappropriate for the parental target range centiles (Ouarezki et al. 2017). Karyotype analysis is indicated in this situation and/or in the context of dysmorphic features, middle ear disease, and cardiac anomalies. Follow-up is required to pre-empt associated problems such as autoimmune thyroiditis, middle-ear disease, learning difficulties, and hypertension and is best provided in designated Turner syndrome clinics, with good hand-over arrangements for specialist adult care.

Noonan syndrome

Noonan syndrome (see Table 3.5, Figure 3.9 and Appendix 2) refers to a heterogeneous group of conditions resulting from various gene mutations, of which four have been identified – *PTPN11* (encoding SHP-2), *SOS1, KRAS*, and *RAF-1*. Sporadic mutations are commonest, affected individuals then transmit the condition in autosomal dominant fashion (see Figure 3.9). Prevalence is estimated at between one in 1000–2500 live births. The principal features of Noonan

Table 3.5 Principal features of Noonan syndrome.

Characteristic facies
- Hypertelorism
- Ptosis
- Low set, posteriorly rotated, prominent ears
Skeletal problems with:
- short stature
- scoliosis
- pectus excavatum
- cubitus valgus
Cardiac defects (usually pulmonary stenosis; also atrial septal defect, hypertrophic cardiomyopathy)
Gonadal problems (cryptorchidism in most males)
Delayed puberty
Lymphoedema (neck webbing)
Mild educational difficulties
Coagulation defect causing bleeding tendency

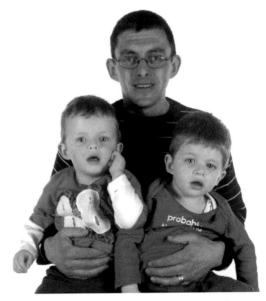

Figure 3.9 Father and twin boys with Noonan syndrome.

syndrome are shown in Table 3.5. Growth is usually affected with height velocity being subnormal and puberty is typically delayed and associated with a blunted adolescent growth spurt. Adult heights are approximately 162 cm in males and 152 cm in females (Ranke et al. 1998).

Williams syndrome

This condition arises from a spontaneous deletion affecting 7q11.23 and may present with short stature in a child with intellectual disability but with aptitude for music, increased fearfulness, engaging behaviour described as 'cocktail party manner', hyperacusis, and characteristic facies – button nose, full lips, and 'elfin' appearance. Associated problems include infantile hypercalcaemia, supravalvular aortic stenosis, pulmonary artery stenosis, hypertension, and scoliosis.

Aarskog syndrome

This condition results from a mutation in the *FGDY1* gene located on Xp11.21. The phenotype – hypertelorism, interdigital webbing, short broad hands, and shawl scrotum in males – is milder in affected females and more pronounced in their sons. Intelligence is normal and the degree of short stature usually insufficient to warrant intervention.

Skeletal dysplasias

This is a varied and complex group of disorders requiring input from colleagues in other disciplines including genetics, radiology, and orthopaedics, as well as endocrinology. Patients may present with severe short stature and obvious disproportion (abnormal upper:lower segment ratio, sitting height, and arm span relative to height), in which case the diagnosis of skeletal dysplasia is obvious. Less severe cases may present with short stature of uncertain cause requiring a diagnosis, and shrewd assessment may be needed to detect mild disproportion. The limbs will be short in disorders principally affecting the long bones, for example, achondroplasia, hypochondroplasia, and metaphyseal dysplasia; the back will be short in disorders affecting the spine as well as the long bones, for example, spondylo-epiphyseal-dysplasia (SED). Table 3.6 shows the key features of three important disorders – achondroplasia, hypochondroplasia, and spondylo-epiphyseal-dysplasia. The following points should be borne in mind:

• Skeletal dysplasia may be only one component of a wider disorder, for example, Turner syndrome, neurofibromatosis, and the mucopolysaccharidoses; careful evaluation of other systems including eyes, hearing, neurodevelopment, and phenotype is therefore important.

• Many skeletal dysplasias are autosomal dominant in inheritance. The clinician should be wary of assuming normal familial short stature when one parent is particularly short.

• Sitting height must be measured, plotting both this and the derived leg length onto standard growth charts in both child and parent.

• Assessment should also include examination of the hands (looking for short, stubby fingers), the proportions of the upper and lower segments of the arms and legs, skull shape and circumference, and the spine for exaggerated lordosis.

• Typically bone age is advanced, and pubertal growth response is blunted.

• Some children display a pattern of mild/no disproportion in the context of short stature with advanced bone age, normal skeletal survey, poor growth response to puberty, and lower adult than childhood height centile. It is possible that some of these cases (currently classified as ISS) will be found to represent mild forms of skeletal dyplasia which are undetectable with standard radiology.

Chronic disease

Chronic illness is a potent cause of impaired linear growth in childhood and adolescence, and pubertal delay (Kao et al. 2018). The child may already be diagnosed, and referred to evaluate the contribution of various components including the disease (e.g. chronic arthritis) and its treatment (e.g. systemic steroids) to the poor growth. By contrast, chronic disease may be an unsuspected cause of short stature. Gastrointestinal disorders, such as coeliac disease and inflammatory bowel disease, can present in this way, while chronic renal disease is notoriously silent. The degree of growth failure varies considerably from a relatively mild effect, usually with constitutional delay, in mild to moderate asthma to potentially severe short stature in Crohn disease and juvenile chronic arthritis. The three principal mechanisms for poor growth and short stature in chronic disease are:

• secretion of pro-inflammatory cytokines, particularly TNF, IL1 and IL6, in conditions such as Crohn disease and juvenile idiopathic arthritis (primary effect of disease);

• undernutrition (secondary effect of disease);

• steroid treatment (iatrogenic effect).

Table 3.6 Key features of achondroplasia, hypochondroplasia, and spondylo-epiphyseal- dysplasia.

Achondroplasia
Activating mutation of *fibroblast growth factor receptor 3* (*FGFR3*) gene (located on 4p16.3) in 99% of cases
Usually de novo mutation; autosomal dominant transmission
Normal intelligence
Severe shortening of long bones
Relatively long trunk with lumbar lordosis
Large head with hypoplastic mid-face
Hypotonia and ligamentous laxity with associated limb pains
Narrow spinal canal with risk of symptoms from cord compression
Childhood height – 5 to – 6 SDS
Adult height approximately 132 cm in males, 125 cm in females

Hypochondroplasia
Activating *FGFR3* mutation in 70% of cases
Autosomal dominant with variable severity
Normal head and face
Mild disproportion with short limbs
Short, broad hands and feet
Characteristic X-ray changes with failure of interpedicular distance to increase in a cephalocaudal direction
Blunted pubertal growth spurt
Approximate adult height 155 cm in males, 142 cm in females

Spondylo-epiphyseal-dysplasia (SED)
Group of conditions including SED congenita due to mutations in the *COL2A1* gene encoding type II collagen (autosomal dominant); and SED tarda which can be X-linked (mutations in *SEDL gene*), dominant or recessive
Shortening of trunk and limbs with disproportionately short back
Relatively normal-sized hands and feet
Atlanto–axial instability

SED congenita
Associated with myopia and hearing loss
Pain, especially in hips and back
Thoracic kyphosis and barrel chest
Coxa vara with waddling gait

SED tarda
Milder form with later presentation

Other factors include delayed maturation and puberty; hypoxia (cyanotic congenital heart disease); metabolic disturbance (glycogen storage disease, renal failure); and partial GH resistance (Crohn disease, renal failure)

Psychosocial deprivation

There is an established relationship between socio-economic status and physical growth. However, it can be difficult to weigh up the contribution of the social environment to short stature and poor growth in the individual. This is because factors such as SGA, poor diet, respiratory illness related to parental smoking, and parental short stature may be contributory and of variable relation to the poor social circumstances.

Adverse family and social factors can delay a child's physical and emotional development. David Skuse and colleagues described a striking variant of psychosocial growth failure featuring abnormal behaviour with hyperphagia and polydipsia. Investigation shows GH insufficiency which is resistant to exogenous GH therapy but is reversible on moving the child to a favourable environment (Skuse et al. 1996).

Psychosocial deprivation should always be considered when a child is referred with short stature, and the clinician must take a thorough family and social history. Careful follow- up of suspected cases, with sequential height and weights, is crucial not only in confirming the diagnosis, but also in documenting the child's needs in terms of future care and placement.

Endocrine disorders

GH insufficiency and deficiency
Definition and cut-offs
These are controversial! *GH insufficiency* can be defined in terms of a peak GH level which is below an agreed arbitrary cut-off level. Assays vary between centres while the intra-patient variability of peak GH secretion is high. Severe GH insufficiency can be defined as a maximum stimulated GH concentration of <3 µg/L), partial GH insufficiency as 3-7µg/L. It is important to recognize that low GH levels can be encountered in virtually any short child and that low levels are not indicative of permanent impairment of the hypothalamo–pituitary (H-P) axis. It follows that GH status should be measured judiciously and carefully interpreted in the clinical context. A significant proportion of peripubertal children with short stature, slow height velocity, and low stimulated GH levels will show normal GH status on retesting once final height is attained. In retrospect, many such children would have been displaying constitutional delay with hypothalamo–pituitary 'dormancy'.

The term *GH deficiency* (as opposed to GH insufficiency) can be used to refer to permanent impairment of the GHRH-GH axis, due to either congenital or acquired disease. According to this nomenclature,

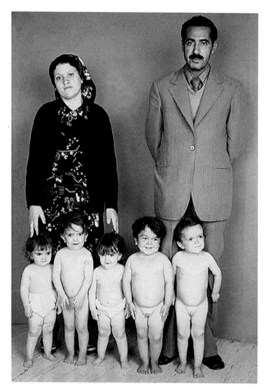

Figure 3.10 Five children aged two to seven years from two consanguineous families (two brothers married two first cousins who were sisters) with severe isolated GH deficiency. One parent from each family is shown in the picture. Note the excess subcutaneous fat, immature appearance and small genitalia in the affected boys. Source: Donaldson et al. 1980, reproduced with kind permission of *British Journal of Medical Genetics*.

Table 3.7 Clinical features of severe and mild GH deficiency.

Severe GH deficiency
Presents before age three years (unless acquired)
Obvious short stature
Subnormal height velocity from birth, becoming more abnormal with age
Neonatal hypoglycaemia and hyperbilirubinaemia
Micropenis
Possible associated anterior pituitary hormone deficiencies (TSH, ACTH, LH, FSH)
Excess subcutaneous fat, increasing with age
Mid-facial hypoplasia (only in extreme cases)
Possible features of septo-optic dysplasia
Delayed skeletal maturation
Maximum stimulated GH concentration < 3 µg/L

Mild GH deficiency
Unlikely to present before school entry
Less severe short stature
Subnormal height velocity documented by careful auxology over minimum interval of 12 months
Isolated GH insufficiency
Normal subcutaneous fat
Delayed skeletal maturation
Delayed puberty
Maximum stimulated GH concentration 3–7 µg/L (3–10 µg/L in some centres)

Abbreviations: ACTH, adrenocorticotrophic hormone; FSH, follicle-stimulating hormone; GH, growth hormone; LH, luteinizing hormone; TSH, thyroid-stimulating hormone.

therefore, GH deficiency is a subset of GH insufficiency. We recommend using the term 'GH deficiency' if actual impairment of GH secretion is either certain or very likely, and the term 'GH insufficiency' when GH levels are low but definite H-P axis abnormality has not been demonstrated.

While classic and severe growth hormone deficiency is clinically easy to diagnose (see Figure 3.10), milder forms are difficult to separate from normal variant short stature. The features of these two ends of the spectrum are shown in Table 3.7 and the causes of GH deficiency are shown in Table 3.8.

Isolated GH insufficiency and deficiency
Idiopathic isolated GH insufficiency

In >80% of cases, GH insufficiency is 'isolated', i.e. not associated with other anterior pituitary

hormone deficiencies and may (see above) turn out to be a transient insufficiency rather than a permanent deficiency, falling into the 'mild' rather than 'severe' category described above. It is now known that the basic defect in most true isolated GH deficiency cases is in the synthesis or release of the hypothalamic peptide GHRH, but the precise pathogenesis is unknown. However, these patients respond to administration of exogenous GHRH by secreting GH, indicating that the somatotroph cells are functional and that the primary defect is in the hypothalamus. Magnetic resonance imaging (MRI) imaging and genetic studies are normal.

True isolated GH deficiency related to genetic and structural MRI abnormalities presents as:
1 *GH deficiency of genetic origin:* These disorders are very rare, occurring in the context of consanguinity

Table 3.8 Principal causes of GH insufficiency.

Transient GH insufficiency: Conditions in which GH levels may be <7 µg/L on initial stimulation testing but normal on retesting
- Constitutional delay in growth and adolescence
- Short stature following smallness for gestational age
- Hypothyroidism
- Psychosocial deprivation

Permanent GH deficiency: Conditions in which GH levels are < 7 µg/L due to impairment of hypothalamo–pituitary axis

Congenital
Inherited causes
- GHRH mutations
- GH-1 mutations (autosomal recessive, autosomal dominant, X-linked)
- Pit-1, Prop-1 mutations

Structural defects
- Septo-optic dysplasia
- Agenesis of corpus callosum
- Holoprosencephaly
- Hypopituitarism with single central incisor

Hypothalamic disorders
- Prader–Willi syndrome

Acquired
Tumours adjacent to hypothalamo–pituitary axis
- Craniopharyngioma
- Suprasellar germinoma
- Optic glioma

Head injury
Surgery to the H-P axis
Cranial radiotherapy (e.g. for medulloblastoma)
Granulomatous disease
- Langerhans cell histiocytosis
- Sarcoidosis

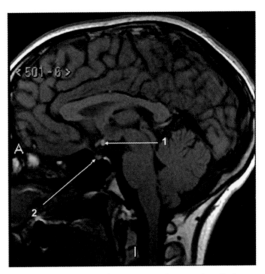

Figure 3.11 MRI scan showing ectopic posterior pituitary gland (1) and small anterior pituitary (2) in a 15-year-old girl with GH deficiency and partial gonadotrophin deficiency.

and closed communities. Severe GH deficiency is the rule. Disorders result from the following:
- GHRH receptor gene mutations.
- Deletions of the *GH-1* gene resulting in four variants of hereditary hGH deficiency:
    type IA (recessive, absent GH, blocking antibodies to hGH develop upon therapy)
    type IB (recessive, low GH, response to hGH therapy)
    type II (dominant, low GH, response to hGH therapy)
    type III (X-linked, low GH, response to GH therapy)

2 *GH deficiency with MRI abnormality:* The following three MRI abnormalities have been well documented in relation to either isolated GH deficiency or multiple pituitary deficiency (Figure 3.11):
- small anterior pituitary;
- interrupted pituitary stalk;
- ectopic posterior pituitary (EPP).

Of these three features, EPP has the lowest inter-observer variability and is the most strongly predictive of GH deficiency.

Multiple anterior pituitary hormone deficiencies
Idiopathic multiple anterior pituitary hormone deficiencies
Multiple anterior pituitary hormone deficiencies may present in the newborn period or early infancy with:
- hypoglycaemia, resulting from a combination of GH and adrenocorticotrophic hormone (ACTH) deficiency, leading to hypocortisolaemia;
- cholestatic jaundice related to low cortisol;
- micropenis –caused mainly by prenatal testosterone deficiency secondary to luteinizing hormone (LH) deficiency and compounded by prenatal GH deficiency.

Hypothyroidism of pituitary origin is likely to be present, becoming manifest later, but usually without intellectual impairment. Low serum IGF-I and IGFBP-3 levels may be suggestive of GH deficiency. Subsequent imaging may show small anterior pituitary/interrupted stalk/EPP.

The treatment of congenital hypopituitarism is a neonatal emergency. It is crucial to give hydrocortisone to prevent persisting hypoglycaemia. If this is not effective, GH therapy must be added. T4 replacement will also be indicated. GH reserve should not be tested, as GH stimulation tests can induce serious and life-threatening hypoglycaemia.

Genetic causes of multiple anterior pituitary hormone deficiencies

Gene mutations affecting the pituitary transcription factors Pit-1 (causing GH, thyroid-stimulating hormone [TSH], and prolactin deficiency) and Prop-1 (deficiency of GH, ACTH, TSH, LH, follicle-stimulating hormone [FSH]) are now well documented in multiple pituitary hormone deficiencies. Genetic defects are rarely found in the structural central nervous system (CNS) defects.

Congenital structural CNS defects

Congenital CNS defects occurring in the mid-line may be associated with GH deficiency, usually with multiple pituitary hormone deficiencies. However, these lesions cause considerable endocrine heterogeneity.

The most frequent is the syndrome of septo-optic dysplasia consisting of two or three components of the triad:
• optic nerve hypoplasia (usually bilateral but may be asymmetrical);
• absent septum pellucidum;
• hypothalamic hypopituitarism.

GH deficiency may be isolated, and evolve during childhood. ACTH and TSH deficiencies are common, vasopressin deficiency affects 20%. Interestingly, LH and FSH secretion is often preserved (and there may even be sexual precocity) but some patients have partial or severe deficiency. Presentation is usually in early infancy with either visual abnormality (roving nystagmus and failure of fixation), or hypopituitarism (neonatal hypoglycaemia, jaundice, poor feeding). Learning disability is a variable associated feature, some patients being of completely normal intelligence, others severely affected. Defects in the *HESX-1* gene have been described in a few cases, mainly familial in nature.

Other congenital defects which can be associated with GH deficiency are agenesis of the corpus callosum, holoprosencephaly, and arachnoid cysts. These conditions can be diagnosed by MRI scan; the risks of general anaesthetic in the hypopituitary infant must be carefully considered.

Acquired causes of multiple anterior pituitary deficiencies
CNS tumours

Craniopharyngioma

Although rare, this is the most common tumour in the hypothalamo-pituitary region in childhood. Although histologically benign, craniopharyngioma is locally invasive, involving adjacent structures, including the hypothalamus, thus affecting the pituitary function, and the optic nerves, and chiasm. The three modes of presentation are:
• raised intracranial pressure;
• visual disturbance because of the proximity of the optic chiasm;
• hypopituitarism with short stature, growth failure, diabetes insipidus.

The management of craniopharyngioma is complex and controversial. The devastating endocrine and psychoneurological morbidity of radical surgery with the removal of hypothalamic tissue is well recognized (De Vile et al. 1996). Complete macroscopic removal is now attempted only if damage to adjacent structures can be avoided. Otherwise the tumour is decompressed and debulked as safely as possible, following which radiotherapy is given.

Germinoma

This may present with diabetes insipidus alone for many years before the tumour itself and other pituitary deficiencies become manifest. Consequently, so-called 'idiopathic' diabetes insipidus must always be viewed with suspicion and investigated with serial MRI of the brain. Bifocal germinoma with suprasellar and pineal lesions may occur. Pituitary stalk thickening may be the first radiological abnormality. Elevation of serum ± cerebrospinal fluid human chorionic gonadotrophin (hCG) and α-feto-protein (AFP) levels are useful tumour markers. Treatment is with chemotherapy and craniospinal radiotherapy.

Optic nerve glioma

Optic nerve glioma, which occurs more commonly in patients with neurofibromatosis, may also be associated with pituitary deficiency and, paradoxically, precocious puberty. Targeted radiotherapy is indicated if vision is threatened but most cases are managed conservatively, giving endocrine therapy as required.

Histiocytosis

The infiltrative lesion of Langerhans cell histiocytosis typically involves the hypothalamus and causes diabetes insipidus. In a proportion of cases, this will be associated with GH deficiency.

Cranial irradiation

This topic is dealt with in Chapter 12. Children who have received CNS irradiation, whether for prophylaxis for leukaemia, for tumours distant from or adjacent to the hypothalamo-pituitary region or during total body irradiation are at risk for the development of GH deficiency, and should receive endocrine monitoring and follow-up.

Diagnosis of GH insufficiency and deficiency

As indicated earlier, most children with GH insufficiency do not have 'severe' GH deficiency (see Table 3.7). A combination of both auxological and biochemical criteria is required to make this diagnosis. GH therapy should not be prescribed without documentation of biochemical GH insufficiency.

Auxology

- Short stature
- Height inappropriately low for parental target range centiles
- Subnormal height velocity (<25th centile for age).

Biochemical diagnosis
Physiological tests

GH profile. GH secretion is pulsatile, with peaks occurring approximately every three hours. A pattern of GH secretion, demonstrating physiological peaks and troughs can be obtained by continuous or 20-minute venous sampling for serum GH levels through an indwelling cannula. This technique, known as GH profiling, is too time-consuming, labour-intensive, and expensive to be recommended for routine clinical practice but remains a valuable research tool.

Serum markers of GH secretion or action. Serum IGF-I and IGFBP-3 reflect the status of GH secretion, provided that the GH receptor is functioning normally. In severe GH deficiency, IGF-I and IGFBP-3 levels are low; however, the large overlap between normal children and children with less severe GH deficiency limits the diagnostic value of IGF-1. Also, low IGF-I in a short child may reflect a negative caloric balance (e.g. in children treated with psychostimulant medication) rather than GH deficiency.

Pharmacological tests

GH stimulation tests. This difficult area has been addressed in the 2016 guidelines by the Paediatric Endocrine Society (Grimberg et al. 2016) and by the British Society for Paediatric Endocrinology and Diabetes (BSPED GH standards document, 2017). The former guidelines caution against 'reliance on GH provocative test results as the sole diagnostic criterion of GHD'. BSPED guidelines recommend that GH stimulation testing should only be carried out by experienced personnel in centres carrying out a minimum of 10 tests per year.

GH stimulation testing is not needed in patients who satisfy these three conditions: (i) auxological criteria for GH deficiency (particularly low height velocity) are met; (ii) MRI scan shows one of the classic triad of defects, or presence of tumour or irradiation affecting the HP-axis; and (iii) at least one other anterior pituitary hormone deficiency has been demonstrated. Neither is testing recommended in newborns with serum GH < 5 µg/L in the context of hypoglycaemia plus *either* deficiency of at least one additional pituitary hormone; *or* one or more classic features on MRI imaging; *or* both.

In other situations, TWO stimulation tests are recommended, five of which are shown in Table 3.9.

Sex steroid priming prior to GH stimulation testing

Between about nine years and the onset of the pubertal growth spurt, the hypothalamo-pituitary axis has become relatively 'dormant' so that height velocity slows and response to GH stimulation is diminished. Boys and girls with constitutional delay may be misdiagnosed as having isolated GH deficiency on direct stimulation testing and are subsequently shown to have normal pituitary function on retesting once pubertal development is complete. This diagnostic trap may be offset by 'priming' the axis with sex steroids prior to stimulation testing from nine years until Tanner stage G3 in boys and Tanner stage B2 in girls.

The counter-argument for carrying out sex steroid priming is that children with functional growth hormone insufficiency during the peripubertal years may benefit from GH treatment both in terms of enhancing short-to-medium term growth; and improving final height. There is thus a *diagnostic* argument in favour of priming and a *therapeutic* argument against priming. Given the expense of growth hormone, and the concerns about subjecting essentially healthy subjects to years of daily injections, we favour sex steroid priming.

Table 3.9 Details of some GH stimulation tests. Absolute requirements *before* all GH stimulation tests are to document normal serum T4 concentration and normal serum cortisol concentration (>100 nmol/L). Note that glucagon and insulin tolerance tests also test adrenal axis while additional cortisol testing is required for the other three methods. Testing is performed after an overnight fast.

Glucagon test	
Dose	15 µg /kg intramuscularly
Sampling	GH, cortisol, glucose at 0, 30, 60, 90, 120, 150, 180 min.
Complication	Hypoglycaemia, particularly in young children; nausea
Requirement	Doctor or specialist nurse in attendance throughout test
Contraindication	Epilepsy in young children
Clonidine test	
Dose	0.15 mg/m² orally
Sampling	GH at 0, 30, 60, 90, 120, 150, 180 min.
Complication	Hypotension
Requirement	BP monitoring
Insulin-tolerance test	
Dose	0.15 units/kg intravenously
Sampling	GH, cortisol, glucose at 0, 20, 30, 60, 90, 120 min.
Complication	Hypoglycaemia
Requirement	Doctor or specialist nurse at bedside throughout test, blood glucose <2.2 mmol/
Contraindication	Age < 5 years, epilepsy
Arginine test	
Dose	0.5 g kg⁻¹ intravenously over 30 min
Sampling	GH at 0, 30, 60, 90, 120, 150 min.
Complication	Nausea; irritation at iv site

Abbreviations: GH, growth hormone.

Choice of stimulation tests

The two most commonly used tests in the United Kingdom are the glucagon and clonidine tests. The glucagon test also stimulates cortisol secretion, which can be an advantage if multiple pituitary hormone deficiencies are suspected but may cause hypoglycaemia, particularly in young children. The insulin-tolerance test (ITT) is avoided by many centres in the United Kingdom because of the risks of serious hypoglycaemia, and should never be used for children under five years, nor should it be performed in a non-specialist environment. However, in the context of an established paediatric endocrine unit, the ITT has been found to be safe and probably provides the best validated stimulus for GH secretion.

Execution of GH stimulation testing

Whichever test is used, secure intravenous access with a good-sized cannula in situ, oxygen and suction facilities, and experienced staff must be available. If hypoglycaemia occurs, the symptoms can be quickly and safely relieved with oral or intravenous administration of glucose.

Other endocrine causes of short stature

Hypothyroidism

This is discussed in Chapter 6. Unless diagnosed early, congenital hypothyroidism leads to severe stunting of growth. The introduction of neonatal screening has eliminated this cause of short stature. By contrast, acquired hypothyroidism caused by autoimmune thyroiditis may present with short stature and growth failure, hence the need to include thyroid function testing in all short children requiring investigation.

Cushing's syndrome

Hypercortisolaemia impairs linear growth. Consequently, most patients with Cushing's syndrome will have a deceleration in height gain, in marked contrast to subjects with simple obesity in whom height velocity is enhanced. Exceptions are cases of Cushing's syndrome where excess adrenal androgens are secreted, which may counteract the growth-suppressive effect of high cortisol. Cushing's syndrome is discussed in Chapter 8.

GH resistance

GH resistance accounts for a very small number of patients with short stature. In its severe form, it presents as Laron syndrome, a rare severe autosomal recessive disorder caused by a homozygous mutation of the GH receptor. Growth failure is extreme in this condition, with an untreated adult height of 120–130 cm. Milder forms of GH resistance may be a cause of short stature, but this has yet to be established.

Idiopathic short stature (ISS)

This is a descriptive rather than a diagnostic category and its definition is controversial. In this chapter, ISS refers to children with height < −2.5 SD in whom the problem is either not attributable to normal familial short stature or constitutional delay, and in which other causes of short stature have been excluded. ISS probably includes a range of conditions including partial GH resistance and subtle skeletal dysplasias which cannot be detected on standard skeletal X-rays.

Treatment of short stature

A limited repertoire of growth-promoting preparations is available for short stature treatment: growth hormone; the weakly androgenic anabolic steroid Oxandrolone; and the sex steroids. GH is licensed for treatment of GH insufficiency, Turner syndrome, Prader-Willi syndrome, short SGA children, and short children with renal failure. Oxandrolone can be used for growth promotion in peripubertal boys and in Turner syndrome. Sex steroid therapy is available for stimulation of pubertal growth. Other therapies, such as GHRH and IGF-I, are not widely used in routine practice.

Constitutional delay of growth and puberty

The cornerstone of management is correct diagnosis, reassurance, and a realistic prognosis for final height, the latter being facilitated by adult height prediction in subjects aged more than 10–11 years. Some families with constitutional growth delay can be discharged after the initial consultation. Others find it helpful to receive regular 6-monthly follow-up until the pubertal growth spurt is well underway. In roughly half the boys seen with constitutional delay, there is no strong demand for therapy, but Table 3.10 shows some features which guide towards intervention.

Aims of treatment

Males

The aims of treatment depend on the age of the patient: growth acceleration in boys aged 10–13 years; and both growth and pubertal acceleration > 13 years.

Oxandrolone is helpful in accelerating growth in boys aged >10 years who are too young for puberty to be induced. Unfortunately, it has not been manufactured in Europe since 2008 but it can be purchased from North America for use in selected cases. Oxandrolone is given in the dose of 1.25 mg orally at night for three to six months in boys aged <12 years and 2.5 mg for boys aged >12 years.

Testosterone esters will accelerate growth and pubertal development. This therapy does not affect final height and simply speeds up the pubertal process. Testosterone cypionate (Sustanon) or enanthate (Primoteston Depot) 50–125 mg by intramuscular injection every four weeks for three to six months are available for use. Testosterone enanthate 125 mg by intramuscular injection for three months only was shown in a Scottish study to be effective and to have no adverse effect on final height in comparison with untreated boys (Kelly et al. 2003). There is a good case therefore for giving testosterone in this dose rather than using lower, less effective doses such as monthly injections of 50 mg. Oral testosterone undecanoate 40 mg daily, increasing to 80 mg daily depending on response, is an effective alternative to intramuscular testosterone (Lawaetz et al. 2015).

Endogenous puberty can be followed by serial measurement of testicular volumes which are unaffected by exogenous testosterone and reflect gonadotrophin activity. If the testes remain at <5–6 ml a year after testosterone treatment, indicating that endogenous puberty is still in the early stages, a second course of testosterone may be given.

Females

In girls with delay of growth and puberty, oral ethinyl-estradiol 2 μg either daily or on alternate days for 6–12 months will induce some growth acceleration, which may be associated with early breast development. However, careful patient selection and evaluation are required in this situation, some specialists electing to 'cover' oestrogen treatment with GH therapy.

GH insufficiency

GH insufficiency can be effectively treated with recombinant GH. Successful treatment is potentially

Table 3.10 Indications for consideration of endocrine therapy in the patient with constitutional delay in growth and adolescence.

Short stature
Low height velocity ($<4\,cm\,yr^{-1}$)
Delayed secondary sexual development
Abnormal body proportions (long legs, short trunk)
Reduced bone mineral density
Psychological distress related to:
• poor self-image
• looking and feeling different or younger than peers
• lack of confidence
• depression
• school refusal
• difficulty participating in sporting activities
• difficulty being admitted to age-appropriate venues (e.g. cinema)
• aggressive behaviour, delinquency
• reduced employment opportunities
Parental concern

Table 3.11 Guidelines for GH therapy in children with GH insufficiency.

Early diagnosis and initiation of therapy; central role of the endocrine specialist nurse
Dose 25–30 µg/kg/day (5 mg/m²/week) given subcutaneously in the evening, 7 days a week
4–6 monthly clinic visits for assessment including auxology and pubertal staging
Enquiry as to the number of injections missed between visits
Input from endocrine specialist nurse if growth response disappointing
6–12 monthly IGF-I measurement to monitor dosage and compliance
Annual bone age
Discontinuation of GH at completion of growth (height velocity < 2 cm/year)
Retesting of GH status prior to adult transfer (IGF-I and stimulated GH levels)
Transition clinic for adult transfer if permanent GH deficiency confirmed

able to normalize height, but this is achieved at a significant economic cost and requires daily subcutaneous injections. The less severe the GH insufficiency, the less the benefit from replacement therapy.

Every child considered for GH therapy must be assessed in detail so that treatment is reserved for those who will unequivocally benefit by an increase in final adult height. Early diagnosis and initiation of therapy in GH deficient children must be the goal of all those involved in growth assessment.

Before starting treatment, auxological assessment for 6–12 months is desirable unless the time available for further growth is limited, or the degree of GH deficiency and short stature is severe. The following conditions should be met:

1 Pubertal assessment and bone age must indicate that growth potential exists.
2 Height velocity must be subnormal before treatment is started.
3 Pre-treatment height velocity assessment should be available so that height velocity after one year of treatment can be interpreted.
4 The family must be fully committed after a detailed discussion (see Table 3.11).

The role of the endocrine nurse specialist is crucial in:
• counselling the families before treatment is started;
• assessing the likelihood of good compliance and the need for support;

• showing a variety of GH brands and devices to the family, and helping parents and child to make an informed choice;
• teaching the technique of daily subcutaneous injection. In Glasgow, the endocrine nurses visit the home to initiate GH treatment, with subsequent follow-up visits as required.

Three- to four-monthly, rather than six-monthly clinic visits are recommended to adequately monitor the response to and compliance with treatment. Measurement of IGF-1 in children receiving GH is a yardstick against which compliance/adherence can be monitored. IGF-1 measurement is also advised for safety, decreasing the GH dose if the IGF-1 level is >2 standard deviations above the age-related laboratory reference range.

Increasing GH dosage at puberty to mimic the physiological increase that occurs during this phase seems logical but is controversial. FDA recommendations are for an increase from 30–50 to 100 µg/kg/day to cover the pubertal years while the Paediatric Endocrine Society guidelines advise against the routine increase in GH dose during this phase of growth.

After linear growth is complete, appraisal of GH status should be according to consensus guidelines (Clayton et al. 2005). When permanent deficiency is certain, e.g. with craniopharyngioma, genetically proven GH deficiency and multiple pituitary hormone deficiency, there is no need to stop treatment. If GH deficiency is highly likely, an IGF-1 level is taken six weeks after stopping treatment, a subnormal value being sufficient to confirm the diagnosis. Otherwise, a formal GH stimulation test is required, using insulin, arginine or glucagon but not clonidine. Many patients with 'idiopathic GH insufficiency' will now have a normal response and can be retrospectively diagnosed as having had constitutional delay.

Subjects with proven GH deficiency should be transferred to an adult endocrine clinic for follow-up. Experience has shown that a transition clinic attended by both paediatric and adult endocrinologists improves the quality of transfer, and the chance of compliance with attendance at the adult clinic.

Adverse events

Recombinant GH has a remarkably good safety record. The complication of Creutzfeldt-Jakob disease associated with pituitary-extracted GH was identified in 1985 and from this time only biosynthetic GH should have been used. Intracranial hypertension, usually seen shortly after the initiation of therapy, resolves with temporary cessation of GH followed by reintroduction at a lower dose. Slipped capital femoral epiphysis and progression of pre-existing scoliosis should be detected by clinical awareness and monitoring, including regular examination of the spine. Any increase in cancer risk among GH-treated patients can be largely related to previous treatment for malignancy, and a direct influence of GH is doubtful. A large study of nearly 24 000 GH-treated patients from eight European countries showed no general increase in cancer risk, but the finding of a slight increase in bone cancer, bladder cancer, and Hodgkin's lymphoma requires ongoing surveillance (Swerdlow et al. 2017).

GH therapy in non-GH-deficient disorders

The availability of recombinant GH, although admittedly at high cost, has led to its use in a number of non-GH-deficient disorders, where its pharmacological properties might benefit growth. Prominent among these are Turner and Noonan syndromes, short stature related to SGA, renal disease, and skeletal dysplasias. Each of these categories will be discussed briefly.

Idiopathic short stature

The use of GH therapy in children with ISS remains controversial and often presents the clinician with a moral dilemma. The efficacy of this treatment has been demonstrated, with several clinical studies showing a positive effect on final height. Indeed, GH therapy was approved in the US for children with this indication in 2003. In the United Kingdom, this indication has not found favour, experience showing that many of the families whose children have short stature and borderline GH levels (which do constitute an indication for treatment) become discouraged by the modest increase in height status after one to two years, and either openly state their wish to discontinue treatment, or demonstrate their lack of enthusiasm by defaulting from the outpatient clinic.

Turner syndrome

While optimizing growth and puberty in Turner syndrome is important, it is essential that other aspects of this complex condition, including cardiovascular, otological, bone, uterine, and psychological health, are not neglected and are well reviewed in the 2017 Cincinnati guidelines (Gravholt et al. 2017).

Mildly affected girls (e.g. some patients with 45,X/46,XX mosaicism) may not require growth-promoting treatment, but short stature is usually sufficiently severe for most families to opt for intervention. GH has been definitively shown to increase final height by approximately 7 cm (Stephure 2005). However, all studies have demonstrated varying responses in individuals, some girls faring much better than others. Because of the skeletal dysplasia component in Turner syndrome, the GH dose required is higher than for classical GH deficiency – 55 µg/kg/day (10 mg/m^2/week).GH can be started when the patient's height falls below the 3rd centile, usually around the age of five years, or sooner if the girl is unusually short, e.g. when IUGR is a feature.

The addition of Oxandrolone 0.05 mg/kg per day (maximum dose 2.5 mg daily) from the age of nine years showed a significant improvement in adult height over placebo in a UK study (Gault et al. 2011). Side effects were not reported with the dose regimen used but virilization has occurred in other studies using larger doses. Since Oxandrolone is not readily available in Europe, it tends to be reserved for girls aged >9 years in whom growth rate on GH is disappointing despite good compliance, as reflected by high/normal IGF-1 levels.

About 90% of girls with Turner syndrome require pubertal induction and the various oral and transdermal regimens are discussed in Chapter 5. The more physiological transdermal regimen might be expected to result in better pubertal growth but this hypothesis remains untested.

In theory, delaying pubertal induction in Turner syndrome might be expected to increase final height. However, the UK Turner study, which randomized girls to receive pubertal induction at 12 or 14 years, found only marginal final height benefit from later induction. Moreover, late induction of puberty in Turner syndrome is now recognized to be undesirable both psychologically and in terms of uterine and bone health. It is now agreed that induction should usually begin at 11–12 years. However, the option of starting induction later in late-diagnosed girls, to allow further time for growth, should be discussed with the patient and family.

The strategy of introducing ultra-low dose oestrogen from five years of age to promote growth (as well as bone, uterine, and cardiovascular health) is currently being investigated.

Noonan syndrome

GH therapy has been used to increase adult height in this condition. To date, robust adult height data are lacking (Giacomozzi et al. 2015). Growth impairment is relatively modest in many patients and in this situation the patient and family may not desire intervention. We recommend reserving GH use for patients with marked short stature (e.g. >-2.5 SD) after discussion with the family. If GH is used to treat children and adolescents with Noonan syndrome, cardiac and skeletal surveillance should be enhanced.

Short stature associated with SGA

GH therapy has been shown to cause a dose-dependent increase in height velocity in short patients with a history of SGA. High-dose therapy for a period of two years induces catch-up growth (De Zegher et al. 1998) and a European licence was granted for the treatment of short SGA children in 2003. The recommended dose varies widely, from 35 µg/kg/day in many European centres to an FDA-approved dose of 67–69 µg/kg/day.

However, evaluation of the safety and efficacy of GH therapy in SGA patients is challenging. The SGA population is heterogeneous and not all patients will have proven IUGR. Growth in response to GH may be restricted by an unusually rapid pubertal growth phase. Final adult height data are still limited and long-term follow-up data on cardiac and metabolic health are needed to evaluate safety, particularly with higher doses of GH.

We recommend careful selection of patients who might benefit from treatment, comprising those with clinical evidence to suggest IUGR rather than SGA, and in whom height by the age of four years is < -2SD without catch-up growth. We suggest a starting GH dose of 35 µg/kg/day, modifying this according to growth response, serum IGF-1 levels, and bone age. Once a decision has been taken to treat with GH, this should be continued until final height is achieved, provided that the family are compliant, since discontinuous treatment is associated with catch-down growth.

Renal disease

Chronic renal failure is a potent cause of poor growth (Tonshoff and Mehls 1999). Treatment with GH has been extensively studied but this modality is used less often now with the advent of effective strategies which include:

- an aggressive approach to optimizing nutrition;
- meticulous treatment of high blood pressure;
- earlier recourse to transplantation;
- keeping time on dialysis to a minimum.

GH is occasionally used post-transplantation, but better graft outcomes and reduced steroid use have decreased its role. Since patients are partially GH-resistant, pharmacological doses of 50 µg/kg/day are required if GH is to be prescribed. The use of GH in renal disease should be monitored in a specialist renal department with experience of this treatment.

Skeletal dysplasias

Patients with skeletal dysplasia have normal GH secretion. GH can improve short-term height velocity in achondroplasia with a typical first -ear response of 2–3 cm (Hagenäs and Hertel 2003). However, the benefit in terms of quality of life (e.g. being able to reach objects, self-dress, etc.) are not well documented and there are no satisfactory data on the final height benefit of continuous treatment. One approach is to give GH in childhood to optimize linear growth, followed by limb lengthening from 13 years of age. However, non-intervention is chosen by many families. The optimal dose is not known, but will be greater than for classic GH deficiency. We do not recommend the routine use of GH in this group of disorders.

Chronic paediatric diseases

Short stature from chronic illness is best managed by treating the primary illness itself. This is dramatically demonstrated in Crohn disease, where successful resection of the inflamed bowel results in spectacular

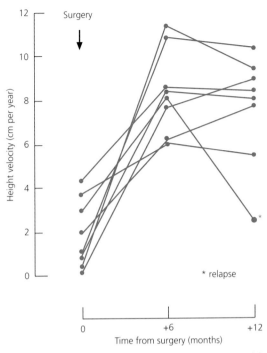

Figure 3.12 Increase in height velocity following successful resection of inflamed bowel in prepubertal and early pubertal patients with Crohn disease. Source: After Walker-Smith (1996).

catch-up growth (Figure 3.12). It is important to optimize nutrition and minimize steroid dosage. Newer treatments including anti-TNFα therapy in Crohn disease and juvenile idiopathic arthritis (JIA) have led to significant improvements in growth. Treatment with GH is reserved for patients in whom growth remains poor despite every aspect of the chronic illness being managed as well as possible. Use of high dose recombinant GH in Crohn disease and JIA significantly increases growth rate but not completely, suggesting a degree of resistance at the level of the growth plate. Long-term data on the benefit of GH therapy for adult height is awaited and ideally patients should only be treated in the context of a prospective clinical trial.

Induction of puberty is indicated in boys aged >14 years and girls aged >13 years with no pubertal development and earlier in selected cases when pubertal progress is slow or when delayed maturation is causing distress to the patient.

Psychosocial deprivation

Psychosocial deprivation may also be regarded as a chronic disease state. The best therapy for associated growth failure is to correct or reverse the disadvantageous home setting or, if this is not possible, to remove the child to a supportive environment. GH therapy is not indicated in this context nor is it effective.

IGF-I

Recombinant IGF-I was developed in the late 1980s and is the only therapy available for treatment of severe genetic GH resistance. It is effective in stimulating growth in Laron syndrome. However, a more common therapeutic indication for IGF-I is still to be found. A compound which complexes IGF-I with IGFBP-3 has also been developed. This physiological approach is logical; however, its clinical efficacy for treatment of growth disorders remains to be demonstrated.

Use of gonadotrophin-releasing hormone (GnRH) analogue therapy to improve growth in GH-treated patients

Gonadotrophin-releasing hormone (GnRH) analogue therapy has been used in conjunction with GH. The rationale of this approach is to suppress gonadotrophin secretion and arrest bone maturation, thus allowing a longer period for GH treatment. A prospective study with GnRH in 21 GH-treated subjects reported an increase in adult height SD (Mericq et al. 2000). This strategy has not found widespread acceptance. However, the combination of early puberty and GH insufficiency, for example after cranial irradiation, constitutes a mandatory indication for combination treatment using GH and GnRH analogue to optimize growth before epiphysial closure. In this situation, puberty should be allowed to continue when an appropriate age is reached, continuing with GH therapy. Controversially, a combination of GH and GnRH analogue can be used to increase adult height in children with simple virilizing congenital adrenal hyperplasia when linear growth is poor despite minimal suppressive treatment with glucocorticoids.

Transition

It is now well established that patients with severe GH deficiency, especially if accompanied by other anterior pituitary hormone deficiencies, require adult follow-up to pre-empt and treat the consequences of adult GH deficiency which include incomplete accretion and/or loss of bone mass with increased fracture risk, decrease in muscle mass, and increased fat mass (particularly visceral fat), disturbance of insulin and lipid metabolism, and increase in cardiovascular morbidity. Patients with the adult GH deficiency syndrome may experience marked fatigue with reduction in strength and exercise tolerance, and hence reduced quality of life.

For this reason, it is essential to organize transitional care to an adult endocrine clinic for GH-deficient adolescents leaving paediatric care (Clayton et al. 2005). The challenge is to convince the patient that this is necessary and beneficial, given that teenagers often view hospital attendance as tedious and non-essential. Experience has shown that the setting up of a transition clinic in the paediatric centre, with quarterly joint clinics attended by the paediatric and adult endocrinologists increases the likelihood of successful long-term follow-up.

Girls with Turner syndrome require transfer to a gynaecologist or adult endocrinologist, preferably in the context of an adult Turner clinic for surveillance of their reproductive, thyroid, bone, cardiac, and ENT/hearing status. If an adult Turner clinic is created then whoever runs it, whether reproductive endocrinologist, gynaecologist, or adult endocrine physician, needs to liaise closely with other disciplines, particularly cardiac and ENT.

When to involve a specialist centre

• Short stature whose cause remains uncertain after clinical assessment and baseline investigations.
• GH insufficiency/deficiency states, including those associated with CNS lesion.
• When GH therapy is contemplated.
• Dysmorphic syndromes associated with short stature.
• Management of Turner syndrome.
• Poor postnatal growth with short stature in SGA, particularly if height < 2nd centile aged two years of more.
• Cranial irradiation associated with GH deficiency.

Future developments

• Alternative methods of GH administration, including a long-acting preparation.
• Growth-promoting preparations, such as IGF-I and IGF-I/IGFBP-3, have been tried as an alternative to GH, but are not currently established as being superior, except in severe genetic GH resistance.
• Combination treatment with IGF-I and GH may be a therapeutic option in JIA and Crohn disease in the future.
• The use of GnRH analogues to delay puberty and possibly increase adult height has been tried but this treatment, except in patients with severe GH deficiency, has not been established to give a better long-term outcome.
• The use of aromatase inhibitors in ISS to delay epiphyseal fusion.
• Genetic studies to identify the molecular basis of individual growth disorders will develop. The essential clinical component of these studies is to establish the precise clinical phenotype in combination with the genetic analysis. It is likely that children currently diagnosed as ISS will gradually be assigned to specific diagnostic categories.

Controversial points

• Treatment of non-GH-deficient children with hGH is an important controversial issue which relates to clinical benefit, risk of therapy, and health economics.
• The optimum organization of growth screening in the community is controversial. In general, community paediatricians favour a smaller number of measurements, whereas paediatric endocrinologists and patient support groups, such as the Child Growth Foundation, favour multiple measurements throughout the preschool period and during school years. The latter view is probably ideal; however, resources are not available for such detailed and comprehensive growth screening.
• Genetic analysis of patients with short stature is growing in frequency. Genetic analysis and identification of gene mutations may contribute to the characterization and understanding of the pathophysiology of growth disorders.
• Treatment of young adults with GH deficiency: A case can be made for the automatic transition from paediatric to adult GH treatment, the latter being given in the initial dosage of about 0.6 mg daily (far lower than in childhood) and adjusted by titrating against serum IGF-I levels. An alternative approach is to be selective, accepting that compliance with adult GH replacement will be poor in asymptomatic young adults, and to reserve treatment for patients who become symptomatic, or in whom problems such as hyperlipidaemia or reduced bone mass are found in the course of monitoring.

Potential pitfalls

• Over-diagnosis of GH deficiency by focusing on biochemical results rather than the history, examination, and auxology.
• Over-reliance on bone age assessment, which is not a diagnostic investigation.
• Reluctance to use testosterone therapy for delayed puberty in males. In short courses, using the appropriate dose, there is no compromising effect on adult height and the psychological benefits are obvious in many boys.

Case histories

Case 3.1
A four-year-old boy was being followed in a joint medical/surgical cryptorchidism clinic and was found to have short stature. He had subtle dysmorphic features with a small mid-face. He was apparently healthy. Both testes were palpable, but the penis was rather small. Height was below the 3rd centile, weight on the 10th centile and height velocity was 3.4 cm per year.

These findings indicated that he was abnormally short (mid-parental height was 75th centile) and that he needed investigation. The results were as follows. Full blood count, erythrocyte sedimentation rate (ESR), electrolytes, creatinine, liver function tests were normal and endomysial antibodies were negative.

TSH 1.8 mU/L [NR 0.3–5.0]
Free T4 6.6 pmol/L [NR 11–25]
[0.53 ng/dL, NR 0.8–2.4]
Cortisol 255 nmol/L [NR 09.00 h, 300–700]
[9.3 μg/dL, NR 8.0–25.0]
Prolactin 286 mU/L [NR up to 360]

Questions and Answers
1 What do these baseline results mean?

They show that he has hypothyroidism of central origin because his TSH level is not elevated.

2 What is the next step?

He needs a GH stimulation test *after* treatment with levo-thyroxine to normalize serum thyroxine concentration.

3 Is this test normal?

Table 3.12 Results of glucagon stimulation test.

Time (min)	GH (mU/L)
0	0.8
60	0.5
90	1.6
120	1.4
150	0.6
180	0.7

After glucagon 15 mg/kg intramuscularly, GH secretion is measured as shown in Table 3.12. All values are < 10 mU/L (<μg/L) indicating GH deficiency.

4 Are any more investigations needed before he starts his GH therapy?

Yes, he needs an MRI scan of the pituitary and hypothalamus to exclude an organic cause of GH deficiency, such as craniopharyngioma. The MRI scan was reported as showing an extremely shallow pituitary fossa with no evidence of pituitary tissue. *The diagnosis is idiopathic hypopituitarism with proven deficiency of GH and TSH.*

5 Are there any other pituitary hormone deficiencies?

Probably. He had cryptorchidism and a small penis which could be caused by gonadotrophin deficiency. This will need investigating at the time of puberty. He started GH therapy at 25 μg/kg/day (a relatively low dose). His height velocity increased in six months from 4.9 to 19.2 cm per year. This was a record for the clinic. At the age of 9.5 years his height was 139.6 cm, i.e. between the 75th and 90th centiles and within his height target range.

Case 3.2
A six-year-old girl was referred with growth failure, poor appetite, recurrent abdominal pain, 'thick custard' stools, and vomiting.

Questions and Answers
1 What is the differential diagnosis of this child's short stature?

Look at Table 3.2 and remember that the paediatrician should always approach the problem of short stature as a generalist and not as an endocrinologist. On examination, her height was below the 0.4th centile and her weight was on the 2nd centile. Her height velocity was 1.8 cm per year (normal is >4 cm per year). This means that she needs baseline investigations for short stature. The results of these investigations were as follows:

Hb 12.2 g/dL
Ferritin 8.0 μ/L [NR 15–300]
Anti-endomysial antibodies were positive
ESR 24 mm/h

2 What is the next investigation needed?

Jejunal biopsy. This showed villous atrophy and lymphocytic infiltrate in the lamina propria with hyperplastic crypts. This confirmed a diagnosis of coeliac disease.

Case 3.3

A seven-year-old girl is referred from the cardiac clinic with short stature. She was born weighing 2.73 kg at 40 weeks' gestation (−1.53 SD) and at nine-week check was found to have a heart murmur, echocardiogram showing aortic stenosis. The girl was asymptomatic and the short stature had always been attributed to her parents being short – mother 151.1 cm, father 162.4 cm – but the disparity between her height and that of her school mates seemed to be increasing.

Questions and Answers

1 What is the differential diagnosis of this child's short stature, and what specific questions should be asked?

Turner syndrome must be seriously considered in a short girl with aortic stenosis and an enquiry should be made about ear infections, middle ear deafness, difficulty with mathematics, and a history of poor feeding, high activity levels, and sleeplessness in infancy and early childhood.

It is of course possible that this is normal familial short stature compounded by constitutional delay, so the childhood stature and pubertal milestones of the family should be ascertained, together with any history of atopy since asthma can be associated with constitutional delay.

The girl had had a couple of ear infections, otherwise her health was good, and there had been no problems in early childhood with feeding or sleeping. She was doing well at school and had no particular difficulty with mathematics. There was no history of delayed puberty in either parent. Examination showed a normal-looking girl measuring 101.4 cm, (−3.8 SDS, compared with the mid-parental height SDS of −1.7) and weighing 18 kg (−1.7 SDS) with only subtle dysmorphism including slightly puffy fingers and pudgy nail folds, high palate, shield chest, and posteriorly rotated ears. Pulses were normal, blood pressure was 86/56 mm per Hg, aortic stenosis murmur noted with carotid thrill and bruit. Ear examination showed no active inflammation of tympanic membranes.

2 What investigations should be done in this girl?

Chromosomes to confirm the diagnosis of Turner syndrome, basal LH and FSH to detect evidence of primary ovarian failure, thyroid function, and thyroid peroxidase antibodies (since Hashimoto's thyroiditis is common in Turner syndrome), full blood count and ferritin, and IGF-I. Pelvic and renal ultrasound examination to assess ovarian, uterine and renal morphology.

Karyotype showed a 46,X,iXq pattern, with duplication of the long arm (q) resulting in an isochromosome and thus loss of the short arm (p). FSH was elevated at 17 U/l consistent with primary ovarian failure, LH normal for age at 0.1 U/l. Thyroid function was normal, and TPO antibodies were negative. Renal ultrasound was normal, uterus slightly hypoplastic, ovaries were not identified.

Comment
The clue that the short stature might not be familial (apart from the associated aortic stenosis), was the mismatch between the girl's height and that of her parents, i.e. she was inappropriately short even for her short family (see Ouarezki et al. 2017). The borderline smallness-for-gestational age is consistent with Turner syndrome. The dysmorphic features were subtle and easily overlooked.

Case 3.4

A boy is referred to the growth clinic aged 10.2 year with short stature. He has been followed up in a general clinic because of the diagnosis of maternal GH deficiency. His height has fallen from the 10th–25th centile at 5.8 years to just below the 3rd centile now. He was born at 39 weeks gestation weighing 6 lb. 1 oz. to a mother who had received pituitary-derived human GH for four years around the age of puberty following the demonstration of low GH levels on stimulation testing. The boy's measurements at the clinic are height 128 cm (−1.80 SDS) and weight 25 kg (−1.68 SDS), mother's height 149.5 cm (−2.09 SDS), father's reported height 6′0″.

Question and Answer

1 What diagnostic possibilities should be considered in this boy?

This could be autosomal dominant GH deficiency. However, one would expect more severe short stature from an earlier age if this were the case. Normal variant familial short stature is a possibility, with the mother going through a phase of GH insufficiency, rather than true GH deficiency, when she was tested. A further possibility is an autosomal dominant skeletal dysplasia, the low levels of GH in the mother at the time she was tested being a 'red herring'.

Careful physical examination shows obvious café au lait patches in the boy consistent with neurofibromatosis. These are also present in the mother. Further history reveals that two maternal aunts and two maternal cousins also have café au lait patches. The boy's visual fields and fundi are normal, blood pressure 110/70. He is followed up in the growth clinic and his height continues to be just below the 3rd centile. At 12.5 years dynamic testing shows a GH peak of 10.2 mU/L in response to insulin (partial GH insufficiency), IGF1 117 μg/L (low/normal for age), pubertal LH response to stimulation with GnRH, and normal thyroid function. The boy receives recombinant GH from 12.3 until 17 years, and does well, going through puberty normally and attaining an adult height of 169 cm (−0.89 SDS). MRI scans of brain show slight bulkiness of the optic nerves, but normal hypothalamus and pituitary.

Comment

This case illustrates the need to consider a dominant growth disorder when one parent is short. The discovery of café au lait patches was made during careful physical examination, as should always be the case with new patient referrals. The short stature that is frequently seen in subjects with neurofibromatosis is in part related to an accompanying skeletal dysplasia, but subjects may also demonstrate a degree of GH insufficiency. This case reinforces the concept that low GH levels – GH insufficiency –constitute a problem and not a diagnosis.

Significant Guidelines/Consensus Statements

Growth Hormone

British Society for Paediatric Endocrinology and Diabetes (BSPED) (2017) Growth Hormone Standards. www.bsped.org.uk/media/1372/gh-standards-document_nov2017.pdf (accessed 13 October 2018).

Cohen, P., Rogol, A.D., Deal, C.L. et al. (2008). Consensus statement on the diagnosis and treatment of children with idiopathic short stature: a summary of the Growth Hormone Research Society, the Lawson Wilkins paediatric Endocrine Society, and the European Society for Paediatric Endocrinology Workshop. *J. Clin. Endocrinol. Metab.* 93 (11): 4210–4217.

Growth Hormone Research Society (2000). Consensus guidelines for the diagnosis and treatment of growth hormone (GH) deficiency in childhood and adolescence: summary statement of the GH Research Society. *JCEM* 85 (11): 3990–3993.

Grimberg, A., DiVall, S.A., Polychronakos, C. et al. Drug and Therapeutics Committee and Ethhics Committee of the Pediatric Endocrine Society (2016). Guidelines for growth hormone and insulin-like growth factor-I treatment in children and adolescents: growth hormone deficiency, idiopathic short stature, and primary insulin-like growth factor-I deficiency. *Horm. Res. Paediatr.* 86: 361–397:https://doi.org/10.1159/000452150.

Small for Gestational Age
Lee, P.A., Chernausek, S.D., Hokken-Koelega, A.C.S., and Czernichow, P. (2003). International SGA Advisory Board consensus development conference statement: management of short children born small for gestational age, April 24–October 1, 2001. *Pediatr.* 111: 1253–1261.

Transition
Clayton, P.E., Cuneo, R.C., Juul, A. et al. (2005). Consensus statement on the management of the GH-treated adolescent in the transition to adult care. *Eur. J. Endocrinol.* 152: 165–170.

Turner Syndrome
Gravholt, C.H., Andersen, N.H., Conway, G.S. et al. (2017). Clinical practice guidelines for the care of girls and women with Turner syndrome: proceedings from the 2016 Cincinnati International Turner Syndrome Meeting. *Eur. J. Endocrinol.* 177 (3): G1–G7:https://doi.org/10.1530/EJE-17-0430.

References

Albertsson-Wikland, K. and Karlberg, J. (1994). Natural growth in children born small for gestational age with and without catch-up growth. *Acta Paediatr. Suppl.* 399: 64–70; discussion 71.

Albin, A.K., Niklasson, A., Westgren, U., and Norjavaara, E. (2012). Estradiol and pubertal growth in girls. *Horm. Res. Paediatr.* 78: 218–225: https://doi.org/10.1159/000343076.

Ankarberg-Lindgren, C. and Norjvaara, E. (2008). Twenty-four hours secretion pattern of serum oestradiol levels in prepubertal and pubertal boys as determined by a validated ultra-sensitive extraction RIA. *BMC Endocr. Disord.* 8: 10:https://doi.org/10.1186/1472-6823-8-10.

British Society for Paediatric Endocrinology and Diabetes (BSPED) (2017) Growth Hormone Standards www.bsped.org.uk/media/1372/gh-standards-document_nov2017.pdf (accessed 13 October 2018).

Brito, N.B., Llanos, J.P.S., Ferrer, M.F. et al. (2016). Relationship between mid-upper arm circumference and body mass index in inpatients. *PLoS One* 11 (8): https://doi.org/10.1371/journal.pone.0160480.

Cizmecioglu, F., Doherty, A., Paterson, W.F. et al. (2005). Measured versus reported parental height. *Arch. Dis. Child.* 90 (9): 941–942.

Clayton, P.E., Cuneo, R.C., Juul, A. et al. (2005). Consensus statement on the management of the GH-treated adolescent in the transition to adult care. *Eur. J. Endocrinol.* 152: 165–170.

Crane, J.L. and Cao, X. (2014). Function of, Matrix IGF-1 in coupling bone resorption and formation. *J. Mol. Med. (Berl.)* 92 (2): 107–115:https://doi.org/10.1007/s00109-013-1084-3.

De Vile, C.J., Grant, D.B., Hayward, R.D., and Stanhope, R. (1996). Growth and endocrine sequelae of craniopharyngioma. *Arch. Dis. Child.* 75 (2): 108–114.

De Zegher, F., Francois, I., Van Helvoirt, M. et al. (1998). Growth hormone treatment of short children born small for gestational age. *Trends Endocrinol. Metab.* 9: 233–237.

Dias, R.P., Bogdarina, I., Cazier, J.-B. et al. (2012). Multiple segmental uniparental disomy associated with abnormal DNA methylation of imprinted loci in silver-Russell syndrome. *JCEM* 97 (11): https://doi.org/10.1210/jc.2012-1980.

Donaldson, M.D.C., Tucker, S.N., and Grant, D.B. (1980). Recessively inherited growth hormone deficiency in a family from Iraq. *J. Med. Genet.* 17 (4): 288–290.

Freeman, J.V., Cole, T.J., Chinn, S. et al. (1995). Cross sectional stature and weight reference curves for the UK. *Arch. Dis. Child.* 73: 17–24.

Gault, E.J., Perry, R.J., Cole, T.J. et al., on behalf of the British Society for Paediatric Endocrinology and Diabetes(2011). The effect of Oxandrolone and timing of pubertal induction on final height in Turner syndrome: a randomised, double blind, placebo controlled trial. *BMJ* 342: d1980: https://doi.org/10.1136/bmj.d1980.

Giacomozzi, C., Deodati, A., Shaikh, M.G. et al. (2015). The impact of growth hormone therapy on adult height in Noonan syndrome: a systematic review. *Horm. Res. Paediatr.* 83 (3): 167–176:https://doi.org/10.1159/000371635.

Gravholt, C.H., Andersen, N.H., Conway, G.S. et al. (2017). Clinical practice guidelines for the care of girls and women with Turner syndrome: proceedings from the 2016 Cincinnati International Turner Syndrome Meeting. *Eur. J. Endocrinol.* 177 (3): G1–G70: https://doi.org/10.1530/EJE-17-0430.

Grimberg, A., DiVall, S.A., Polychronakos, C. et al. Drug and Therapeutics Committee and Ethhics Committee of the Pediatric Endocrine Society(2016). Guidelines for growth hormone and insulin-like growth factor-I treatment in children and adolescents: growth hormone deficiency, idiopathic short stature, and primary insulin-like growth factor-I deficiency. *Horm. Res. Paediatr.* 86: 361–397: https://doi.org/10.1159/000452150.

Hagenäs, L. and Hertel, T. (2003). Skeletal dysplasia, growth hormone treatment and body proportion: comparison with other syndromic and non-syndromic short children. *Horm. Res.* 60 (suppl 3): 65–70:https://doi.org/10.1159/000074504.

Jones, K.L. (1997). *Smith's Recognizable Patterns of Human Malformation*. Philadelphia, PA: W.B. Saunders.

Kao, K.T., Ahmed, S.F., and Wong, S.C. (2018). Growth in childhood chronic conditions. In: *Encyclopedia of Endocrine Diseases* (ed. I. Huhtaniemi), 102–117. Elsevier.

Karlberg, J. (1989). A mathematical model breaking down linear growth from birth to adulthood into 3 components that reflect the different hormonal phases of the growth process. *Acta Paediatr. Suppl.* 350: 70–94.

Kelly, B.P., Paterson, W.F., and Donaldson, M.D.C. (2003). Final height outcome and value of height prediction in boys with constitutional delay in growth and adolescence treated with intramuscular testosterone 125 mg per month for 3 months. *Clin. Endocrinol.* 58: 267–272.

Lawaetz, J.G., Hagen, C.P., Mieritz, M.G. et al. (2015). Evaluation of 451 Danish boys with delayed puberty: diagnostic use of a new puberty Nomogram and effects of oral testosterone therapy. *JCEM* 100: 1376–1385.

Lee, H., Tajmir, S., Lee, J. et al. (2017). Fully automated deep learning system for bone age assessment. *J. Digit. Imaging* 30 (4): 427–441: https://doi.org/10.1007/s10278-017-9955-8.

Mericq, M.V., Eggers, M., Avila, A. et al. (2000). Near final height in pubertal growth hormone (GH)-deficient patients treated with GH alone or in combination with luteinizing hormone-releasing hormone analog: results of a prospective, randomized trial. *JCEM* 85 (2): 569–573.

Ouarezki, Y., Cizmecioglu, F.M., Mansour, C. et al. (2017). Measured parental height in Turner syndrome—a valuable but underused diagnostic tool. *Eur. J. Pediatr.* 177: 2, 171–179. https://doi.org/10.1007/s00431-017-3045-2.

Ranke, M.B. (1998). Turner and Noonan syndromes: disease specific growth and growth-promoting therapies. In: *Growth Disorders: Pathophysiology and Treatment* (ed. C.J.H. Kelnar, M.O. Savage, et al.), 623–639. London: Chapman & Hall Medical.

Ranke, M.B., Stubbe, P., Majewski, F., and Bierich, J.R. (1998). Spontaneous growth in Turner's syndrome. *Acta Paediatr.* 77: 22–30. https://doi.org/10.1111/j.1651-2227.1988.tb10796.x.

Rose, S.R., Municchi, G., Barnes, K.M. et al. (1991). Spontaneous growth hormone secretion increases during puberty in normal girls and boys. *JCEM* 73 (2): 428–435.

Sardar, C.M., Kinmond, S., Siddique, J. et al. (2015). Short stature screening by accurate length measurement of infants with birthweight <9th centile. *Horm. Res. Paediatr.* 83: 400–407:https://doi.org/10.1159/000376611.

Skuse, D., Albanese, A., Stanhope, R. et al. (1996). A new stress-related syndrome of growth failure and hyperphagia in children, associated with reversibility of growth-hormone insufficiency. *Lancet* 10348 (9024): 353–358.

Stephure, D.K. (2005). Impact of growth hormone supplementation on adult height in Turner syndrome: results of Canadian randomized controlled trial. *JCEM* 90: 3360–3366:https://doi.org/10.1210/jc.2004-2187.

Swerdlow, A.J., Cooke, R., Beckers, D. et al. (2017). Cancer risks in patients treated with growth hormone in childhood: the SAGhE European cohort study. *JCEM* 102 (5): 1661–1672:https://doi.org/10.1210/jc.2016-2046.

Tanner, J.M. (1986). Normal growth and techniques of growth assessment. In: *Growth Disorders, Clinics in Endocrinology and Metabolism*, vol. 3, 411–451. London: W.B. Saunders.

Tanner, J.M. and PWS, D. (1985). Clinical longitudinal standards for height and height velocity for North American children. *J. Pediatr.* 107 (1): 317–328.

Tanner, J.M., Goldstein, H., and Whitehouse, R.H. (1970). Standards for children's height at age 2–9 years allowing for height of parents. *Arch. Dis. Child.* 45: 755–762.

Tonshoff, B. and Mehls, O. (1999). Growth retardation in children with chronic renal disease: pathophysiology and treatment. In: *Current Indications for Growth Hormone Therapy* (ed. P.C. Hindmarsh), 118–127. Basel: S. Karger.

Voss, L.D., Bailey, B.J., Cumming, K. et al. (1990). The reliability of height measurement (the Wessex growth study). *Arch. Dis. Child.* 65 (12): 1340–1344.

Walker-Smith, J.A. (1996). Management of growth failure in Crohn's disease. *Arch. Dis. Child.* 75: 351–354.

Further Reading

Cooke, D.W., DiVall, S.A., and Radovick, S. (2016). Normal and aberrant growth in children. In: *Williams Textbook of Endocrinology*, 13e (ed. S. Melmed, K.S. Polonsky, P. Reed Larsen and H.M. Kronenberg), 964–1073. Philadelphia, PA.: Elsevier.

Cowell, C.T. (1995). Short stature. In: *Clinical Paediatric Endocrinology* (ed. C.G.D. Brook), 136–172. Oxford: Blackwell Science.

Delemarre-van de Waal, H.A. (2007). Delay of growth and puberty. In: *Growth Disorders*, 2e (ed. C.J.H. Kelnar, M.O. Savage, P. Saenger and C.T. Cowell), 595–603. London: Hodder Arnold.

Donaldson, M.D.C. and Paterson, W. (2007). Abnormal growth: definition, pathogenesis and practical assessment. In: *Growth Disorders: Pathophysiology and Treatment*, 2e (ed. C.J.H. Kelnar, M.O. Savage, P. Saenger and C.T. Cowell), 185–207. London: Hodder Arnold.

Hindmarsh, P.C. (2007). Endocrine assessment and principles of endocrine testing. In: *Growth Disorders*, 2e (ed. C.J.H. Kelnar, M.O. Savage, P. Saenger and C.T. Cowell), 219–229. London: Hodder Arnold.

Hintz, R.L. (2005). Growth hormone treatment of idiopathic short stature. *Growth Horm. IGF Res.* 15: S6–S8.

Mortier, G.R., Graham, J.M., and Rimoin, D.L. (2007). Short stature syndromes. In: *Growth Disorders*, 2e (ed. C.J.H. Kelnar, M.O. Savage, P. Saenger and C.T. Cowell), 259–280. London: Hodder Arnold.

Tanner, J.M., Healy, M.J.R., Goldstein, H. et al. (2001). *Assessment of Skeletal Maturity and Prediction of Adult Height (TW3 Method)*, 3e. London.: W.B. Saunders.

Tanner, J.M., Whitehouse, R.H., Cameron, N. et al. (1983). *Assessment of Skeletal Maturity and Prediction of Adult Height (TW2 Method)*, 2e. London: Academic Press.

Useful Information for Patients and Parents

The Restricted Growth Association offers support to a range of short stature conditions, particularly achondroplasia and other causes of disproportionate short stature.

Website: www.restrictedgrowth.co.uk (accessed 3 October 2018).

The Turner Syndrome Support Society (TSSS) has excellent information for parents, children and teenagers with Turner syndrome. Website: www.tss.org.uk (accessed 3 October 2018).

The Child Growth Foundation (CGF) offers support to children and adults with growth problems and their families, and also to healthcare professionals with an interest. CGF provides a superb range of 15 booklets on growth and hormone problems including IUGR, GH deficiency, GH deficiency in adults, constitutional delay, Turner syndrome, and craniopharyngioma disorders including GH deficiency. Website: http://www.childgrowthfoundation.org (accessed 3 October 2018).

European Society for Paediatric Endocrinology Parent and Patient provides pamphlets on a wide variety of growth disorders in English, French, Italian, Spanish and Turkish.

Website: http://www.eurospe.org/patient/index.html (accessed 3 October 2018).

4 Tall Stature

Tall stature is defined as height greater than two standard deviations above the mean (equivalent to >97th centile) for the general population. It may accompany disorders such as sexual precocity and simple obesity, and not be the prime concern. When tall stature per se is the principal reason for referral, the family will wish an estimate of final height and possible treatment to be discussed. Tall stature is a much less common cause of referral than short stature, being more acceptable to families than the latter unless the degree of tallness is particularly marked, especially in a girl.

Pathogenesis and differential diagnosis

Tall stature is usually associated with one of four broad aetiological categories. In order of frequency these are: (i) familial tall stature/constitutional advance in growth; (ii) simple obesity; (iii) syndromic tall stature, which has usually been present since infancy; and (iv) endocrine causes. The differential diagnosis is shown in Table 4.1 and a helpful diagnostic algorithm is also recommended (Davies and Cheetham 2014). The European Society for Paediatric Endocrinology (ESPE) provides a more comprehensive classification (Wit et al. 2007).

Most tall stature conditions are rare. An idea of their relative frequency as the principal reason for referral can be gained by examining the following breakdown of referrals to one consultant in Glasgow from 1989 to 2009: normal genetic tall stature (81); constitutional advance in growth and adolescence (49); tall stature due to simple obesity (70); dysmorphic syndromes: 47,XYY (3), 47,XXY (11), 47,XXX (1), Marfan syndrome (18), Sotos syndrome (5), Weaver syndrome (1), Beckwith-Wiedemann syndrome (3), unclassified dysmorphic syndromes (22); sexual precocity (19); thyrotoxicosis (2), and growth hormone excess (2).

Assessment of the child or adolescent with tall stature

The key aspects of clinical assessment of a child or adolescent referred with tall stature are given in Table 4.2. With a combination of auxology, careful history taking, and physical examination followed by serial measurements of height, laboratory investigations will not usually be needed. If there are dysmorphic features, particularly in the context of learning difficulties, a clinical geneticist should be invited to see the child and advise on specific molecular genetic studies. Since the phenotype of Marfan syndrome (see Table 4.5) can be mild, it is wise to carry out a screening cardiac ultrasound in children who are taller than expected for parental heights, or in whom one parent is particularly tall.

Investigations

Children whose height falls above the parental target range centiles in the absence of a family history of constitutional advance and/or an enhanced growth rate will require investigation, as shown in Table 4.3. The combination of tall stature and developmental

Practical Endocrinology and Diabetes in Children, Fourth Edition. Malcolm D.C. Donaldson, John W. Gregory,
Guy Van Vliet, and Joseph I. Wolfsdorf.
© 2019 John Wiley & Sons Ltd. Published 2019 by John Wiley & Sons Ltd.

Table 4.1 Differential diagnosis of tall stature.

1 Normal familial tall stature
   • Normal genetic tall stature
   • Constitutional advance in growth and adolescence
2 Simple (exogenous) obesity
3 Dysmorphic syndromes associated with tall stature
   (i) With X or Y aneuploidy
       • 47,XYY
       • 47,XXY (Klinefelters syndrome)
       • 47,XXX
       • Other aneuploidy syndromes
   (ii) With metabolic/skeletal abnormality
       • Marfan syndrome
       • Homocystinuria
       • Total lipodystrophy
       • Other
   (iii) With symmetrical overgrowth
       • Fragile X syndrome
       • Sotos syndrome
       • Weaver syndrome
       • Other syndromes
   (iv) With asymmetrical overgrowth
       • Beckwith–Wiedemann syndrome
       • Klippel–Trenaunay–Weber syndrome
       • Proteus syndrome syndrome
       • Other syndromes
4 Endocrine causes
   (i) Sexual precocity (e.g. virilizing congenital adrenal hyperplasia, true central precocious puberty; see Chapter 5)
   (ii) Thyrotoxicosis (mostly in prepubertal children)
   (iii) GH excess (very rare)
       • GHRH tumour/dysregulation
       • GH secreting adenoma ± MEN1, McCune–Albright syndrome
   (iv) Familial glucocorticoid deficiency (rarely a presenting complaint)
   (v) Endocrine abnormalities causing delayed epiphyseal closure (e.g. aromatase deficiency and oestrogen receptor defect).

Table 4.2 Clinical assessment of tall stature.

Auxology
Height, weight, height velocity
Heights of parents and siblings
Bone age and (if appropriate) height prediction

History
Pattern of growth including age when tall stature recognized
Birth weight, head circumference and (if available) birth length
Family patterns of childhood growth and puberty
Neurodevelopment, academic performance and behaviour

Examination
Presence of dysmorphic features
Pubertal staging including assessment of testicular volume
Fundoscopy to assess optic discs
Systematic examination

Table 4.3 Baseline investigations for tall stature.

Cardiac ultrasound

Karyotype

Fibrillin-1 gene for Marfan syndrome

FMR1 gene analysis for Fragile X syndrome in boys with tall stature and learning difficulties

DNA for specific syndromes (after assessment by clinical geneticist)

Thyroid function tests

IGF-I

Bone age assessment and (where appropriate) height prediction

delay should always prompt a search for an underlying syndrome. If physical examination is completely normal and the child comes from a tall family, investigations are usually not indicated and regular height measurements will be sufficient. Further investigations will be dictated by the results of the baseline tests. If the rare diagnosis of excess growth hormone (GH) secretion caused by a GH-secreting pituitary adenoma is considered, investigation should proceed as shown in Table 4.4.

Table 4.4 Assessment for possible growth hormone excess.

GH suppression test using oral glucose load

MRI of hypothalamus and pituitary

Visual fields

9.00 a.m. cortisol

Prolactin

Testosterone, LH, FSH (depending on age)

Protocol for GH suppression test with glucose

This test involves giving 1.75 g/kg carbohydrate orally (up to maximum of 75 g = two glasses of Lucozade) as for the glucose tolerance test, and measuring serum GH at: -30, 0, 30, 60, 90, 120 and 150 minutes together with an insulin-like growth factor IGF-I level at baseline. Normal GH suppression is a value of <4 mU/L at some time during the test.

NB: It is wise to put in the request for this test as 'GH suppression test with glucose' rather than 'glucose tolerance test' – if the latter term is used, the day ward is likely to take samples for glucose and not GH!

Causes of tall stature

Familial tall stature and constitutional advance in growth and adolescence

Physiological tall stature can be sub-classified into familial tall stature and constitutional advance in growth – the counterpart of familial short stature and constitutional delay (see Chapter 3). As with familial short stature and constitutional delay, there is considerable overlap between familial tallness and constitutional advance. Also, as with short stature, the clinician needs to guard against the pitfall of assuming that tallness in one parent is necessarily normal – dominantly inherited tall stature disorders (e.g. Marfan syndrome) can be mistaken for normal tall stature.

Normal tall stature is the most common cause of referral in tall children and adolescents, and the patient is usually a girl. In this case, it is frequently the mother who, having suffered herself from being unusually tall as a child and adolescent, is concerned about her daughter. In groups of tall children, GH secretion has been shown to be statistically elevated when compared to children with normal or short stature. However, in an individual child, excess GH secretion is not usually apparent. The tall stature is usually noticeable by primary school entry. It is helpful to ask the parents about their childhood height and age of onset of puberty. The history of one parent being particularly tall as a child, having an early adolescence, and being relatively less tall as an adult, is indicative of familial constitutional advance, and the diagnosis is supported by bone age advance in the child. Physical examination is normal although advanced adolescence may be noted in girls >9 years. In girls and boys with normal tall stature, prediction of final height from skeletal maturity and current height may be helpful from around 11 years upwards. However, the accuracy of final height prediction in tall stature varies between populations and with the prediction method used, hence should not be used to assess any treatment effect. The likelihood of an earlier-than-average puberty should be explained to parents whose children are still prepubertal. Reassurance and growth monitoring are the principles of management.

Simple obesity

Children with simple (exogenous) obesity are relatively tall in relation to their parental height centiles, with increased height velocity and moderately advanced bone age (Buckler 1994). This increase in height status may, depending on familial heights, be sufficient to put the child above the 97th centile for height, or to compound existing tall stature.

Syndromes associated with tall stature

The combination of tall stature and developmental delay should always prompt a search for an underlying dysmorphic syndrome. Boys with learning difficulties should be screened for Fragile X syndrome irrespective of stature. The typical phenotype in this condition includes long face, large and prominent ears, increased head size, and (especially after puberty) enlarged testes. Of the aneuploidy syndromes, the 47,XYY syndrome is the most likely to present as tall stature (with long legs) and, in most cases, both phenotype and intelligence are normal although some individuals show behavioural problems. The principal phenotypic features of three important tall stature syndromes which may present to the growth clinic – Marfan, Sotos, and Beckwith-Wiedemann syndrome – are given in Table 4.5.

Marfan syndrome and related disorders are a complex and phenotypically variable group of conditions caused by mutations in the *FBN1* gene which encodes fibrillin-1 (Pepe et al. 2016). In suspected cases, the revised Ghent scoring system (Loeys et al. 2010) is useful in helping both to avoid over-diagnosis and to distinguish classic Marfan syndrome from allied conditions, such as the mitral valve prolapse, aortic enlargement, skin and skeletal (MASS) variant. In MASS, lens dislocation does not occur and the risk of aortic dissection is lower.

Sotos syndrome is considered when tall stature is accompanied by mild learning difficulties and characteristic facial/skull appearance. Bone age is usually advanced so that adult final height is not markedly increased, with values of 184.3 cm for men and 172.9 cm for women in one study (Agwu et al. 1999).

Table 4.5 Principal features of Marfan, Sotos, and Beckwith-Wiedemann syndromes.

Marfan syndrome
Genetics
- Autosomal dominant; spontaneous mutation in ~ 25%
- Mutations in *FBN1* gene (encoding the glycoprotein fibrillin-1)

Clinical features
- Characteristic phenotype – tall thin build, arachnodactyly, long face, high palate
- Joint laxity with hypotonia, kyphoscoliosis, pes planus
- Eye problems – upward lens subluxation, myopia, retinal detachment
- Cardiac problems – aortic root dilatation leading to rupture, mitral valve prolapse

Diagnosis
Clinical, supported by cardiac ultrasound and eye findings, confirmed by genetic studies
N.B.: Phenotype may be mild.

Sotos syndrome
Genetics
- *NSD1* gene (located 5q35) defect in 80%
- Sporadic in 95%, commoner in boys; autosomal dominant transmission

Clinical features
- Accelerated prenatal and infantile growth with large head size
- Tall childhood stature with bone age advance, adult height not excessive
- Variable degree of learning difficulties (50% need learning support)
- Hypotonia and poor coordination
- 'Inverted pear' head shape – long narrow face with high-bossed forehead, prominent jaw, down-slanting eyes

Diagnosis
- Suggested by triad of typical facies, overgrowth, and learning difficulties
- Confirmed by molecular genetic studies

Beckwith–Wiedemann syndrome
Genetics
- Two-thirds of patients have demonstrable abnormalities affecting imprinted genes in 11p15.5 region including paternal disomy; abnormal DNA methylation; maternal translocations/inversion with break points
- Sporadic in 85%, autosomal dominant in 15% with incomplete penetrance
- Closely linked with Wilms' tumour gene (*WT2*)
- Imbalance between maternally imprinted IGF-II growth enhancer gene and paternally imprinted H19 growth suppresser gene

Clinical
- Foetal overgrowth with birth weight and length > 90th centile and postnatal overgrowth during first 4–6 yr; macroglossia; large kidneys; hemihypertrophy
- Midline abdominal wall defects – omphalocoele, umbilical hernia
- Transient neonatal hyperinsulinaemic hypoglycaemia due to pancreatic hyperplasia
- Ear lobe creases and pits
- Predisposition to tumours, especially Wilms' (7%)
- Mild learning difficulties in some patients

Diagnosis
- Presence of 3/5 major criteria (large birth size, abdominal wall defect, macroglossia, ear creases, neonatal hypoglycaemia)
- Genetic studies support rather than exclude diagnosis.

The typical genetic defect is in the *NSD1* gene, but Sotos has reported a new form of the condition caused by heterozygous mutations in the Nuclear Factor 1,X type (*NFIX*) gene on 19p13.3 (Sotos 2014).

In Beckwith-Wiedemann syndrome, tall stature is an accompanying rather than presenting feature. Diagnosis is important so that appropriate management and surveillance can be implemented, particularly for tumour development (Weksberg et al. 2010)

Endocrine causes of tall stature

Sexual precocity, thyrotoxicosis, and familial glucocorticoid deficiency (see Chapter 8) do not usually present with tall stature alone, while aromatase deficiency/oestrogen receptor defects are extremely rare. Children with suspected GH excess will require hormone investigations to confirm the abnormality; specialist referral at this stage is recommended.

Pituitary gigantism

A GH-secreting tumour causes tall stature and gigantism in childhood and adolescence, and acromegaly in adult life. An association with McCune–Albright syndrome is recognized. Because of its extreme rarity in childhood, this disorder should be managed jointly with an adult endocrinologist with experience of managing acromegaly.

Management of pituitary gigantism should be according to the Endocrine Society guidelines (Katznelson et al. 2014). Trans-sphenoidal surgery is the treatment of choice, with either medical therapy or radiotherapy (preferably stereotactic) if tumour removal is incomplete or not feasible. Medical therapy comprises daily subcutaneous injections of the growth hormone receptor antagonist Pegvisomant, which has been shown to decrease height velocity in gigantism. This may be used in conjunction with the long-acting preparation of the somatostatin antagonist Octreotide which is initially given as a deep subcutaneous injection every month.

Treatment of familial (constitutional) tall stature

This is a controversial area. In the US, very few otherwise healthy girls are currently treated with high dose oestrogen to reduce adult height. This is partly because tall stature is now seldom regarded as a problem requiring intervention. Moreover, apart from ethical concerns about intervention in a physiological situation, there are also long-term health concerns (see below). Despite this, the degree of anxiety surrounding advanced growth, may be sufficient for treatment to be given. The aim is to try to slow down growth and therefore reduce final height by reducing the prepubertal rather than the pubertal component of growth, Three forms of therapy have either been used or are under consideration:
- high-dose sex-steroid therapy;
- GH-suppressive therapy using a somatostatin analogue;
- GH receptor antagonist therapy.

Sex-steroid therapy
The indication for the use of sex steroids to reduce final height is based on evidence that abnormally high circulating levels will advance skeletal maturation and eventually cause early epiphyseal fusion. The most extensive results have been published by a group from the Netherlands (De Waal et al. 1996). In girls, Ethinylestradiol 100–300 μg/day orally combined with cyclical progesterone (i.e. norethisterone 5 mg/day for days 1–14 of each calendar month), reduced final height by up to 7 cm. In boys, testosterone 250–1000 mg monthly caused a similar reduction. An early age of onset of treatment (bone age 10 years in girls, 12.5 years in boys) was associated with the best results.

However, further work from the Netherlands has raised fertility concerns following high dose oestrogen treatment in childhood and adolescence. A study on 125 tall women found time to first pregnancy to be increased in the 95 subjects who had been treated with high dose Ethinylestradiol compared with the untreated women. Also, those treated with 200 μg daily

took longer to conceive than the women receiving 100 μg, suggesting a dose effect (Hendriks et al. 2012).

In Glasgow, our experience of tall stature treatment has been virtually limited to selected girls with Marfan syndrome, using lower doses (50–100 μg daily) of Ethinylestradiol (Kalkan Ucar et al. 2009). In boys, high dose intramuscular testosterone therapy (250 mg every two weeks) can be given to accelerate epiphyseal fusion but, in practice, few centres employ this strategy.

Somatostatin analogue and GH receptor antagonist therapy
Treatment with Lanreotide, a long-acting preparation of the somatostatin analogue Octreotide, has been reported (Carel et al. 2009). The GH receptor antagonist Pegvisomant is known to reduce growth velocity in pituitary gigantism and would thus be expected to reduce final height in tall girls and boys. However, experience remains limited and not all clinicians are comfortable giving therapy of this invasive nature to essentially normal subjects. At present we advise against use of either treatment unless the circumstances are exceptional. Where possible, such experimental therapy should be conducted within a prospective research setting.

Surgical treatment
Epiphysiodesis, in which the knee epiphyses are ablated by percutaneous drill and curettage, is an established treatment for leg length inequality, the longer limb being treated. This technique has also been applied to tall girls and boys. A study from Sweden reported the outcome of bilateral percutaneous epiphysiodesis in 12 girls and 9 boys with tall stature in which final height was 4.1 and 6.4 cm below the predicted height (Benyi et al. 2010). The long-term safety of this technique remains unclear. Also, assessment of its efficacy is difficult because of small patient numbers, and the questionable validity of the height prediction model in exceptionally tall (and short) subjects.

Future developments

- Molecular analysis of tall stature and overgrowth syndromes continues to identify new genetic causes of these disorders.
- Prospective multicentre studies to assess the safety and efficacy of new treatment protocols.
- Experience with somatostatin and GH receptor antagonist therapy in pituitary gigantism is likely to accumulate.

When to involve a specialist centre

- Dysmorphic syndromes associated with tall stature.
- Tall stature associated with excess GH secretion.
- Tall stature in which intervention is contemplated, either with high dose oestrogen, surgery, or somatostatin/GH antagonist therapy.

Controversial points

- The treatment of tall stature in girls remains controversial with ethical and long-term safety concerns regarding high dose oestrogen therapy, the invasive nature and expense of Octreotide and Pegvisomant, and relative lack of experience with epiphysiodesis.
- As tall stature has become more acceptable and is better tolerated by society, there seems to be less indication for therapy.
- Rare conditions, such as GH-secreting pituitary tumours, are rarely seen in paediatric practice. These patients should be managed jointly with an adult endocrine unit.

Potential pitfalls

- Assuming that tall stature is normal familial in nature when it could be due to a dominant growth disorder such as Marfan syndrome. This diagnosis has important implications, for these patients need lifelong cardiovascular surveillance.
- Failure to consider the diagnosis of, or examine the patient carefully enough for, dysmorphic features suggestive of a syndrome to be appreciated.
- Failure to recognize that tall stature and delayed puberty are an unusual combination. An important differential diagnosis is Klinefelter syndrome, which should be considered.

Case histories

Case 4.1

A nine-year-old girl was referred because of tall stature. She was in good health with no learning problems. On examination there were no dysmorphic features. Her height was just above the 97th centile and her parents' heights were on the 90th and 97th centiles. Pubertal development

was: breast, stage 2; pubic hair, stage 3; and no menarche. Baseline investigations (Table 4.3) were all normal.

Consequently, an endocrine cause of her advanced growth was not identified. Bone age was 12.4 years and final height prediction was 188 cm. The parents, particularly the mother who had suffered as a result of her own tall stature, enquired about treatment. The child was not particularly concerned. Treatment was not advised.

Question and Answer

1 Are any further investigations indicated?

Probably not. She had occasional headaches so a magnetic resonance imaging (MRI) scan of the pituitary was performed which showed a pituitary gland with a convex upper border but no suprasellar extension. She also had a height velocity of 9.2 cm per year. She therefore had an oral glucose test for GH suppression. Her GH levels during the glucose test suppressed to 0.5 mU/L, indicating that there was no evidence of increased GH secretion. *Diagnosis*: Familial tall stature with constitutional advance.

Case 4.2

A 20-year-old Chinese girl was referred with concern as to her tallness compared with the rest of the family, and lack of secondary sexual development. She had mild to moderate learning difficulties and had attended a special needs school in the past. On examination she measured 167.8 cm (0.96 SDS) whereas the mid-parental (target) height is 154.2 cm (−1.30 SDS) and had some dysmorphic features including triangular, rather concave facies with long mandible, large hands and feet, and claw toes. There was scanty pubic hair (P2) but no significant breast development.

Question and Answer

1 What is the most likely diagnosis?

An underlying dysmorphic syndrome with overgrowth, learning difficulties, and gonadal impairment would explain the clinical features. Failure of epiphyseal fusion would contribute to the relative tall stature. Investigations showed a bone age of 13.8 years, 46,XX karyotype, elevated FSH and LH, 21.7 and 5.2 units/L, respectively, and hypoplastic uterus with streak ovaries. Treatment with low dose ethinyloestradiol was started to induce puberty, adding in Norethisterone later on. The genetic department was unable to make a specific diagnosis for her underlying syndrome.

Case 4.3

A boy was seen in the dermatology department aged four years with a soft tissue swelling on the forehead. He was noted to be very tall and hence referred to the growth clinic. He was born at 40 weeks' gestation weighing 3.75 kg and was noted to be large from the age of 6 months. His mother's height was 156.8 cm (just below 25th centile), father 182 cm (75–90th centiles). On examination at 4.4 years, the child was extremely very tall – height 128.1 (5.18 SDS), weight 41 kg (5.93 SDS) – and looked more like a seven-year-old than a boy aged four. He was darker-skinned than the rest of the family, prepubertal with 2–3 ml testes, BP 115/70 mm Hg. Fundoscopy showed slight optic nerve pallor on the left.

Questions and Answers

1 What is the most likely diagnosis and what investigations should be done?

Pituitary gigantism is likely. Formal ophthalmology assessment, brain imaging, and an IGF-I level are indicated. The ophthalmologist confirmed the fundoscopic findings, and found slight left visual field constriction with visual acuity 6/9 in the left eye and 6/6 in the right. IGF-I level was elevated at >500 μg/L, GH failed to suppress below 8.6 mu/L after a glucose load, overnight GH profile showed loss of normal pulsatile secretion with failure of GH to fall below 10 mu/L although the highest level was only 55 mu/L, and prolactin was mildly elevated at (600–1300 mu/L). CT scan showed a possible suprasellar tumour. Surgical exploration and biopsy showed that this was a chiasmal and left optic nerve glioma, and histochemistry indicated that it was not secreting any anterior pituitary hormones, including GH.

2 How could a non-secreting optic nerve glioma result in pituitary gigantism?

Subsequent MRI scan of brain showed extension of the glioma into the somatostatin-rich temporal lobes, and it was concluded that the GH excess was secondary to loss of somatostatin modulation of GH releasing hormone.

3 What are the treatment options? What complications of the optic nerve glioma should be pre-empted?

The lesion could not be removed surgically, and radiotherapy was judged undesirable in a child of this age in the absence of progressive visual loss or other pressure effects. The boy was treated with subcutaneous octreotide injections, initially daily, and then monthly when a long-acting preparation became available. His vision was carefully monitored in the ophthalmology clinic and his pubertal status was regularly checked in anticipation of him going into puberty early. Predictably, he developed testicular enlargement (4 ml) at 6.1 years and GnRH test confirmed true puberty, which was treated with long-acting three-monthly GnRH analogue until 11.5 years following which normal puberty ensued. His vision has fortunately remained stable, and his IGF-I normalized on long-acting Octreotide, remaining normal when this was discontinued at 16.5 years. His final height was 191 cm (2.45 SDS) and at 18 years he was referred to the adult clinic for surveillance. Intracranial neurofibromatosis was suspected but not confirmed, biopsy of the subcutaneous frontal skin lesion showing simple fatty tissue rather than a neurofibroma.

Case 4.4

A seven-year-old girl is referred because of tall stature associated with Marfan syndrome. Her maternal grandmother, mother, and maternal aunt are affected, with eye problems but no cardiac involvement. The mother has suffered from cataract due to previously dislocated lenses but is not especially tall – 171.9 cm (1.65 SDS). The father's reported height is 180 cm (0.80 SDS). On examination, the child has long fingers and toes, and a high palate but does not look particularly Marfanoid. Heart examination is normal, blood pressure 100/60. Her height aged 7.3 years is 137 cm (2.69 SDS) and weight 27.4 kg (0.87 SDS).

Questions and Answers

1 Are any genetic or endocrine investigations indicated at this stage?

Genetic studies confirmed a point mutation in exon 3 of the fibrillin gene on chromosome 15 in daughter and father. Bone age estimation at this age is of limited value in giving a guide as to final height, and formal height prediction is not appropriate in a child with a growth disorder, as opposed to normal tall stature. The girl merits cardiac ultrasound which showed mild aortic root dilatation, requiring surveillance, and follow-up of her growth. At 10.9 years the girl measured 160.4 cm (2.48 SD), the bone age was 12.1 years and her pubertal stage was B2P2A1.

2 What are the treatment options?

The options include no treatment, oestrogen therapy to close the epiphyses earlier than usual, and (possibly) somatostatin analogue and GH receptor antagonist. In this case, the family were advised that an adult height of around 180 cm (5′11″) was possible, and they requested treatment. Ethinyloestradiol was given from 11.0 to 16.5 years gradually increasing the dose to 100 µg daily during the first year, decreasing the dose to 50 µg during the second year, and giving Loestrin 30 (containing 30 µg of Ethinyloestradiol) thereafter. Blood pressure was monitored 3-monthly and remained normal, cardiac ultrasound was performed annually and was satisfactory. During the first two years, Norethisterone 5 mg daily for the first five days of each calendar month was also given to induce a monthly bleed. The family were pleased with her final height of 175 cm (2.13 SDS) and she was discharged to long-term cardiac follow-up.

References

Agwu, J., Shaw, N., Kirk, J. et al. (1999). Growth in Sotos syndrome. *Arch. Dis. Child.* 80 (4): 339–342.

Benyi, E., Berner, M., Bjernekull, I. et al. (2010). Efficacy and safety of percutaneous epiphysiodesis operation around the knee to reduce adult height in extremely tall adolescent girls and boys. *Int. J. Pediatr. Endocrinol.* 2010: 740629. https://doi.org/10.1155/2010/740629.

Buckler, J.M.H. (1994). Interpretation of weight. In: *Growth Disorders in Children*, 37–46. London: BMJ Publishing Group.

Carel, J.-C., Blumberg, J., Bougeard-Julien, M.R. et al. (2009). Long-acting lanreotide in adolescent girls with constitutional tall stature. *Horm. Res.* 71: 228–236.

Davies, J.H. and Cheetham, T. (2014). Investigation and management of tall stature. *Arch. Dis. Child.* 99: 772–777. https://doi.org/10.1136/archdischild-2013-304830.

De Waal, W.J., GreynFokker, M.H., Stijnen, T. et al. (1996). Accuracy of final height prediction and effect of growth reductive therapy in 362 constitutionally tall children. *JCEM* 81: 1206–1216.

Hendriks, A.E., Drop, S.L., Laven, J.S. et al. (2012). Fertility of tall girls treated with high-dose estrogen, a dose-response relationship. *JCEM* 97: 3107–3714.

Kalkan Ucar, S., Paterson, W.F., Donaldson, M.D.C., and Young, D. (2009). Ethinyl estradiol treatment for growth limitation in girls with Marfan's syndrome—experience from a single center. *Endocr. Res.* 34 (4): 109–120:https://doi.org/10.3109/07435800903207283.

Katznelson, L., Laws, E.R., Melmed, S. et al. (2014). Acromegaly: an Endocrine Society clinical practice guideline. *JCEM* 99 (11): 3933–3951.:https://doi.org/10.1210/jc.2014-2700.

Loeys, B.L., Dietz, H.C., Braverman, A.C. et al. (2010). The revised Ghent nosology for the Marfan syndrome. *J. Med. Genet.* 47: 476–485.

Pepe, G., Giusti, B., Sticchi, E. et al. (2016). Marfan syndrome: current perspectives. *Appl Clin. Genet.* 9: 55–65: https://doi.org/10.2147/TACG.S96233.

Sotos, J.F. (2014). Sotos syndrome 1 and 2. *Pediatr. Endocrinol. Rev.* 12 (1): 2–16.

Weksberg, R., Shuman, C., and Beckwith, J. (2010). Beckwith-Wiedemann syndrome. *Eur. J. Hum. Genet.* 18: 8–14. https://doi.org/10.1038/ejhg.2009.106.

Wit, J.M., Ranke, M.B., and Kelnar, C.J.H. (eds.) (2007). ESPE classification of paediatric endocrine diagnosis. *Horm Res* 68 (suppl 2): 10–12.

Further Reading

Drop, S.L.S. and de Muinck, Keizer-Schrama, S.M.P.F. (2007). Medical management of tall stature. In: *Growth Disorders*, 2e (ed. C.J.H. Kelnar, M.O. Savage, P. Saenger and C.T. Cowell), 655–666. London: Hodder Arnold.

Patten, M.A. and Rahman, N. (2007). Genetic and dysmorphic syndromes with increased stature. In: *Growth Disorders*, 2e (ed. C.J.H. Kelnar, M.O. Savage, P. Saenger and C.T. Cowell), 281–290. London: Hodder Arnold.

Venn, A., Hosmer, T., Bruinsma, D. et al. (2008). Oestrogen treatment for tall stature in girls: estimating the effect on height and the error in height prediction. *Clin. Endocrin.* 68: 926–929.

Weimann, E., Bergmann, S., and Bohles, H.J. (1998). Oestrogen treatment of constitutional tall stature: a risk–benefit ratio. *Arch. Dis. Child.* 78: 148–151.

Useful Information for Patients and Parents

Child Growth Foundation (CGF) supports families with tall stature and is the umbrella organisation for the Sotos syndrome support group. Website: http://www.childgrowthfoundation.org (accessed 3 October 2018).

The Marfan Association UK provides information and support to patients and families, particularly those in whom the diagnosis has been made recently.

Website: http://www.marfan-association.org.uk (accessed 3 October 2018).

High and Mighty (website: www.highandmighty.co.uk) and Long Tall Sally (website: www.patient.co.uk/support/Long-Tall-Sally.htm) sell clothing and accessories for tall men and women, respectively (accessed 3 October 2018).

5   Puberty

Physiology of normal puberty

Puberty occurs when the secretion of gonadotrophin-releasing hormone (GnRH) by the hypothalamus, which is largely but not entirely suppressed during childhood, increases so that pulsatile secretion of luteinizing hormone (LH) increases, resulting in sufficient sex steroid production to induce secondary sexual development (see Figure 5.1).

In boys
• LH stimulates the Leydig cells to produce testosterone which induces penile growth. Human chorionic gonadotrophin (hCG) has similar structure and action to LH.
• Follicle-stimulating hormone (FSH) binds to receptors on the Sertoli cells, enhancing spermatogenesis.
• Spermatogenesis depends on the complex interaction of various paracrine factors; qualitatively normal spermatogenesis can occur without FSH and LH but production of normal quantities requires gonadotrophins.
• Testosterone modulates LH secretion.
• Inhibin B produced by the Sertoli cells exerts a negative feedback effect on FSH secretion.

• Sex hormone-binding globulin (SHBG) levels fall so that free androgen levels rise.

In girls
• LH stimulates the proliferation of follicular and thecal cells, and during the follicular phase of the menstrual cycle induces androgen secretion by theca cells.
• FSH induces proliferation of granulosa cells; increases expression of LH receptors on granulosa cells; enhances aromatase activity so that androstenedione is converted to oestradiol (E2); and increases progesterone production.
• E2 acts on FSH receptors on the granulosa cells to cause proliferation of the follicular cells, in addition to inducing secondary sexual development and menses.
• Inhibin B is produced by granulosa cells in small antral follicles, inhibin A by large antral follicles and by the corpus luteum. Inhibins may have a role in inhibiting FSH secretion and in dominant follicle selection.
• Ovulation results from interaction of LH, FSH and E2 on the developing primordial follicle (see section 'Clinical aspects of normal puberty').
• SHBG levels decrease only slightly.

Practical Endocrinology and Diabetes in Children, Fourth Edition. Malcolm D.C. Donaldson, John W. Gregory,
Guy Van Vliet, and Joseph I. Wolfsdorf.
© 2019 John Wiley & Sons Ltd. Published 2019 by John Wiley & Sons Ltd.

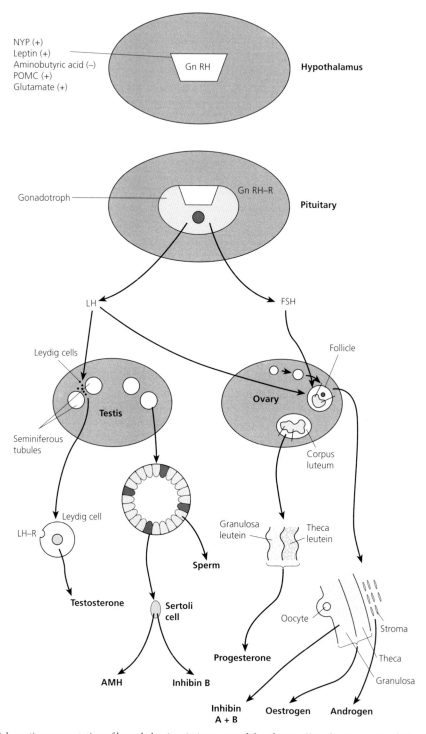

Figure 5.1 Schematic representation of hypothalamic–pituitary–gonadal pathways. (See also Figure 3.4 of Chapter 3). Abbreviations: +, stimulatory effect; −, inhibitory effect; NPY, neuropeptide Y; POMC, pro-opiomelanocortin C; GnRH, gonadotrophin-releasing hormone; LH, luteinizing hormone; FSH, follicle-stimulating hormone; LH-R, luteinizing hormone receptor; AMH, anti-Müllerian Hormone.

In both sexes

• Growth hormone (GH) and insulin-like growth factor (IGF-I) secretion are markedly enhanced because of increased levels of sex steroids and insulin.
• Insulin secretion rises and is accompanied by an increase in insulin resistance.

Physiology of the menstrual cycle

During embryogenesis the primordial germ cells migrate to the ovary and develop into primordial follicles. In the foetus, the pool of primordial follicles reaches a peak of around 7 million germ cells at 20 weeks gestation, falling to 1–2 million at birth, 500000 at menarche, and about 100 at menopause. FSH levels reflect the size of the primordial follicle pool at any given time. Each follicle contains an oocyte arrested in the prophase of the first meiotic division.

Follicular Phase (Approximately 14 Days, but Variable in Duration)

• At the beginning of the menstrual cycle, 15–20 primordial follicles develop, of which only one ultimately develops into a Graafian follicle, the rest becoming atretic.
• On day 1 of the follicular phase, FSH levels increase as a result of decreased inhibition from the falling levels of E2 and progesterone (P) at the end of the previous cycle.
• FSH stimulates the follicles to secrete E2 by increasing androstenedione secretion by the thecal cells and inducing aromatase expression in the granulosa cells. Increasing E2 levels causes a decrease in LH and FSH secretion.
• During this time one follicle emerges as dominant, with more FSH receptors than the others; it therefore recruits more of the diminishing supply of FSH, thus secreting more and more E2.
• At this crucial moment, E2 feedback on the pituitary changes from negative to positive, inducing the preovulatory LH surge.

Luteal Phase (Always 14 Days)

• LH stimulation results in the ovum entering the final phase of first meiotic division to become a secondary oocyte. The follicle swells and ruptures, releasing the ovum into the peritoneal cavity, thence into the Fallopian tube.
• LH induces luteinization of granulosa and thecal cells of the follicle to form the corpus luteum. This results in increased P synthesis; P induces swelling and secretion of the endometrium.

• Progesterone levels peak five to seven days post ovulation, exerting a negative effect on GnRH secretion and cause a decrease in pulse frequency.
• As GnRH pulse frequency falls, FSH and LH secretion decrease, causing the corpus luteum to lose its receptors.
• In the absence of pregnancy, the corpus luteum becomes atretic (corpus albicans), levels of P and E2 fall, and FSH levels start to rise as the new cycle begins.

Onset of puberty

The GnRH-secreting neurons are under the influence of controlling neurons of both an excitatory (glutamate) and an inhibitory (gamma-aminobutyric acid, GABA) nature. In 1999, a paternally imprinted gene was described, encoding Makorin ring finger protein 3 (MKRN3) (Jong et al. 1999). This protein has an inhibitory effect on GnRH secretion which wanes with the onset of puberty.

GnRH neurons are also under the control of glial cells which are excitatory in effect. At the time of puberty, changes in trans-synaptic neurotransmission and glial inputs (such as that provided by prostaglandins released by astrocytes) result in the pulsatile secretion of GnRH and hence the pubertal cascade.

Two points should be noted:
• In girls, the hypothalamus is more prone to 'break free' of suppression than in boys. Thus, idiopathic precocious puberty is more common in girls, and girls exposed to cranial irradiation and with central nervous system (CNS) disorders, such as hydrocephalus, are more prone than boys to develop precocious and early puberty.
• Exposure of the hypothalamus to high levels of sex steroids (e.g. in poorly controlled salt-wasting 21-hydroxylase deficiency) may activate puberty; this phenomenon is known as 'priming'.

Clinical aspects of normal puberty

Pubertal staging

This involves an assessment of breast (B) development in girls, genital (G) development and testicular volume in boys, and pubic (P) and axillary (A) hair development in both sexes. This is the staging system, modified after Tanner and with Tanner's original pictures shown in Figure 5.2.

Breast Staging

B1 Prepubertal
B2 Breast budding (barely visible under a tee-shirt)

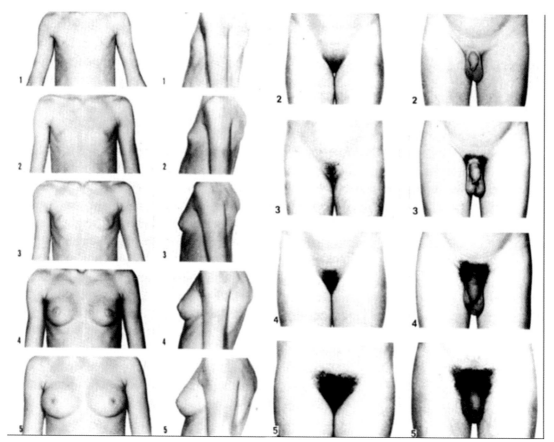

Figure 5.2 Tanner staging showing breast stages 1–5, pubic hair and genital stages 2–5. See text for key to stages (Tanner, 1962).

B3 Development of actual breast mound (NB: in obese girls it can be difficult to distinguish between B1 and B3. Examining the patient in the supine position facilitates this distinction.)

B4 Areola projects at an angle to breast mound; 'a mound on a mound' (NB some girls remain at this stage)

B5 Adult configuration

Genital Staging

G1 Prepubertal penis (unstretched length 2.5–6 cm), scrotum undeveloped and testes ≤3 ml volume

G2 Testes 4 ml scrotal laxity, but no penile enlargement

G3 Penile lengthening and increased mid-shaft diameter with further development of testes and scrotum

G4 Penile lengthening and broadening, further development of the testes (volume usually 10–12 ml)

G5 Adult genitalia, testes usually 15–25 ml

N.B. Testicular volume should be gauged using the Prader orchidometer. The orchidometer allows adolescents who refuse to be examined to self-assess their testicular volume. If an orchidometer is not available, length and breadth can be measured using a paper tape measure and assuming that breadth and depth are the same and employing the formula for a prolate ellipsoid, volume can be calculated as 'length × breadth × depth × π/6.

Penile size (useful for serial staging and important if hypogonadism is suspected) is measured from the base of the penis to tip of the glans (not the foreskin). In obese individuals, it is important to push back the suprapubic fat to obtain the true penile length.

Pubic Hair Staging

P1 No pubic hair

P2 Fine hair over labia or base of the penis

P3 Adult type hair (coarse, curly) but distribution confined to pubis

P4 Extension to near adult distribution

P5 Adult

Axillary Hair Staging
A1 No axillary hair
A2 Hair present but not adult amount
A3 Adult

Milestones of puberty

Boys enter puberty roughly six months later than girls. Mean ages of breast (B) and genital (G) stages in girls and boys with corresponding height velocities including peak height velocity (PHV) are shown in Table 5.1 (girls) and Table 5.2 (boys).

In girls, breast budding is accompanied by acceleration in growth rate with PHV at B2–3 and usually marked deceleration in height velocity after menarche.

In boys, at G2, growth rate is either the same as or slower than at G1. The increase in growth rate coincides with testicular volumes of 8–12 ml.

In both sexes, the age of onset and duration of pubertal development are subject to marked individual variation. Early puberty is associated with a higher PHV, and delayed puberty with a lower PHV.

The 13 cm difference in height between adult males and females relates to the following three factors:
1 The difference in age of PHV – 12 years in girls and 14 years in boys – means that boys have 2 extra years of 'childhood' growth.
2 The intensity of the growth spurt is greater in boys than girls.
3 Boys are slightly taller than girls during the childhood years.

Table 5.1 Mean ages of breast (B) stages in girls with corresponding height velocities including peak height velocity (PHV).

	Age (yr)	Height velocity (cm yr^{-1})
B1	Prepuberty	approx 4–7 from 7 yr
B2	11.2	7
PHV	12.1	8.3 (6.2–10.4).
B3	12.2	8.2
B4	13.1	5
Menarche	13.5	3.6
B5	15.3	?1

Breast budding is accompanied by acceleration in growth rate with PHV at B2–3 and usually marked deceleration in height velocity after menarche.
Source: Data from Tanner and Whitehouse (1976).

Table 5.2 Mean ages of genital (B) stages in boys with corresponding height velocities including peak height velocity (PHV).

	Age (yr)	Height velocity (cm year)
G1	Prepuberty	approx. 4–7 from 7 yr
G2	11.6	5
G3	12.9	6.3
G4	13.8	9.3
PHV	14.0	9.5 (7.2–11.7)
G5	14.9	6.2

At G2 growth rate is either the same as or slower than at G1.
Increase in growth rate coincides with testicular volumes of 6–10 ml.
Source: Data from Tanner and Whitehouse (1976).

Pubertal assessment

Clinical Evaluation
As for short stature examination, this involves meticulous auxology followed by the taking of a focused history and carrying out an appropriate physical examination which includes pubertal staging

Auxology
• Height
• Mid-parental height and target range
• Height velocity

History and Examination
• See Chapter 3 on short stature. Details of pubertal milestones are elicited, including onset of menses and pattern of periods (where applicable).
• Pubertal staging: the importance of following a well-defined procedure.

In the context of current concerns about child and adolescent safe-guarding, it is very important that the clinician approaches the issue of pubertal staging in a sensitive, open and honest manner.

After the history taking and *before* the clinician rises from his/her seat to conduct the examination, the family are informed of the desirability of examining underarm and pubic hair in both girls and boys; breast development in girls; and penis and testicles in boys. The clinician explains to the family why the examination is needed, indicates that this is a matter of good clinical practice, but stresses that it can only be done if the patient and family/carer agree. Where possible, girls should be examined by a trained female member of staff and boys by a trained male staff member (neither of whom need to be medical). Where this is not feasible, a male examiner offers a girl the choice of her mother, or a female nurse as chaperone, while a female examiner offers the choice of a male chaperone or the father. In practice, boys tend to prefer to be examined in privacy (i.e. behind the screen or curtain) but with the parent present in the room.

If the patient is initially unsure or unwilling to be pubertally staged, it is helpful to offer the family some time outside the consulting room to discuss the matter while the clinician sees the next patient. If necessary, examination can be rescheduled for when an appropriate member of staff is able to attend. Self-assessment for pubertal staging has been recommended as an alternative option but we advise against making clinical decisions based on this. In those rare instances where a patient refuses examination by any member of staff, measurement of gonadotrophins and sex steroids will help to indicate if puberty has started.

Diagnostic Imaging

Bone Age
- Useful for documenting the degree of advance or delay in physical maturity; valuable for height prediction in healthy boys and girls with constitutional delay but not in pathological conditions.

Pelvic Ultrasound
- Uterine size, shape, and endometrial thickness reflect the effect of oestrogen.
- Ovarian penile size (useful for serial volumes and the size/number of follicles identified reflect gonadotrophin effect.

Findings should be compared with normative data (e.g. Griffin et al. 1995).

Laboratory Assessment
This is required where there is diagnostic uncertainty and/or when treatment is contemplated. The investigation of puberty may include the following tests:
- Karyotype.
- Basal LH and FSH.
- GnRH, also known as luteinizing hormone-releasing hormone (LHRH) 100 μg intravenous (IV) with LH and FSH sampling at 0, 30, and 60 minutes.
- Serum testosterone/oestradiol.
- SHBG.
- In boys, serum testosterone measurement four days after single subcutaneous (sc) injection of hCG 100 units/kg (maximum 1500 units).

- Measurement of serum androstenedione, 17-hydroxy progesterone (17-OHP) and dehydroepiandrosterone sulphate (DHEAS) together with testosterone or oestradiol basal gonadotrophins are of limited value in diagnosing puberty, but elevation of FSH (10 units/L) indicates primary gonadal failure.
- Prepubertal GRH test shows LH peak <5–7 units/L, with LH response less marked than FSH response.
- A pubertal GnRH test shows LH peak 5–7 units/L, LH response usually > FSH response.
- In countries/centres where GNRH is not available, a basal LH value of ≥0.5 u/L is strongly suggestive of true puberty while values of <0.1 u/L indicate prepubertal status (or pseudoprecocious puberty).
- A prepubertal GnRH test is indistinguishable from central hypogonadism with GnRH or LH and FSH deficiency.

Normative data are shown in Table 5.3.

Sexual precocity

Definitions
Sexual precocity: A general term meaning early sexual development of any kind, with no aetiology implied (Table 5.4).

True central precocious puberty (CPP): CPP is defined as normal puberty, resulting from activation of the hypothalamus, and following a normal sequence, but occurring abnormally early. In the United Kingdom, the age cut-offs are before 8 years in girls and before 9 years in boys.

Any such definition should take account of population norms and demographic change. A study from the United States Pediatric Research in Office Settings network highlighted concern that standard cut-offs for defining precious puberty were outdated and that evaluation of either breast development or pubic hair was indicated, should this occur in white girls aged <7 years and black girls aged <6 years (Kaplowitz and Oberfield 1999). In the United Kingdom, age at menarche has changed little but there is evidence that onset of breast development is earlier. A study by O'Connor showed that age at menarche decreased by 0.30 years between 1948 and 2005, while age at onset of breast development decreased by one year (O'Connor 2013). Since assessment of breast development can be difficult in overweight and obese girls, caution is needed in interpreting data which suggests an increase in the prevalence of female early/precocious puberty.

Table 5.3 Normative data for LH and FSH before (basal) and after (peak) stimulation with 100 µg intravenous LHRH, derived for 85 subjects aged 3–17 years with no evidence of endocrine disease.

	LH (units l^{-1})		FSH (units l^{-1})			
Tanner stage	Basal	Peak	Basal	Peak	Testosterone (nmol l^{-1})^a	Estradiol (pmol/l)^a
			Girls			
B1	0.5 (0.5–2.4)	2.4 (0.5–4.9)	2.0 (0.2–5.0)	12.0 (2.2–26.4)		<50
B2	0.55 (0.5–2.6)	9.7 (1.6–16.4)	3.3 (0.5–8.9)	9.9 (6.8–22.2)		
B3–4	1.6 (0.5–4.8)	23.6 (6.1–50.6)	5.8 (2.5–7.0)	14.3 (12.0–26.7)		
			Boys			
G1	0.5 (0.2–0.5)	2.0 (0.5–5.11)	1.0 (0.2–4.7)	4.4 (1.0–11.6)	<0.3	
G2	1.1 (0.5–2.0)	8.3 (4.4–13.8)	1.7 (0.3–4.2)	2.5 (0.9–11.2)		
G3–5	1.9 (1.9–4.0)	16.6 (10.4–21.1)	3.2 (1.8–10.6)	6.3 (2.8–17.0)		
Adult					8.7–35.0	180–1500

Reference range for testosterone and estradiol is from the Institute of Biochemistry, Glasgow Royal Infirmary.
^{a} To convert testosterone to ng/d and estradiol to pg/m used these conversion factors: testosterone nmol × 28.8 = ng/dL; estradiol pmol/L divide by 3.671 = pg/ml.

Precocious pseudopuberty: Sexual precocity caused by the abnormal secretion of sex steroids independent of hypothalamo–pituitary control.

Thelarche: Isolated breast development, common in infants and preschool children, in the absence of other symptoms and signs of sexual precocity.

Thelarche variant: This term was first used by Richard Stanhope and Charles Brook from London to describe girls in whom thelarche is persistent or slowly progressive, often associated with a moderate increase in height velocity and bone age, and sometimes vaginal bleeding, but the GnRH test shows a prepubertal response (Stanhope and Brook 1990).

Exaggerated adrenarche: In some individuals, adrenarche, a term which refers to the activation of adrenal androgen production normally occurring between six and eight years is associated with sufficient androgen secretion to cause symptoms and signs of sexual precocity. This phenomenon is often mistakenly referred to as 'premature adrenarche' – a term which should be confined to adrenarche occurring before six years of age.

Premature pubarche: A descriptive term simply meaning early onset of pubic hair development which usually occurs in the context of exaggerated adrenarche.

Premature menarche: Cyclical uterine bleeding (confirmed by identifying an endometrial echo on pelvic ultrasound at the time of vaginal bleeding) in the absence of other symptoms and signs of sexual precocity.

Clinical assessment and diagnosis of boys and girls with sexual precocity

Tables 5.4 and 5.5 show the types and causes of sexual precocity in boys and girls. The data illustrate that:
- CPP in girls is usually idiopathic (this is the case in >90% of cases);
- idiopathic CPP is rare in boys;
- precocious pseudopuberty is rare;
- in secondary precocious puberty, the underlying cause is usually self-evident (e.g. known CNS disorder);
- exaggerated adrenarche is more common in girls than boys.

History
The following two key aspects must be addressed:
1 Symptoms relating to sex steroid production.
2 Features suggesting aetiology of sexual precocity.

Symptoms related to sex steroid production

Androgen-Related
- Greasy skin
- Acne
- Greasy hair
- Body odour

Table 5.4 Types of sexual precocity encountered at Royal Hospital for Sick Children, Glasgow, 1989–2009.

	Girls	Boys
Central precocious puberty:		
Idiopathic	122	5
Secondary	39	15
Precocious pseudopuberty	10[a]	9[b]
Exaggerated adrenarche	251	50
Thelarche	104	
Thelarche variant	44	
Isolated premature menarche	29	

[a] Caused by: feminizing adrenal adenoma (1), feminizing ovarian tumour (1), virilizing adrenal adenoma (1), virilizing ovarian tumour (1), McCune–Albright syndrome (2), simple virilizing 21-hydroxylase deficiency (1), 11-hydroxylase deficiency (1), cause unknown (2).
[b] Simple virilizing 21-hydroxylase deficiency (3), gonadotropin-independent precocious puberty (testotoxicosis) (1), virilizing adrenal adenoma (2), Oxymetholone therapy for aplastic anaemia(2), iatrogenic (accidental absorption of paternal testosterone gel) (1)

- Pubic and/or axillary hair
- Enlargement of penis or clitoris
- Deepening of voice
- Increase in growth rate
- Mood swings/behaviour problems
- Aggression

Oestrogen-Related
- Breast tenderness and development (often asymmetrical initially)
- Mood swings/behaviour problems
- Vaginal discharge
- Cyclical vaginal bleeding
  NB Mood swings and behaviour changes are important in deciding whether or not to treat precocious puberty, but must be gauged carefully, and where possible, separated as far as possible from 'normal' difficult behaviour.

Features Suggesting the Cause of Sexual Precocity
- Family history of early puberty.
- Excessive weight gain or obesity in infancy and early childhood.
- International adoption.
- History of headache, vomiting, or visual disturbance (suggestive of intracranial tumour).

Table 5.5 Aetiology of true central precocious puberty (onset ≤8 years in girls and ≤9 years in boys) in 189 patients seen at RHSC, Glasgow, 1989–2009.

	Girls	Boys
Idiopathic	122	5
Cranial irradiation		
ALL	2	0
Medulloblastoma	1	0
Other tumour	1	0
NHL	0	0
Tumour		
Optic nerve glioma (NF)	6 (4)	5 (3)
Craniopharyngioma	1	1
Hypothalamic hamartoma	3	1
Germinoma	0	1
3rd ventricle cyst	1	1
Neurological disorder		
Learning disability +/− epilepsy	8	4
Hydrocephalus/spina bifida	11	1
Tuberculous meningitis	1	0
Cerebral palsy	5	0
Priming		
11-OHD	1	0
SV 21-OHD	1	3
Oxymethalone	0	2
Testotoxicosis	0	1

Abbreviations: ALL, acute lymphoblastic leukaemia; NF, neurofibromatosis; NHL, non-Hodgkin's lymphoma; 11-OHD, 11-hydroxylase deficiency; SV21-OHD, simple virilizing 21-hydroxylase deficiency.

- Perinatal problems including: periventricular haemorrhage with hydrocephalus; low birth weight/small for gestational age.
- Neurological deficit (e.g. cerebral palsy).
- Cranial irradiation.
- Drug therapy, for example oxymetholone (a synthetic androgen used to treat anaemia).

Physical Assessment
- Auxology (see section 'Auxology').
- Pubertal status, including examination of the genitalia in girls with a history suggestive of androgen excess.
- Blood pressure.
- Examination of fundi and visual fields.

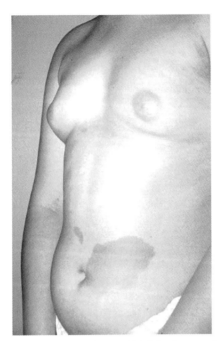

Figure 5.3 Precocious puberty with B4 development in a seven-year-old girl with neurofibromatosis and optic nerve glioma.

- Systemic examination.
- Examination for café au lait patches (seen in neurofibromatosis (Figure 5.3) and McCune-Albright syndrome) and axillary freckling (seen in neurofibromatosis).

Diagnosis and management of sexual precocity in girls

Oestrogen-mediated sexual precocity

True Central Precocious Puberty
Clinical features
In a straightforward case, there will be a history of breast development followed by other features of normal puberty including an increase in growth rate, development of pubic and axillary hair, vaginal discharge, mood swings, and sometimes vaginal bleeding (Table 5.5). Examination will show a girl who looks older than her chronological age, with a height centile above the parental target range and features of normal puberty.

Investigations
- GnRH test to confirm pubertal response – peak LH >5-7 u/L; or basal LH ≥0.5 u/L if GnRH unavailable.
- Serum oestradiol.

- Thyroid function tests, serum and urine steroid measurements in selected cases, where precocious pseudopuberty is suspected.
- Bone age (depending on duration of the process, in CPP, this will often be advanced by ≥2 years).
- Pelvic US (in CPP, the ovaries usually enlarge to above 3 ml in volume and contain multiple (>6) follicles that are >4 mm in diameter and the uterus changes from a tubular type structure to a pear-shaped one with the fundal diameter exceeding that of the cervix. Oestrogenization leads to thickening of the endometrium but menarche does not occur until the endometrial thickness is approximately 6–8 mm.
- Pituitary imaging if CPP confirmed.
- Genetic studies. A study from Boston, USA, showed that of 15 families (40 patients) with CPP, patients of both sexes from five of the families showed the *MKRN3* mutation, which was paternally inherited in all cases (Abreu et al. 2013). This is an important discovery, enabling cases of familial CPP to be confirmed and managed more effectively.

Magnetic resonance imaging (MRI) focusing on the hypothalamic–pituitary area and looking for a tumour or hamartoma is the investigation of choice, since resolution is better than with computed tomography (CT) scanning and MRI does not expose the child to ionizing radiation.

The likelihood of finding a tumour or hamartoma in girls with an onset of puberty between the ages of six to eight years who are otherwise healthy with no neurological symptoms or signs was about 2% in a French study (Chalumeau et al. 2002). Therefore, an MRI may be unnecessary in this group depending on the clinical situation. The younger the child, the greater the chance of finding a cranial lesion with an incidence of 20% when the onset of puberty is <6 years.

Management
The object of treatment is to prevent early epiphyseal closure with compromise in final height, and to alleviate psychosocial problems in the child and family. In some cases, the pubertal manifestations will remain static or even regress and no treatment will be necessary. In other cases, because the child's age is borderline (i.e. seven to eight years) and the family is coping well or because the progress of puberty is very slow, treatment may not be indicated. Some families do not wish to have treatment that they perceive as interfering with the natural course of events, especially if the CPP is familial.

- If treatment is to be undertaken, the drug of choice is a GnRH analogue which, when given in pharmacological doses, initially leads to a brief initial period of stimulation but is then followed by down-regulation of the GnRH receptors, thus inhibiting LH and FSH secretion and leading to a fall in their levels in two to four weeks. Available preparations are:

- Goserelin 3.6 mg sc monthly or long-acting preparation giving 10.8 mg sc three-monthly.
- Leuprorelin 3.75 mg sc or intramuscular (im) monthly (half this dose is sometimes used in children <20 kg) or long-acting preparation 11.25 mg sc or im three-monthly.
- Triptorelin 3.75 mg sc or im monthly (a smaller dose is given in those <30 kg, an additional single injection is given on day 14 of treatment), or long-acting preparation giving 11.25 mg im. This is the only medication licensed in the United Kingdom for the treatment of CPP.

A withdrawal bleed can occur in the first four weeks following the start of treatment due to an initial agonist effect of GnRH analogue and by the fall in the oestrogen levels. Provided that families are warned of this possibility, there is usually no need to give pre-emptive treatment. However, in selected cases, patients can be treated with cyproterone acetate, starting three days before and continuing for the first two weeks after giving GnRH analogue.

Occasionally treatment can be associated with headaches and menopausal symptoms such as hot flushes. Local problems such as erythema and sterile abscesses at the injection site may also sometimes occur.

Rarely, the CPP is secondary to a tumour in the hypothalamic–pituitary area. In such cases, the histology determines the prognosis. Gliomas tend to be more aggressive than astrocytomas whereas hamartomas are benign. Treatment of the causal lesion usually has no effect on the course of puberty. Hypothalamic hamartomas should not be removed surgically to treat the precocious puberty since this can be treated with GnRH analogues. However, hamartomas causing mass effect or gelastic seizures (epileptic fits characterized by laughing) may require surgical management.

Follow-up

Treatment can be expected to prevent or stop menses, to improve mood swings, and to decrease height velocity. Usually, treatment maintains the patient at the same pubertal stage as at diagnosis although occasionally there may be a small reduction in breast size. The parents should be told that treatment does not reverse adrenarche so that pubic hair may continue to develop. In a minority of girls, puberty continues to progress and in those the monthly preparation of GnRH analogue can be given three-weekly, or the three-monthly preparation can be given 9–10-weekly.

The child should initially be seen three-monthly for clinical assessment and auxology, and then six-monthly once the symptoms have largely settled and the tempo of puberty is clear. Some centres perform regular pelvic ultrasounds and gonadotrophin measurement but we believe that clinical symptoms, breast development stage, and growth rate are better reflections of pubertal status. Bone age should be performed annually.

In girls with very slowly progressive CPP, there will be little impact on final height. Many girls with untreated CPP reach a final adult height within the adult reference range. However, these heights may be towards the lower end of the reference range with final heights of 151–155 cm being not uncommon. Final height in treated girls with CPP will depend on when puberty started and when treatment was commenced. Data on final height suggests that treatment does not fully recover lost height potential and children often do not attain their mid-parental height, possibly because the growth spurt suppressed by treatment does not resume when treatment is stopped. In one study of girls treated till an average age of 11 years, the mean adult height was 160 cm.

The timing of stopping GnRH therapy should be discussed with the family. We have found that menses occurs approximately 12–18 months after discontinuing the injections. This has led us to recommend stopping therapy in the middle to end of the last year of primary school so that menses usually start during the first year of secondary school. Families whose girls have learning disabilities may wish to continue treatment for longer but suppressive therapy beyond 11–12 years of age carries the theoretical risk of preventing normal calcium accretion by the skeleton, and so we are reluctant to continue beyond this age.

Psychological sequelae of precocious puberty

A large cohort study from the US has shown an important link between early menarche and subsequent problems with depression during and beyond adolescence, and anti-social behaviour (Mendle et al. 2018). The authors of this study highlighted the importance of follow-up beyond the paediatric age range.

It is evident that the mental health of girls with CPP has tended to be overlooked in the past, with too much focus on diagnosis and medical treatment. Awareness of the psychological vulnerability of these girls is important in pre-empting and managing emotional problems.

Precocious Pseudopuberty: Feminizing

The diagnosis is suspected when there is progressive feminizing precocity associated with a prepubertal GnRH test or more often undetectable LH and FSH throughout the test (see Table 5.4). Causes include adrenal adenoma, granulosa cell tumour of the ovary, and McCune–Albright syndrome. The last disorder may present with breast development and vaginal bleeding in a girl with café au lait patches and bony symptoms or signs on X-ray. Rarely, severe and protracted primary hypothyroidism results in cross-reaction between elevated thyroid-stimulating hormone (TSH) levels and gonadotrophin receptors, leading to breast development and vaginal bleeding (Van Wyk and Grumbach 1960).

Investigations

Serial imaging of the ovaries by pelvic ultrasound, adrenal ultrasound, and CT, urine steroid analysis in selected cases, GnRH test, measurement of the tumour markers – α foeto-protein and β hCG – and a skeletal survey may be required.

Treatment

Surgery is the treatment of choice for adrenal and ovarian tumours. Medical treatment for precocious pseudopuberty is directed at restricting or antagonizing sex steroid production. Useful agents include the following:
- Androgen receptor blockers – Cyproterone acetate, Flutamide, and Spironolactone
- 5α-reductase inhibitors – Finasteride
- Testosterone biosynthesis inhibitors – Ketoconazole
- Aromatase inhibitors – Testolactone, Anastrozole, Letrozole

Secondary true puberty resulting from priming of the hypothalamus will require additional GnRH therapy.

NB: Experience with these agents in the management of sexual precocity is necessarily limited because of the rarity of the conditions concerned. These medications should therefore be prescribed only by specialist centres.

Thelarche
Clinical features

Premature thelarche is usually seen in preschool girls (Figure 5.4). Sometimes the breast development has been present from birth. More commonly, the mother notices breast development, often asymmetrical and with a tendency to wax and wane, from the age of 6–12 months. There are no other features of sexual precocity and height

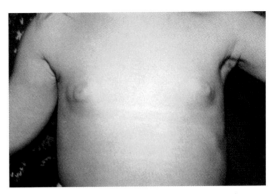

Figure 5.4 Premature thelarche with Tanner stage 3 breast development.

velocity is normal. The bone age and pelvic ultrasound are consistent with chronological age.

Investigations

Bone age and pelvic ultrasound may be waived in mild cases of premature thelarche. In more florid cases, these together with an GnRH test should be performed. The FSH response is often pronounced, with 30- or 60-min. values of up to 25 units/L while LH values are below 4 units/L. Plasma oestradiol is usually unrecordable using standard assays.

Treatment

None is required.

Follow-up

Three- or four-monthly clinic visits over a one-year period to confirm that breast development is static or regressing.

Thelarche variant

Girls with thelarche variant are usually between five and eight years of age and present with breast development which persists and may progress slightly in association with slight increase in height velocity and modest advance in bone age. Vaginal bleeding sometimes occurs. Pelvic ultrasound may show an oestrogen effect on the uterus, but is less marked than for CPP. Ovaries may show some enlargement with an increase in follicular activity.

Diagnosis

Thelarche variant is diagnosed in the context of persistent but mildly progressive sexual precocity in conjunction with a prepubertal GnRH test, modest bone age advance and uterine development, normal imaging of the adrenal glands, and an indolent clinical course. Thelarche variant probably includes a variety of conditions including CPP that is too mild to be detected on the GnRH test, and subtle alterations in responsiveness of the ovaries to normal prepubertal LH and FSH levels.

Management

Usually, no treatment is required but the girls must remain under surveillance and undergo serial auxology, pubertal staging, and pelvic ultrasound examination. Rarely, girls may show unacceptable progression of symptoms and signs so that treatment is requested. Under these circumstances, specialist referral is recommended. Peripheral antagonists, such as cyproterone, may be tried.

Premature Menarche

This condition occurs in girls usually between four and eight years of age in whom cyclical vaginal bleeding occurs in the absence of other features of sexual precocity. The diagnosis is made by identifying an endometrial echo on pelvic ultrasound when the child is experiencing vaginal bleeding.

Diagnosis

It is essential not to diagnose premature menarche unless the above criteria are satisfied and other causes of vaginal bleeding have been excluded. These include recurrent vulvovaginitis, foreign body, child sexual abuse, other causes of trauma, and vaginal tumours (e.g. rhabdomyosarcoma).

Investigations

Pelvic ultrasound examination is usually sufficient but an GnRH test may be required if there is any suspicion of symptoms other than vaginal bleeding.

Treatment

No hormone treatment required.

Follow-up

Three- to four-monthly review to confirm normal auxology and no development of other features of sexual precocity.

Androgen-mediated sexual precocity

Exaggerated Adrenarche
Clinical features

This is by far the most common cause of androgenicity in girls, and presents from six years of age with a history of body odour, greasy skin and hair, weight gain, and sometimes mood disturbance, usually in association with some pubic and/or axillary hair development. The distribution of the pubic hair is characteristic over the labia majora rather than the mons pubis.

Diagnosis

Adrenarche must be distinguished from simple virilizing and non-classical 21-hydroxylase deficiency, and androgen-secreting tumours of the adrenal glands or ovaries. This is usually easy on clinical grounds as the symptoms and signs of adrenarche are relatively mild and in particular there is no clitoromegaly. Bone age may be advanced by one year, sometimes more if obesity is an accompanying feature.

Investigations

In all but the mildest cases, blood should be taken for serum testosterone, androstenedione, 17-OHP and DHEAS (see Chapter 8 for normal values), preferably at 8 a.m. to detect mild 21-hydroxylase deficiency. If baseline androgens are elevated or clinical features are particularly marked, then further investigation with a standard Synacthen test and adrenal imaging are indicated to exclude non-classical congenital adrenal hyperplasia (CAH) or an adrenal tumour.

Treatment and follow-up

No treatment is required. If the serum androgens show a mild elevation, particularly of androstenedione and DHEAS, then one further clinic visit in four to six months to confirm normal growth rate and lack of progressive virilization is sufficient before discharge. Although a link between exaggerated adrenarche and low birth weight/smallness-for-gestational age and subsequent hyperandrogenism (e.g. polycystic ovary syndrome [PCOS]) has been described (Ibáñez et al. 1998), the majority of girls examined in Scotland were of normal birth weight and clinical features of androgen excess were mild (Paterson et al. 2010). We do not normally, therefore, recommend long-term follow-up in these patients.

Precocious Pseudopuberty: Virilizing

Simple virilizing 21-hydroxylase deficiency is suggested by the combination of advanced growth, clitoromegaly, pubic/axillary hair development and bone age advance, especially if the girl is younger than six years (see Table 5.4). Virilizing tumours of the adrenal or ovary are suggested by a shorter history, so that features such as tall stature have not usually had time to become manifest (Figure 5.5).

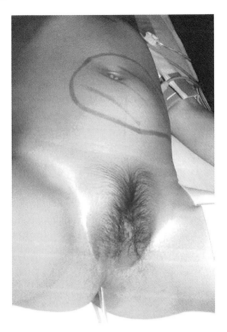

Figure 5.5 Virilizing ovarian tumour (outline shaded on skin) causing pubic hair and clitoromegaly in a three-year-old girl.

Investigations

Measurement of serum testosterone, 17-OHP, androstenedione, and DHEAS under basal conditions and in selected cases after stimulation with Synacthen will demonstrate any abnormalities in serum androgens. Urine steroid analysis and/or molecular studies may be required to help identify an adrenal enzyme defect. Adrenal MRI or CT may be required as well as careful evaluation of the ovaries on ultrasound. If, despite imaging, a tumour cannot be identified, then selective venous sampling from the adrenal veins should be carried out at a specialist centre.

Treatment and monitoring

Simple virilizing 21-hydroxylase deficiency is discussed in Chapter 8. Virilizing tumours of the adrenal glands and ovaries are treated surgically.

Follow-up

This involves three- to four-monthly assessment to oversee regression of the features of sexual precocity and a normal growth rate. Depending on availability, MRI (preferable), CT scanning or ultrasound scanning of the adrenals or ovaries should be performed annually. Long-term follow-up is needed to pre-empt the development of CPP because of priming.

Diagnosis and management of sexual precocity in boys

Androgen-mediated sexual precocity

True Central Precocious Puberty

This condition is rare in boys, and its occurrence must prompt a search for an underlying cause (Figure 5.6) (see Table 5.5). The prevalence of a brain tumour in boys is 40–90%. Clinical symptoms include rapid growth rate, behaviour disturbances, a deepening of the voice, and enlargement of the genitalia. Examination will demonstrate symmetrical enlargement of the testes to volumes ≥4 ml.

Diagnosis

The combination of sexual precocity with bilateral testicular enlargement makes the diagnosis of CPP in boys easy. If the testes are prepubertal in volume and/or asymmetrical, the causes of precocious pseudopuberty must be sought (see section 'Precocious pseudopuberty').

Investigations

A GnRH test to confirm true puberty, with measurement of serum testosterone, followed by imaging of the hypothalamic–pituitary area by MRI. The tumour markers – β hCG and α foetoprotein should be measured to detect germinomas.

Treatment

Treatment is with a GnRH analogue as described for girls with CPP. Any underlying cause should be treated.

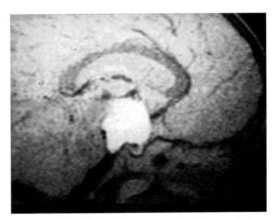

Figure 5.6 Hypothalamic hamartoma in a six-year-old boy, causing gelastic seizures and central precocious puberty.

Monitoring

This is as for CPP in girls. In cases where no brain tumour is found on initial imaging, serial imaging at 6–12-monthly intervals for a 2–3-year period is required to detect an evolving lesion. Testicular size can be expected to diminish and genital development may show some regression. There should also be a reduction in any aggressive behaviour and in the number of erections.

Precocious Pseudopuberty

Simple virilizing 21-hydroxylase deficiency will result in excessive androgen secretion from the adrenal glands (see Table 5.4). Adrenal tumours may be androgen-secreting. In the testes an activating LH receptor mutation affecting all the Leydig cells (germline) causes a condition known as gonadotropin-independent precocious puberty ('testotoxicosis'). An activating LH receptor mutation affects only a single cell (somatic) and results in a Leydig cell tumour (Figure 5.7). Precocious pseudopuberty may be seen in boys receiving the anabolic steroid Oxymetholone which exerts a direct androgenic effect (as well as priming the hypothalamus and causing true precocious puberty).

Common to all these rare conditions are testes that are either prepubertal in volume (in the case of adrenal disorders or an exogenous cause), modestly and symmetrically enlarged (i.e. 3–4 ml in testotoxicosis and hCG-secreting tumours), or unilaterally enlarged with contralateral atrophy (in Leydig cell tumours). By contrast, in CPP, both testes are at least 4 ml in volume.

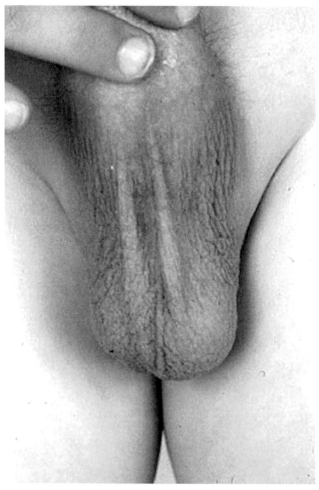

Figure 5.7 Leydig cell tumour causing slight enlargement of left testis with contralateral atrophy, and precocious pseudopuberty in a five-year-old boy.

Investigations

The GnRH test will show suppressed LH and FSH values in precocious pseudopuberty unless the primary disorder has activated the hypothalamus. Investigations of the underlying cause may include β-hCG and α-foetoprotein measurement; serum testosterone, 17-OHP, androstenedione, and DHEAS before and, in selected cases, following Synacthen stimulation; urine steroid analysis; testicular ultrasound; and adrenal MRI or CT.

Treatment

Surgery is the treatment of choice for tumours. Medical treatments include Ketoconazole, Cyproterone, Testolactone, and Flutamide.

Adrenarche

Adrenarche is less common in boys than girls, but is still the most common cause of androgenicity. The clinical diagnosis, investigations, and management are as for girls.

Oestrogen-mediated sexual precocity

Feminizing tumours of the adrenal glands and testes are extremely rare. Gynaecomastia, caused either by enhanced oestrogen production from aromatization of testosterone at puberty, or by increased tissue sensitivity to normal circulating oestrogen levels, is a relatively common problem in boys and is discussed below.

Delayed puberty and pubertal failure

Definitions and classification

Delayed puberty: This is arbitrarily defined as absence of signs of secondary sexual development in a girl aged 13 years or a boy aged 14 years. A more practical and helpful definition is delay in the onset, progression or completion of puberty sufficient to cause concern to the adolescent, parents, or physician.

Absent or arrested puberty: Puberty that either does not begin, or having begun, does not progress (in which case the term 'mid-pubertal arrest' is often used).

Delayed menarche: First period after 15 years.

Primary amenorrhoea: Failure of periods to begin.

Secondary amenorrhoea: Cessation of established periods.

Oligomenorrhoea: Infrequent periods (e.g. occurring > every 35 days or < 4–9 per year).

Delayed puberty be classified simply as *central* or *peripheral*, depending on whether the site of the problem lies in the hypothalamo–pituitary axis or in the gonads. Central delayed puberty can be further subdivided into *delay with intact hypothalamo–pituitary axis*, and *delay caused by impairment of the hypothalamo–pituitary axis*. Table 5.6 gives a working classification of delayed puberty and its causes.

Clinical assessment of boys and girls with delayed puberty

Almost all boys and most girls with delayed puberty have simple constitutional delay in growth and adolescence (CDGA). In pathological delayed puberty, the cause may be obvious from the past medical history. The challenge is to diagnose the occasional case of pathological delay in puberty in which the cause is not evident, and the more complicated cases with a multifactorial aetiology (e.g. constitutional, nutritional, social).

History

• *Growth pattern*. The history of long-standing short or borderline short stature followed by a widening gap in height status between the patient and peer group from secondary school entry onwards is suggestive of CDGA.

• *General health*. An enquiry should be made for any symptoms of chronic ill-health. Asthma may be associated with delayed puberty, especially when inhaled steroids have been used.

• *Features/associations with gonadal impairment*. These include a previous history of cryptorchidism, orchidopexy, and gonadal irradiation. An idea of sense of smell can be determined by asking if the adolescent can smell toast burning or unpleasant odours such as rotten eggs.

• *Family patterns*. An enquiry should be made concerning age at menarche in the mother and delayed growth spurt/voice breaking in the father or continued growth after completion of high school. Where applicable, the pubertal milestones of siblings should be sought.

• *Social and educational aspects*. A tactful enquiry as to the occupation and lifestyle of the family may indicate social disadvantage. The presence of learning disability is established by asking about the need for learning support in mainstream or special education. Learning disability may be a component of

Table 5.6 Classification of delayed and abnormal puberty (including delayed/absent menarche).

Central (both sexes)

Intact H–P axis	CDGA Chronic systemic disease Poor nutrition (including anorexia nervosa) Psychosocial deprivation Steroid therapy Hypothyroidism
Impaired H–P axis	Tumours adjacent to H–P axis • Craniopharyngioma • Optic glioma • Germinomas, astrocytomas, • prolactinoma Congenital anomalies • Septo-optic dysplasia • Congenital hypopituitarism Irradiation • Pituitary tumour/optic glioma • Craniospinal axis for medulloblastoma Trauma • Surgery, e.g. for craniopharyngioma • Head injury GnRH/LH/FSH deficiency • Congenital (genetic or idiopathic) • Kallmann syndrome • Prader–Willi syndrome • Laurence–Moon–Bardet–Biedl syndrome

	Boys	*Girls*
Peripheral	Bilateral testicular damage • Cryptorchidism • Failed orchidopexy with testicular atrophy/necrosis • Atresia • Torsion Syndromes associated with cryptorchidism • Noonan's • Prader–Willi • Laurence–Moon–Bardet–Biedl Disorders of sex development (DSD) • Klinefelter and other aneuploidy syndromes (normal pubertal timing but incomplete testicular growth) • Other forms of 46,XY DSD Irradiation/chemotherapy • Testicular irradiation • Total body irradiation • Cyclophosphamide	Disorders of sex development • Turner syndrome • Pure gonadal dysgenesis • 46,XY DSD (including CAIS) Irradiation/chemotherapy • Ovarian irradiation (e.g. with Wilms' tumour) • Total body irradiation • Cyclophosphamide, Polycystic ovary syndrome Toxic damage Galactosaemia Other metabolic diseases (notably mitochondrial) • Thalassaemia

Abbreviations: CAIS, complete androgen insensitivity syndrome; CDGA, constitutional delay in growth and adolescence; FSH, follicle-stimulating hormone; GnRH, gonadotrophin-releasing hormone; H–P, hypothalamo–pituitary; LH, luteinizing hormone.

dysmorphic syndromes associated with delayed puberty (e.g. Noonan syndrome).

Examination
- Height, weight
- Measured or (much less reliable!) reported parental heights
- Measured or reported sibling heights
- Pubertal staging
- Nutrition
- Dysmorphic features
- General examination with particular attention to:
  - clubbing;
  - blood pressure;
  - fundi.

Investigations
(If indicated.)
- Bone age
- Karyotype
- Basal FSH and LH and serum oestradiol/testosterone
- Serum prolactin
- Pelvic ultrasound in girls
- GnRH test
- Serum testosterone four days after hCG 100 units kg (max 1500 units)
- Urinalysis for blood and protein
- Test of sense of smell

Causes of delayed or absent puberty and pubertal failure

Central delay with intact axis

Constitutional Delay in Growth and Adolescence in Boys
By far the most common cause of delayed puberty, CDGA is usually easily diagnosed by the history of long-standing short/borderline short stature during childhood. Following secondary school entry at 11 years, there is a decline in height status so that the boy becomes relatively shorter for age. Commonly, there is a family history of delayed puberty. Frequently, the boy expresses distress to his parents, sometimes related to teasing, but more often because of discomfort at being small and young-looking for age. There is frequently embarrassment about taking showers at school. In boys of 13 years and over, the testes usually show some enlargement (4 ml), but no penile enlargement (i.e. Tanner stage G2).

Diagnosis
CDGA should usually be a positive diagnosis and not one of exclusion. However, the presence of possible contributory factors such as poor nutrition, socio-economic and psychological difficulties, and chronic ill health (e.g. severe asthma) can render assessment difficult. Endocrine disturbance is suggested when the boy is not short or borderline-short; when the short stature and delayed puberty are out of context with the family pattern; when the testes are undescended or abnormal; when there are symptoms and signs such as headache or optic atrophy suggestive of craniopharyngioma; or when penis and testes are hypoplastic, especially in association with impaired sense of smell (Kallmann syndrome).

Investigation
None is necessary in CDGA except for bone age estimation which usually shows delay.

Management
The boy should be reassured that he is normal, simply a late developer. Prediction of adult height is helpful, providing that a single experienced observer performs the bone age assessment. The following medical treatments can be offered to enhance growth rate and expedite the features of puberty without affecting final height outcome:
- In boys aged 11.5–13.5 years, Oxandrolone 1.25–2.5 mg at night for three to six months may be helpful in maintaining a reasonable prepubertal height velocity (4–6 cm per year). Occasionally, such treatment may increase the height velocity to 6–7 cm per year. However, this treatment is now not available in many countries.
- In boys over 13.5 years of age, testosterone therapy may be offered. This can be given as Sustanon 100 mg or Testosterone enanthate 125 mg intra-muscularly once a month for three months, as testosterone cypionate or enanthate 50 mg intra-muscularly monthly for six months, or as testosterone undecanoate 40 mg orally daily for three months. As indicated in Chapter 3, such treatment simply accelerates growth and puberty, without influencing adult height (Kelly et al. 2003). Treatment should only be given if the clinician is confident that the delay in puberty is physiological, and not a manifestation of underlying disease (e.g. Crohn's disease).

Follow-up
Six-monthly visits to the clinic may be helpful in reassuring untreated boys. Boys treated with Oxandrolone or testosterone should be seen six-monthly for two visits following treatment to ensure satisfactory progress. Occasionally, a repeat course of testosterone is indicated. If there is any doubt about the diagnosis of

CDGA, it is prudent to keep the boy under observation until testicular volumes are 10 ml.

Constitutional Delay in Growth and Adolescence in Girls

CDGA in girls is less common than in boys but remains the most common cause of delayed puberty (Figure 5.8). Characteristically, the tempo of puberty, when it starts, is slower and a gradual increase in height rather than a discernible adolescent growth spurt is observed (Figure 5.8).

Diagnosis

CDGA in girls must be distinguished from Turner's syndrome as well as other pathological causes of delayed puberty. In doubtful cases, the chromosomes and basal gonadotrophins should be checked and a pelvic ultrasound performed. It should be noted that failure to identify one, and occasionally both, ovaries may occur in normal girls.

Treatment

In contrast to boys, who can be given a sizeable dose of testosterone with no ill effect on final height, oestrogen therapy in girls is both less effective and more likely to cause premature epiphyseal closure.

Occasionally, pubertal delay is so marked and growth rate so slow that there is a need for treatment. In these circumstances, GH levels should be measured. Daily ethinyloestradiol 2 µg for a 1–2-year period can be given, with concurrent GH administration if stimulation testing shows GH insufficiency.

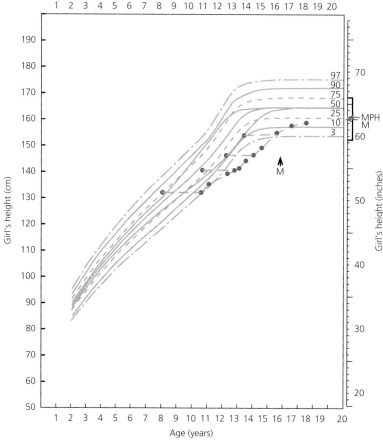

Figure 5.8 Growth chart of girl with delay in growth and adolescence showing attenuated and late growth spurt with menarche at 15 years of age. Final height is equal to the mid-parental height (MPH). M, menarche.

Delayed puberty caused by chronic disease

Sometimes the chronic disease is obvious, and the child is referred simply to confirm that no other pathology is responsible and to advise as to possible treatment. The clinician must assess the severity of the chronic disease and confirm that the severity of the delay in growth and adolescence matches the severity of the chronic condition. If this is not the case, then further investigation is indicated.

A small proportion of girls and boys presenting with delayed puberty will be found to have chronic disease as the underlying cause. Gastrointestinal conditions, such as coeliac disease and Crohn's disease, can be notoriously silent. The following screening investigations are of value in selected cases:
- Thyroid function test (TFT), LH and FSH, cortisol, prolactin (screening for endocrine disease).
- Full blood count (FBC), ferritin, red cell folate, erythrocyte sedimentation rate (screening for gastrointestinal disease).
- IgA tissue transglutaminase antibodies (screening for coeliac disease).
- Creatinine, urea and electrolytes, calcium, phosphate, alkaline phosphatase, urinalysis and culture, renal ultrasound (screening for renal disease).
- Chromosomes in girls.

Impairment of the hypothalamo–pituitary–gonadal axis in boys

Central

Some adolescents have clear evidence of damage to the hypothalamo–pituitary axis (e.g. craniopharyngioma) and will clearly not enter or complete puberty without treatment (see Table 5.6). Adolescents with delayed puberty who do not fulfil the criteria of CDGA pose some difficulty, for the GnRH test cannot distinguish between physiological central delay and true GnRH or gonadotrophin deficiency.

A history of impaired sense of smell, testicular maldescent and/or surgery and assessment of academic performance must be sought. Examination includes a search for dysmorphic features, systemic examination, and detailed examination of the external genitalia. Investigations are detailed above.

Management

In doubtful cases, it is best to induce puberty with testosterone from the age of 13–14 years onwards until either full secondary sexual development has occurred or spontaneous testicular development to 10 ml has taken place (indicating intact endogenous gonadotrophin secretion). If spontaneous testicular enlargement has not occurred by the age of 16–18 years, replacement therapy should be discontinued and the gonadal axis fully re-evaluated.

Peripheral

Table 5.6 classifies delayed or abnormal puberty. Primary hypogonadism is suggested by the combination of:
- history compatible with testicular injury (bilateral cryptorchidism, testicular surgery, testicular irradiation, total body irradiation, bilateral torsion);
- behaviour and learning difficulties (suggestive of an underlying syndrome, e.g. Klinefelter);
- abnormal genital examination with one or both testes cryptorchid or abnormally small;
- testicular volumes which are inappropriate for genital and pubic hair stage (e.g. 4 ml testes in the context of G4, P4, as in Klinefelter syndrome).

Investigations

These will show elevated FSH (above 10 units/L). An hCG test may show impaired testosterone rise, or no rise in severe cases.

Management

Anorchic subjects will clearly require therapy, as will individuals with arrested secondary sexual development, particularly if testosterone levels are low with poor response to hCG. By contrast, boys with low testicular volumes but normal genital and pubic hair development and acceleration of linear growth will not require treatment. As with central hypogonadism, it is best to treat doubtful cases pre-emptively rather than waiting, which carries the risk that development may not progress satisfactorily, resulting in distress to the patient.

Treatment of Hypogonadism

The available treatments for delayed puberty and hypogonadism in males in the United Kingdom are summarized in the British Society for Paediatric Endocrinology and Diabetes guidelines (El-Khairi et al. 2016).

Intramuscular preparations include:
- Sustanon 250 which contains a mixture of testosterone proprionate (30 mg), phenylproprionate (60 mg), iso-caproate (60 mg) and decanoate (100 mg) = 250 mg/ml;

- Sustanon 100 = 100 mg/ml;
- testosterone enanthate 250 mg/ml;
- testosterone undecanoate (Nebido) 1000 mg/4 ml.
  The oral preparation is:
- testosterone undecanoate (Restandol) 40 mg capsules.
  Other preparations include:
- Testogel 1% transdermal preparation and Striant SR, a buccal preparation. Paediatric experience with these is limited although early experience with Testogel in pubertal induction is encouraging (Chioma et al. 2018).

Pubertal induction

The following regimen will bring about satisfactory secondary development in hypogonadal boys over three years:
- Sustanon 125 mg (half a 250 mg ampoule) every six weeks for the first year.
- Sustanon 125 mg every four weeks for the second year.
- Sustanon 250 mg every four weeks for the third year.

Maintenance treatment

Nebido 1 g intramuscularly every 12 weeks, modifying the dose according to clinical response, is an effective treatment for maintaining secondary sexual development in hypogonadal males. The injection is given by the family practitioner or nurse and renders compliance/adherence less of a problem than with oral replacement. The large 4 ml volume of the preparation may be best given as 2 ml into each buttock rather than a single injection and some adults prefer monthly Sustanon 250 mg rather than the larger three-monthly injection.

An alternative to intramuscular testosterone is oral testosterone undecanoate 40 mg per day for the first year, 80 mg per day for the second year and 120 mg per day thereafter.

Impairment of the hypothalamo–pituitary–gonadal axis in girls

Central

The causes of hypothalamic and pituitary gonadotrophin deficiency in girls are similar to boys, although isolated GnRH and gonadotrophin deficiency are rarer. Investigations will show low LH and FSH levels and management is as for boys.

Peripheral

Gonadal dysgenesis as a result of Turner syndrome or iatrogenic damage from total body irradiation are the main causes of primary gonadal failure in girls.

Investigation

Basal FSH and LH will be elevated in frank ovarian failure, with FSH values of ≥ 10 u/L indicating significant impairment. A GnRH test may be required to demonstrate milder germ cell damage. Anti-Müllerian hormone (AMH) is secreted by the granulosa cells of the ovary in girls and serves as an index of ovarian reserve (Visser et al. 2013), values of <0.05 ng ml (<0.36 pmol/L) indicating absence of ovarian tissue. Pelvic ultrasound may show a less-developed uterus than would be expected from the pubertal stage, while ovaries may be small or unidentifiable.

Management

In doubtful cases, pubertal induction should be offered from 12 to 13 years.

Treatment

Pubertal induction

It is important for oestrogen replacement to be gradual, not only to avoid premature fusion of the epiphyses, but also to prevent unsightly overdevelopment of the areolae of the breast. Until recently the three-year oral induction regime most commonly used in the United Kingdom used Ethinyl estradiol, giving 2 µg per day for the first year, 4 µg per day for the second year and then 6, 8 and 10 µg per day during the third year, in four-monthly steps.

Recent consensus statements have recommended a more physiological approach with transdermal rather than oral oestrogen for pubertal induction (Gravholt et al. 2017) and the use of natural 17β-estradiol rather than synthetic oestrogens (Matthews et al. 2017). The oral and transdermal regimens proposed by Matthews et al. are given in Tables 5.7 and 5.8.

Table 5.7 Regimen for pubertal induction using 25 µg/24 hours of 17β-estradiol matrix patches applied once or twice weekly and left in situ for three to four days.

Monday to Thursday	Friday to Sunday	Duration (mo)
¼ patch:	No patch	6
¼ patch	¼ patch	6
½ patch	¼ patch	6
½ patch	½ patch	6
1 patch	1 patch	6

Source: Reproduced from Matthews et al. (2017) with kind permission from *Archives of Disease in Childhood*.

Table 5.8 Regimen for pubertal induction using 1 mg 17β-estradiol tablets.

Dose	Tablets	Frequency	Equivalent daily dose	Duration (mo)
0.5 mg	½	Alternate days	0.25 mg	12
0.5 mg	½	Daily	0.5 mg	6
0.5 mg/1 mg	½, 1	Alternate days	0.75 mg	6
1 mg	1	Daily	1 mg	6

Source: Reproduced from Matthews et al. (2017) with kind permission from *Archives of Disease in Childhood*.

Progesterone is usually introduced in the final 12 months of induction. It is important not to start this treatment too soon, in order to maximize the time for uterine and breast development. When breakthrough bleeding occurs, therefore, a pelvic ultrasound examination should be carried out. If the uterus is under-developed with a thin endometrium, then progesterone treatment should be postponed; but started if adequate uterine development with a thick endometrium is demonstrated. Preparations include Norethisterone 5 mg, Utrogestan 200 mg, and medroxyprogesterone acetate 5 mg, all given orally once daily for the first 12 days of each calendar month.

Postpubertal maintenance
Following successful pubertal induction, maintenance treatment is required. Administration of a low-dose combined contraceptive pill, e.g. Loestrin 20 (21 days on and 7 days off) is convenient but has the disadvantage of rendering the patient untreated with oestrogen for three months of the years.

A more physiological approach is to administer either oral 17β-estradiol 2–3 mg daily or twice-weekly transdermal 17β-estradiol for days 1–25 of each calendar month, adding in a progesterone preparation for days 12–14, to mimic the natural cycle (Christin-Maître 2017). Post induction oestrogen replacement should always be given in consultation with a gynaecology, reproductive endocrine, or adult endocrine colleague. It is very important for late adolescent/early adult patients to be carefully counselled concerning the benefits and the importance of good adherence to hormone replacement, since this affects not only sexual but bone, cardiac, and mental health.

Other pubertal disorders

Prolactinoma

Prolactin-secreting pituitary adenomas are rare in childhood and adolescents. They are classified according to size into microadenomas (≤10 mm diameter) and macroadenomas (>10 mm diameter). Clinical features may be endocrine-related, the high prolactin levels causing galactorrhoea, gynaecomastia, and primary or secondary amenorrhoea; related to tumour mass with headache and visual field defect; or to both hormonal and mass effects. Prolactin levels are usually markedly above the reference range of <440 mIU/L (<25 μg/L) in women and <350 mIU/L (<20 μg/L) in men; a study of 26 children and adolescents showed median (range) prolactin 94 (70–500) μg/L in 11 patients with microadenoma and 720 (145–3300) μg/L in 15 with macroadenoma (Colao et al. 1998). Milder hyperprolactinaemia may be associated with stress and with anti-psychotic medication. Treatment of prolactinoma is with the dopamine agonist Cabergoline, starting at 0.25 mg weekly and increasing depending on the response of prolactin levels and tumour size, is now the treatment of choice. Bromocriptine 1.25 mg nightly increasing to 2.5 mg twice daily can also be used. The usual shrinkage of tumours and excellent biochemical control with these agents means that other treatments such as surgery and radiotherapy are rarely needed and reserved for refractory cases. Patients should be managed jointly with an experienced adult endocrinologist.

Menstrual problems
The most common complaint is that of irregular, prolonged, and heavy uterine bleeding, sometimes associated with considerable discomfort. This is related to immaturity of the hypothalamic–pituitary–ovarian axis and to anovulatory cycles after onset of the menses, and should be considered a normal phenomenon during the first two years following menarche. Maintaining a menstrual diary will help assess the severity of the problem. Usually, no treatment is required other than simple analgesia such as mefenamic acid. The antifibrinolytic drug, tranexamic acid, can also be used during episodes of bleeding to

diminish blood loss. However, the symptoms may be severe and affect schooling and further treatment may be required.

The following strategies may help:

• Medroxyprogesterone 10 mg per day for the first 5–10 days of menstrual bleeding. This medication may not stop the acute bleeding episode but should produce a normal bleeding episode following withdrawal. It acts by stopping endometrial cell proliferation and allowing organized sloughing of the cells following withdrawal. It will lead to regular cyclic withdrawal bleeding until the hypothalamic–pituitary–ovarian axis has matured.

• Low-dose contraceptive pill such as Loestrin 20 for a 6–12-month period.

Prior to prescribing the above two medications, hypertension and a family history of deep vein thrombosis should be excluded. Caution should also be exercised in patients with epilepsy and liver dysfunction.

In cases of severe and frequent dysfunctional uterine bleeding and when bleeding is so heavy that it is accompanied by clots, one should consider undiagnosed underlying causes such as von Willebrand's disease. An FBC to exclude anaemia and thrombocytopaenia, and iron and coagulation studies may be required. Dietary advice and iron supplements may also be required.

If there is no improvement in the dysmenorrhoea, alternative diagnoses such as endometriosis or obstruction of the lower genital tract should be considered and the patient should be seen by a gynaecologist.

Amenorrhoea and oligomenorrhoea are commonly seen as part of normal delayed puberty, and are particularly likely to occur in the context of a low body mass caused by extreme physical training, poor nutrition, and eating disorders, such as anorexia nervosa. It is rare for girls to start their periods if their body weight is <40 kg. A minimum of three to four periods a year are required to ensure adequate oestrogenization and to minimize the risk of osteoporosis. If the patient has a completely normal physical examination with secondary amenorrhoea, consider administering medroxyprogesterone, 10 mg once daily for 5 to 10 days to diagnose anovulation as the cause of the amenorrhoea and to see if a withdrawal bleed will occur (progesterone challenge test). If bleeding occurs, then adequate levels of endogenous oestrogen and a normal anatomy can be inferred.

Primary amenorrhoea is seen in girls with absent puberty, anatomical disorders of the reproductive tract (e.g. imperforate vagina or Rokitansky syndrome, in which there is congenital absence of the uterus and some or all of the vagina) and in the syndrome of complete androgen insensitivity (see Chapter 7).

Investigation

None is required where the history and examination indicate the diagnosis. Pelvic ultrasound assessment and blood samples for chromosomes, gonadotrophins, and sex steroids are helpful in selected cases.

Hirsutism and hypertrichosis

There is an overlap between hirsutism (inappropriate/excessive hair growth in androgen-dependent sites such as moustache and beard area, chest, etc.) and hypertrichosis (generalized increase in body hair).

Hirsutism may be seen in the following instances:

• certain ethnic groups, for example Mediterranean, Indian subcontinent;

• caused by androgen secretion by ovarian or adrenal tumours and adrenal enzyme disorders;

• as part of the PCOS;

• idiopathic, presumably caused by increase in end-organ sensitivity.

Hypertrichosis may be seen in the following instances:

• certain ethnic groups as for hirsutism;

• primary hypothyroidism;

• Cushing's syndrome, especially iatrogenic;

• certain dysmorphic syndromes;

• secondary to drugs such as diazoxide and cyclosporin A;

• idiopathic.

Diagnosis and Management

Androgen excess can be gauged by accompanying features such as tall stature, bone age advance, clitoromegaly, etc. PCOS is suggested by accompanying oligomenorrhoea and/or obesity.

Investigations

These are unnecessary if the hirsutism is mild and the cause obvious (e.g. racial). In selected cases, investigations should be performed as for PCOS.

Treatment

Treatment is directed at the underlying cause, and where this is not possible, cosmetic strategies include bleaching of facial hair, removal of hair by electrolysis, and referral to a dermatologist for consideration of laser treatment.

Polycystic ovary syndrome

Endocrine Society guidelines from the USA continue to support the diagnosis of PCOS being made in the presence of two out of three key criteria (Legro et al. 2013). These are:

- ovulatory dysfunction with oligo-ovulation or anovulation;
- androgen excess;
- polycystic ovaries.

The latter are defined according to the Rotterdam consensus criteria (2004) as at least one ovary with either 12 or more follicles of 2–9 mm diameter and/or a volume of >10 ml in an ovary with no dominant follicle >10 mm, and after exclusion of other causes of androgen excess or related disorders. Ovaries are often bilaterally enlarged with peripheral distribution of the follicles and an increased in stromal density.

PCOS may occur in postmenarcheal teenagers and, very occasionally, in premenarcheal girls. The clinical features of PCOS include obesity, hirsutism, greasy skin and hair, acne, oligo/amenorrhoea, and subfertility.

Polycystic ovaries are not a prerequisite for the diagnosis of PCOS, and are found in approximately 25% of normal women. Laboratory features include elevated serum androgens (particularly testosterone, free testosterone, and androstenedione), LH hypersecretion (with an LH to FSH ratio of 3 : 1 or more), and hyperinsulinism with low SHBG levels. Frequently, only some of the clinical and laboratory features are present.

PCOS can be regarded as a disease complex which is heterogeneous in nature and in which there is no single underlying cause. Insulin resistance and consequent hyperinsulinaemia in association with obesity are commonly seen in women with PCOS but some patients are slim. The frequent association of PCOS with obesity may have a cumulative deleterious effect on glucose homeostasis through hyperinsulinaemia, with an increased prevalence of type 2 diabetes. Ovarian hyperandrogenism results from the action of high insulin levels on the insulin receptor; cross-reaction with the IGF-1 receptor; and synergism with LH hypersecretion. Hyperinsulinaemia also decreases the synthesis of SHBG, leading to an increase in circulating free testosterone. Genetic and environmental factors contribute to the development of PCOS, affecting women from South Asia more severely, with an increased risk of type 2 diabetes.

Diagnosis and management

In a girl with a history suggestive of PCOS, investigations are directed at confirming the diagnosis and excluding conditions such as non-classical CAH and other causes of hyperandrogenism. The full investigation of PCOS with the exclusion of CAH consists of:

- pelvic ultrasound;
- basal LH, FSH, and oestradiol;
- serum testosterone, SHBG, androstenedione, and DHEAS;
- 17-OHP (if 8.00 a.m. 17-OHP is raised, a standard Synacthen test [250 μg] is indicated to exclude non-classical CAH due to 21-hydroxylase deficiency);
- fasting glucose, insulin, HbA1c, cholesterol, and triglycerides;
- TFTs.

Testosterone levels are elevated in PCOS but levels of >5.0 nmol l^{-1} are unusual and suggest an androgen-secreting tumour of the adrenal gland or ovary. An MRI should rule out adrenal pathology and the pelvic ultrasound should have ruled out an ovarian tumour. DHEAS and androstenedione levels are also often elevated. Thyroid dysfunction can lead to amenorrhoea and hirsutism.

Treatment

Mild cases do not require treatment, nor do girls with polycystic ovaries but who are not showing any features of the condition. The cornerstone of non-medical management in obese individuals is weight reduction (by dietary measures and exercise) which reduces the hyperinsulinism and the risk of type 2 diabetes.

Medical treatment is directed at the hyperinsulinaemia and hyperandrogenism. Metformin is used in hyperinsulinaemic girls, especially in the context of obesity. It increases insulin sensitivity and may help to regulate periods. Periods can be regulated with the oral contraceptive pill which will also aid the skin problems. In those with hirsutism, the combination of an oestrogen with an anti-androgen will help combat signs of androgen excess as well as regulating periods. Dianette which contains the anti-androgen cyproterone and ethinyloestradiol and the newer combined contraceptive pill Yasmin which contains drosperidone and ethinyloestradiol can help in this regard. Both preparations have been linked with depression and should not be used lightly. It is important to manage PCOS in collaboration with an adult endocrine physician or a gynaecologist experienced in the field. PCOS is associated with psychological morbidity and an impaired quality of life, and referral to a psychologist or psychiatrist may be indicated.

Breast problems

Breast problems can be divided into gynaecomastia in boys and either asymmetrical or symmetrical smallness or largeness of breast size in girls.

Boys with Gynaecomastia

Apparent gynaecomastia results from an unfortunate emphasis in fat distribution towards the breast area, particularly in obese boys. Exaggerated breast development at puberty is the most common cause of true gynaecomastia in boys. This is usually mild, and transient. More severe gynaecomastia is fortunately less common and almost always idiopathic (Figure 5.9). Normal genital and testicular development should be verified. In severe or doubtful cases, chromosomes for Klinefelter syndrome, basal gonadotrophins, and serum oestradiol should be checked. Occasionally, drugs (prescribed, such as spironolactone, or recreational, such as cannabis) will cause gynaecomastia.

Treatment

If gynaecomastia is severe and causing distressing problems (see Figure 5.9), for example, the boy will not participate in physical activities or have showers in front of his peers, then plastic surgery referral is indicated with a view to mammary reduction by either liposuction or subareolar incision and removal of excess tissue.

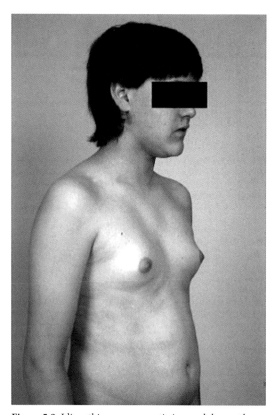

Figure 5.9 Idiopathic gynaecomastia in an adolescent boy.

Girls with Asymmetrical or Symmetrical Smallness or Largeness of Breasts
Symmetrical enlargement

Occasionally, breast size is unacceptably large to the girl and family, in which case referral to a plastic surgeon for consideration of reduction mammoplasty is indicated.

Symmetrical smallness

Girls with delayed puberty will have smaller breasts than their peers and can be reassured accordingly. Poor breast growth may occur in girls who have received chest irradiation for cancer (e.g. lung metastases). Once optimal breast size has been attained by waiting for endogenous puberty to complete, or by oestrogen administration in girls with gonadal failure, referral for augmentation mammoplasty should be discussed with the family. If there is reluctance to inject foreign material, such as silicone, into the breasts of teenage girls on the part of the plastic surgeon, then reconstructive surgery should be considered.

Asymmetrical largeness or smallness

Asymmetrical breast development is very common in the early stages of puberty, particularly in girls with sexual precocity. Occasionally, postpubertal girls present with an unacceptable discrepancy in breast size. Investigation is unhelpful and referral to a plastic surgeon is indicated for either reduction mammoplasty on one side or augmentation mammoplasty on the other.

Future developments

- The role of the *MKRN3* gene in precocious puberty will become better defined as more centres look for mutations in their patient populations.
- Transdermal regimens for oestrogen induction and maintenance of puberty are likely to become more widely used. A previous UK survey showed that the oral contraceptive pill was still the most common form of maintenance replacement in adolescents and young adults with Turner syndrome (Gault and Donaldson 2009). A further survey to assess changes in practice is now due.
- Assessment of bone, uterine, and cardiac health in adolescents and young adults requiring sex steroid replacement will be carried out more systematically before and after pubertal induction. The use of dual

X-ray absorptiometry (DXA), MRI of pelvis and cardiac MRI is likely to increase.

• There is interest in offering males with central hypogonadism, who have completed pubertal induction with testosterone, therapy with LH and FSH to increase testicular volume and thereby facilitate fertility at a later stage.

• The psychological assessment and counselling of children with sexual precocity; and adolescents/young adults with hypogonadism and infertility are important areas for further development.

Potential pitfalls

• Girls with apparent breast development in association with weight gain, tall stature, and pubic hair may be considered to have precocious or early puberty when the actual diagnosis is that of exaggerated adrenarche in association with simple obesity (causing increased growth rate) and giving the impression of true breast development. Pelvic ultrasound is useful in showing a prepubertal uterus, but a GnRH test may be required to clarify the diagnosis in some cases.

• Failure to carry out adequate pubertal staging in boys, to spare the patient embarrassment, causing diagnostic error.

Controversial points

• What is the preferred option for the hormonal treatment of CDGA in boys?

• What hCG regimen (dose, number of injections, and time scale) should be used in the gonadal assessment of boys?

• What hormonal treatment can be offered to girls with CDGA?

• Optimal regimens for inducing and maintaining puberty in both sexes.

When to involve a specialist centre

• Girls with sexual precocity when
  • the diagnosis is unclear; or
  • treatment is contemplated.
• All boys with sexual precocity.
• Hypogonadism in both sexes.
• PCOS.
• Primary and secondary amenorrhea

Case histories

Case 5.1

A seven-year-old girl presents with breast enlargement and slight vaginal discharge, together with moodiness and body odour. There is no relevant past history and she is well with no headaches, visual disturbance, or polydipsia. Her mother and two elder sisters had early menarche at 10–11 years. At the age of 7.8 years, the girl looks more like an 11-year-old and bone age is advanced at 10.8 years. Height is on the 90th centile and mid-parental height on the 50th centile. Examination shows Tanner stage B3, P2, A1. Pelvic ultrasound shows heart/pear-shaped uterus with 4-mm endometrial echo, uterine length 5 cm. Ovaries are 3.5 ml in volume with 5–6 6 mm follicles in each. GnRH test shows basal/stimulated values of 2.6/20 units/L for LH, and 3.2/15 units/L for FSH.

Question and Answer

1 What is the diagnosis, what further investigations should be carried out, and what treatment should be offered?

This girl has central (true) precocious puberty – onset of pubertal development before the age of eight years in a girl with a pubertal GnRH test. Idiopathic CPP is the likeliest cause but it is now regarded as good practice to carry out pituitary imaging with MRI in girls as well as boys with CPP. Given the age of the girl, the intensity of pubertal tempo and the behaviour disturbances, most clinicians would recommend suppressive therapy with an GnRH analogue but this must be carefully discussed with the family.

Case 5.2

A boy of 14 is referred with short stature and concern over pubertal development. He is a somewhat reticent historian but systematic inquiry reveals a fall-off in school attendance and performance over the past year. Further questioning indicates that he has been experiencing some diarrhoea and abdominal pain. On examination, the boy does not look unwell, but weight has dropped from 42 kg at clinic three months ago to 39.2 kg now. Height at 138 cm is below the 3rd centile (mid-parental height 25th centile).

There is mild finger clubbing. The testes are enlarged (4 ml) with scrotal laxity but prepubertal penis and no pubic or axillary hair. Examination is otherwise unremarkable, blood pressure 110/70. Bone age is delayed at 11.2 years.

Question and Answer

1 What is the pubertal stage in this boy? What is the clinical diagnosis? What (if any) investigations should be carried out. What treatment should be offered?

The pubertal stage is Tanner stage G2, P1, A1. While physiological delay in puberty is by far the most common cause of short stature and delayed puberty in boys, the vague abdominal symptoms, poor school performance, and finger clubbing suggest that the boy should be investigated for chronic disease. A barium meal and follow-through showed extensive abnormality in the small bowel, particularly the terminal ileum and the diagnosis of Crohn's disease was subsequently confirmed.

This case illustrates the importance of history taking and general examination in endocrine practice. It would be inappropriate to carry out a height prediction on this boy, whose delayed puberty was caused by illness. Successful treatment of the underlying disease, rather than testosterone therapy, is indicated here.

Case 5.3

A girl of 14 years is seen in the joint oncology/endocrine clinic with concern over delayed menarche. She developed acute lymphoblastic leukaemia aged 10 years, relapsed 18 months after treatment and was successfully managed with autologous bone marrow transplantation. Total body irradiation in the dose of 1400 cGy and cyclophosphamide were given as part of her conditioning pre-transplant. On examination, she is on the 25th centile for height (mid-parental height 75th centile), Tanner stage B3, P3, A2. Pelvic ultrasound shows a cylindrical uterus measuring 3.2 cm with no endometrial echo, ovaries 1.2 and 1.8 ml in volume with no follicles seen. Basal FSH is 58 units/L, LH 20 units/L, oestradiol <50 pmol/L.

Question and Answer

1 What is the diagnosis, what further data are required, and how should this girl be managed?

This girl has primary ovarian insufficiency caused by total body irradiation, resulting in mid-pubertal arrest. Pelvic ultrasound shows reduced uterine size and immature configuration attributable to oestrogen insufficiency. She will require oestrogen replacement, but before instituting this, her bone age and stimulated GH level should be tested. Bone age was 11.6 years and peak GH level 14 mU/L following insulin hypoglycaemia. Treatment with GH therapy was declined by the girl and her family but she agreed to starting low-dose ethinyloestradiol aiming for a full replacement dose within 18 months.

Case 5.4

A 15-year-old girl presents to the emergency department with heavy periods. Her general practitioner (GP) has done an FBC which has shown haemoglobin of 5.2 g/dL with a normal white cell and platelet count. Her periods started at the age of 11 years and are regular at 4 weekly intervals but are heavy with some clots. She says she feels a little tired. She has no bleeding or bruising elsewhere and there is no family history of heavy periods or bleeding disorders. She is otherwise well. The family are vegetarians. On examination, she looks pale. Respiratory rate is 20/min and her chest is clear. Pulse rate is 96/min and there is a grade 2/6 ejection systolic murmur heard loudest to the left of the sternal edge. There is no hepatomegaly and there are no other cardiac signs.

Questions and Answers

1 What is the likeliest cause of the heart murmur?

The likeliest cause of the heart murmur is anaemia which can lead to a hyperdynamic circulation and a subsequent flow murmur. In the absence of any cardiological symptoms and any other cardiac signs, it could be kept under review as it is likely to disappear once anaemia has resolved.

2 What investigations should be performed?

A ferritin, and in the appropriate racial groups, a haemoglobinopathy screen, should be performed. This girl's ferritin was low at 12 ng/ml (normal range 20–300 ng/ml) due to heavy bleeding (the presence of clots denotes heavy bleeding) and her vegetarian diet. A clotting screen should also be done to try and rule out conditions such as von Willebrand's disease. However, the absence of heavy periods in her mother and bleeding disorders in the family makes this diagnosis unlikely. A pelvic ultrasound would also be useful to confirm that the reproductive organs are normal. A gynaecological opinion would also be helpful.

3 What treatment should be instituted?

Although she is severely anaemic, she has no significant symptoms. Her respiratory and pulse rate are within normal limits and she is not in heart failure. The onset of anaemia is likely to have been slow over several months. A blood transfusion is therefore not indicated and iron tablets should be prescribed. She does not eat meat which is the best dietary source of iron, but green vegetables and cereals are also good sources. Tranexamic acid (an antifibrinolytic agent) can also be used on the days when there is bleeding to diminish the blood loss. If heavy periods persist, then a low dose contraceptive pill could be used to decrease the bleeding.

References

Abreu, A.P., Dauber, A., Macedo, D.B. et al. (2013). Central precocious puberty caused by mutations in the imprinted gene MKRN3. *N. Engl. J. Med.* 368 (26): 2467–2475. https://doi.org/10.1056/NEJMoa1302160.

Chalumeau, M., Chemaitilly, W., Trivin, C. et al. (2002). Central precocious puberty in girls: an evidence-based diagnosis tree to predict central nervous system abnormalities. *Pediatr.* 109 (1): 61–67.

Chioma, L., Papucci, G., Fintini, D., and Cappa, M. (2018). Use of testosterone gel compared to intramuscular formulation for puberty induction in males with constitutional delay of growth and puberty: a preliminary study. *J. Endocrinol. Invest.* 41 (2): 259–263. https://doi.org/10.1007/s40618-017-0726-7.

Christin-Maitre, S. (ed.) (2017). Use of hormone replacement in females with endocrine disorders. *Horm. Res. Paediatr.* 87: 215–223. https://doi.org/10.1159/000457125.

Colao, A.M., Loche, S., Cappa, M. et al. (1998). Prolactinomas in children and adolescents. clinical presentation and long-term follow-up. *J. Clin. Endocrinol. Metab.* 83: 2777–2780. https://doi.org/10.1210/jcem.83.8.5001.

El-Khairi R, Shaw N, Crowne EC (2016) Testosterone replacement therapy: BSPED Clinical Committee Clinical Guideline. BSPED. https://www.bsped.org.uk/media/1375/testosteronereplacementguideline.pdf (accessed 13 October 2018).

Gault, E.J. and Donaldson, M. (2009). Oestrogen replacement in Turner syndrome: current prescribing practice in the UK. *Clin. Endocrinol.* 71: 752–755.

Gravholt, C.H., Andersen, N.H., Conway, G.S. et al. (2017). Clinical practice guidelines for the care of girls and women with Turner syndrome: proceedings from the 2016 Cincinnati International Turner Syndrome Meeting. *Eur. J. Endocrinol.* 177 (3): G1–G70. https://doi.org/10.1530/EJE-17-0430.

Griffin, I.J., Cole, T.J., Duncan, K.A. et al. (1995). Pelvic ultrasound measurements in normal girls. *Acta Paediatr.* 84: 536–543.

Ibáñez, L., Potau, N., Francois, I., and de Zegher, F. (1998). Precocious pubarche, hyperinsulinism, and ovarian hyperandrogenism in girls: relation to reduced fetal growth. *J. Clin. Endocrinol. Metab.* 83 (10): 3558–3562.

Jong, M.T., Gray, T.A., Ji, Y. et al. (1999). A novel imprinted gene, encoding a RING zinc-finger protein, and overlapping antisense transcript in the Prader-Willi syndrome critical region. *Hum. Mol. Genet.* 8 (5): 783–793.

Kaplowitz, P.B. and Oberfield, S.E. (1999). Reexamination of the age limit for defining when puberty is precocious in girls in the United States: implications for evaluation and treatment. Drug and Therapeutics and Executive Committees of the Lawson Wilkins Pediatric Endocrine Society. *Pediatr.* 104: 936–941.

Kelly, B.P., Paterson, W.F., and Donaldson, M.D.C. (2003). Final height outcome and value of height prediction in boys with constitutional delay in growth and adolescence treated with intramuscular testosterone 125 mg per month for 3 months. *Clin. Endocrinol.* 58: 267–272.

Legro, R.S., Silva, A., Arslanian, S.A. et al. (2013). Diagnosis and treatment of polycystic ovary syndrome: an Endocrine Society Clinical Practice Guideline. *J. Clin. Endocrinol. Metab.* 98: 4565–4592.

Marshall, W.A. and Tanner, J.M. (1969). Variations in pattern of pubertal changes in girls. *Arch. Dis. Child.* 44: 291–303.

Marshall, W.A. and Tanner, J.M. (1970). Variations in the pattern of pubertal changes in boys. *Arch. Dis. Child.* 45: 13–23.

Matthews, D., Bath, L., Högler, W. et al. (2017). Hormone supplementation for pubertal induction in girls. *Arch. Dis. Child.* 102 (10): 975–980. https://doi.org/10.1136/archdischild-2016-311372.

Mendle, J., Ryan, R.M., and KMP, M.K. (2018). Age at menarche, depression, and antisocial behavior in adulthood. *Pediatr.* 141 (1): e20171703. https://doi.org/10.1542/peds.2017-1703.

O'Connor C (2013) Female pubertal development in the United Kingdom: trends in onset, progress and duration from 1948 to the present. Thesis, Durham University. http://etheses.dur.ac.uk/10620 (accessed 10 October 2018).

Paterson, W.F., Ahmed, S.F., Bath, L. et al. (2010). Exaggerated adrenarche in a cohort of Scottish children: clinical features and biochemistry. *Clin. Endocrinol.* 72 (4): 496–501.

Stanhope, R. and Brook, C.C. (1990). Thelarche variant: a new syndrome of precocious sexual maturation? *Acta Endocrinol.* 123 (5): 481–486.

Tanner, J.M. (1962). *Growth at Adolescence*, 2e. Oxford: Blackwell.

Tanner, J.M. and Whitehouse, R.H. (1976). Clinical longitudinal standards for height, weight, height velocity, weight velocity and stages of puberty. *Arch. Dis. Child.* 51: 170–179.

Van Wyk, J.J. and Grumbach, M.M. (eds.) (1960). Syndrome of precocious menstruation and galactorrhea in juvenile hypothyroidism: an example of hormonal overlap in pituitary feedback. *J. Pediatr.* 57,: 416–435.

Visser, J.A., Hokken-Koelega, A.C., Zandwijken, G.R. et al. (2013). Anti-Müllerian hormone levels in girls and adolescents with Turner syndrome are related to karyotype, pubertal development and growth hormone treatment. *Hum. Reprod.* 28 (7): 1899–1907.

Rotterdam ESHRE/ASRM-Sponsored PCOS Consensus Workshop Group (2004). Revised 2003 consensus on diagnostic criteria and long-term health risks related to polycystic ovary syndrome (PCOS). *Hum. Reprod.* 19: 41–47.

Styne, D.M. and Grumbach, M.M. (2016). Physiology and disorders of puberty. In: *Williams Textbook of Endocrinology*, 13e (ed. S. Melmed, K.S. Polonsky, P. Reed Larsen and H.M. Kronenberg), 1074–1218. Philadelphia, PA.: Elsevier.

Tsilchorozidou, T., Overton, C., and Conway, G.S. (2004). The pathophysiology of polycystic ovarian disease. *Clin. Endocrinol.* 60 (1): 1–17.

Useful Information for Patients and Parents

The UK Child Growth Foundation, www.childgrowthfoundation.org, publishes 15 growth disorder booklets including Constitutional Delay of Growth and Puberty (http://www.childgrowthfoundation.org/CMS/FILES/10_Constitutional_Delay_of_Growth_and_Puberty.pdf) and Premature Sexual Maturation (http://www.childgrowthfoundation.org/CMS/FILES/04) (accessed 13 October 2018).

Turner Syndrome Support Society (TSSS) https://tss.org.uk publishes information on puberty, hormone replacement, and adult care (accessed 13 October 2018).

European Society of Paediatric Endocrinology publishes information booklets (https://www.eurospe.org/patients/english-information-booklets) in English, French, Italian, Spanish, and Turkish on topics including precocious puberty and delayed puberty (accessed 3 October 2018).

Further Reading

Bulun, S.E. (2016). Physiology and pathology of the female reproductive axis. In: *Williams Textbook of Endocrinology*, 12e (ed. S. Melmed, K. Polonsky, P. Reed Larsen and H.M. Kronenberg), 590–663. Elsevier.

Carel, J.C., Eugster, E.A., Rogol, A. et al. (2009). Consensus statement on the use of gonadotropin-releasing hormone analogs in children. *Pediatr.* 123 (4): e752–e762.

Griffen, J.E. and Wilson, J.D. (1998). Disorders of the testes and male reproductive tract. In: *Williams Textbook of Endocrinology*, 9e (ed. J.D. Wilson, D.W. Foster, H.M. Kronenberg and P. Reed Larsen), 819–876. Philadelphia, PA: W.B. Saunders.

Herman-Giddens, M.E., Slora, E.J., Wasserman, R.C. et al. (1997). Secondary sexual characteristics and menses in young girls seen in office practice: a study from the Pediatric Research in Office Settings network. *Pediatr.* 99 (4): 505–512.

6 Thyroid Disorders

Embryology, anatomy, and physiology of the thyroid gland

Embryology and anatomy

The thyroid gland develops from the floor of the pharynx at four weeks gestation in the form of a diverticulum which travels caudally leaving the thyroglossal tract in the neck. The latter normally disappears but cystic remnants may remain and form a thyroglossal cyst. The diverticulum becomes bi-lobed and fuses with the ventral aspect of the fourth pharyngeal pouch. By 10 weeks gestation, the gland has a butterfly-shaped structure with its two lobes connected by the isthmus.

The genetic mechanisms controlling thyroid organogenesis are incompletely understood but four transcription factors NKX2-1 (TTF1), FOXE1 (TTF2), PAX8, and HHEX are known to be involved from 20 days post-fertilization onwards. Integrity of the thyroid stimulating hormone receptor (TSHR) is also known to affect thyroid development since bi-allelic loss-of-function mutations results in thyroid hypoplasia.

Physiology

The main function of the thyroid gland is to synthesize thyroxine (T4) and triiodothyronine (T3).

Control of thyroid metabolism

The hypothalamus secretes thyrotropin-releasing hormone (TRH), which stimulates the anterior pituitary to secrete thyroid stimulating hormone (TSH). TSH acts on the thyroid follicular cell by binding to a specific receptor (TSHR) as shown in Figure 6.1. The occupied receptor activates the G stimulatory protein, which then stimulates the thyroid metabolism via the adenylate cyclase, calcium, and phospholipase C pathways.

T4 synthesis

Figure 6.2 shows the main steps in T4 synthesis. Dietary iodine is actively transported into the follicular cells by the sodium iodide symporter (NIS) and from the cells to the colloid by Pendrin and other apical transporters. Iodine is oxidized to iodide by thyroid peroxidase (TPO). The hydrogen peroxide (H_2O_2) required for this process is generated by the dual oxidase 2 enzymes (DUOX2 and DUOXA2). Tyrosyl residues on the thyroglobulin molecule are then iodinated to form monoiodotyrosine (MIT) and diiodotyrosine (DIT). MIT and DIT are coupled to form T3 and T4. Iodide is recycled from uncoupled MIT and DIT by iodotyrosine dehalogenase. Inactivating mutations at any of these steps result in dyshormonogenesis. The thyroid gland is the sole

Practical Endocrinology and Diabetes in Children, Fourth Edition. Malcolm D.C. Donaldson, John W. Gregory, Guy Van Vliet, and Joseph I. Wolfsdorf.
© 2019 John Wiley & Sons Ltd. Published 2019 by John Wiley & Sons Ltd.

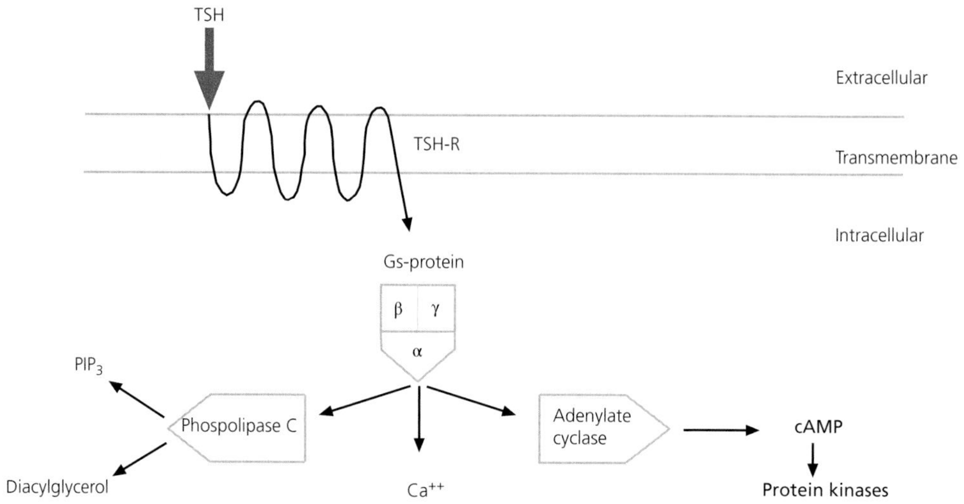

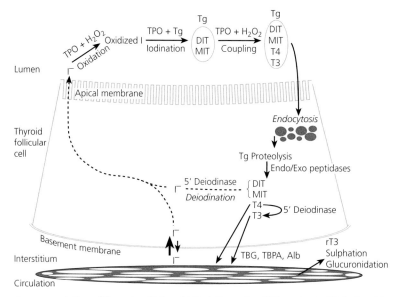

Figure 6.1 Schematic representation of TSH receptor, TSHR, and intracellular pathways. Gs-protein, G stimulatory protein; PIP_3, phosphatidyl inositol triphosphate.

Figure 6.2 Schematic representation of thyroxine (T4) and triiodothyronine (T3) synthesis. TPO, thyroid peroxidase; H_2O_2, hydrogen peroxide; Tg, thyroglobulin; MIT, monoiodotyrosine, DIT, diiodotyrosine; TBG, thyroxine binding globulin; TBPA, thyroid binding pre-albumin; Alb, albumin; rT3, reverse T3. ↑ refers to the sodium iodide symporter (NIS).

producer of T4, essentially a prohormone, which is mostly deiodinated to the bioactive T3 in peripheral tissues.

T4 metabolism

After T4 is secreted by the thyroid gland, it is metabolized by the tissue enzymes deiodinase type I, II and III. Type II deiodinase catalyzes T4 to T3 conversion

by outer ring deiodination (ORD) (Figure 6.3). Type III deiodinase converts T4 to the inactive reverse T3 (rT3) by inner ring deiodination (IRD) while type I deiodinase catalyzes both ORD and IRD. Seventy per cent of circulating T4 and 50% of circulating T3 are bound to thyroxine-binding globulin (TBG), the remainder to other proteins, primarily albumin. Only 0.03% of circulating T4 and 0.3% of T3 are

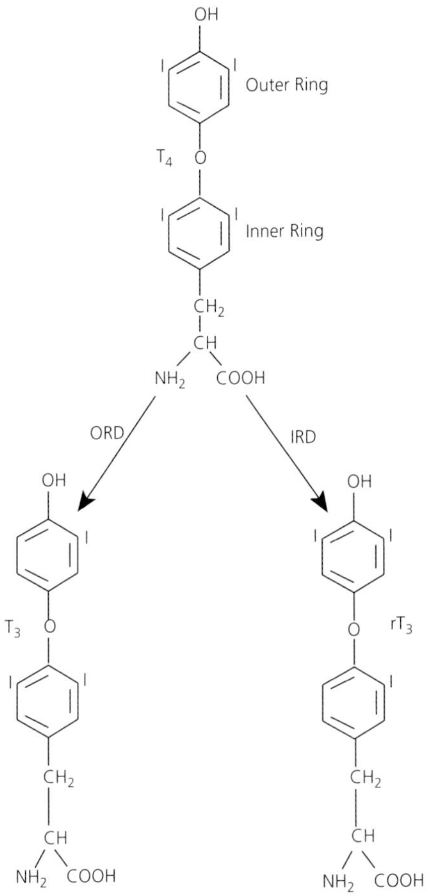

Figure 6.3 Conversion of thyroxine (T4) to tri-iodothyronine (T3) by outer ring deiodination (ORD) and to reverse T3 (rT3) by inner ring deiodination (IRD).

unbound (i.e. free to act on target cells). Total T4 and T3 concentrations therefore reflect TBG concentration, so that measurement of free thyroid hormones gives a more accurate assessment of thyroid function.

Action of the thyroid hormones

The thyroid hormones have profound effects on growth, neurological development, metabolism, and cardiovascular function. T4 and T3 bind to α1, β1, and β2 receptors in the target tissues, for example, heart and skeletal muscle (α1), brain, liver, and kidney (β1), hypothalamus and pituitary (β2). Binding of thyroid hormones to their receptors results in stimulation of target cells with an increase in oxygen consumption, altered protein carbohydrate and lipid metabolism, and potentiation of the action of catecholamines.

Foetal and neonatal thyroid metabolism

Foetal thyroid metabolism

During the first trimester the foetus is largely dependent on small amounts of maternal T4 and T3 that cross the placenta. Levels of TSH start to rise from the second trimester onwards. T4 and T3 concentrations are low in foetal plasma since T4 and T3 are predominantly inactivated, but they are present in relatively high concentrations in target tissues, such as the brain. Some maternal T4 crosses the placenta in late gestation, which explains why cord serum T4 from athyreotic newborns is 20–50% of normal. Iodine freely crosses the placenta so that the intellectual disability seen in the offspring of iodine-deficient mothers can be readily prevented by prenatal iodine administration.

Thyroid function in term neonates

At birth, there is an acute release of TSH. This postnatal TSH surge, which is presumably of physiological benefit, results in high T4 and T3 levels (Figure 6.4). The ratio of T4 and T3 to rT3 rises, corresponding to preferential ORD of T4 and decreased thyroid hormone inactivation. Levels of T4 and T3 are high by 7 days, falling thereafter so that by 14 days of age concentrations are similar to those found in infancy and childhood.

Thyroid function in preterm neonates

The preterm infant, especially below 34 weeks gestation, shows the foetal pattern of low plasma T3 and T4 with high rT3. Factors contributing to this pattern include immaturity of the hypothalamic–pituitary axis, premature interruption of the small but significant maternal contribution to circulating thyroid hormone levels, persistence of the foetal tendency towards inactivation of T4 and T3 and a negative iodine balance. It is uncertain whether or not the preterm thyroid state should be regarded as physiological, or pathological and requiring intervention. The situation is complicated by the knowledge that concentrations of thyroid hormones in the tissues may be substantially different to those found in the plasma. The issue of low T4 levels in preterm infants is discussed further below.

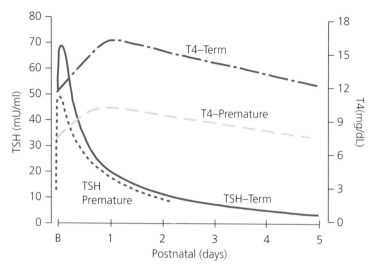

Figure 6.4 Changes in serum TSH and T4 concentrations in full term and premature infants during the first five days of life. Source: From Fisher and Klein 1981, copyright 1981 Massachusetts Medical Society.

Thyroid function tests (TFTs)

Table 6.1 shows the normal values for the commonly measured thyroid function tests (TFTs). Free T4 (FT4) or T4 and TSH measurements are the mainstay of assessment in hypothyroidism, with TSH the most sensitive indicator of primary disease. In primary hyperthyroidism, TSH is suppressed and there is preferential conversion of T4 to T3, so that measurement of both hormones is helpful in the management of thyrotoxicosis. TBG measurement is redundant if FT4 is measured. Measurement of antibodies to TPO or to thyroglobulin (Tg) may be used to confirm autoimmune thyroiditis. Stimulatory TSH receptor antibodies are positive in Graves' disease. Tg is a 660 kDa protein synthesized exclusively in the thyroid gland so that the presence of thyroid tissue can be inferred if it is detectable in the serum. Thyroglobulin is of value in diagnosing the cause of congenital hypothyroidism (see section 'Congenital hypothyroidism') and in the monitoring of patients following thyroidectomy and ^{131}I ablation for thyroid cancer. In pituitary and hypothalamic diseases, TSH levels will be inappropriately low for the low FT4 (or T4) level. TRH, the response to which helps distinguish hypothalamic from primary and pituitary hypothyroidism, is no longer routinely available for testing. Magnetic resonance imaging (MRI) may show anterior pituitary hypoplasia or ectopic posterior pituitary in children with central congenital hypothyroidism.

Table 6.1 Suggested reference ranges for common thyroid function tests, after values from Royal Hospital for Children, and Glasgow Royal Infirmary, Glasgow, UK. Thyroglobulin values are from 29 iodine-sufficient term infants from Czech Republic, analysed at Glasgow Royal Infirmary (Neumann et al. 2018). NB. Reference ranges for TSH receptor antibody vary widely according to the assay used.

	Newborn period	
TSH	1.2–10.5 mU/L	
Free T4	15–40 pmol/L	1.17–3.1
Thyroglobulin (cord blood)		11–127 µg/L
Thyroglobulin (day 3)		62–400 µg/L[1]
	Antibody tests – all ages	
TSH	0.5–5.5 mU/L	
Free T4	9–26 pmol/L	0.79–2.0 ng/dL
Total T4	80–160 nmol/L	6.2–12.4 µg/L
Free T3	4.0–7.5 pmol/L	2.6–4.9 pg/ml
Total T3	1.5–3.4 nmol/L	97.6–221.3 ng/dL
	Antibody tests	
TPO antibodies	<35 mU/L	
TSH receptor antibodies	≤14 u/L (Thybia assay)	

T3, triiodothyronine; T4, thyroxine; TSH, thyroid stimulating hormone; TPO, thyroid peroxidase.

Definition and classification of thyroid disorders

Hypothyroidism is defined as a state in which the hypothalamic–pituitary–thyroid axis is failing, or is in danger of failing, to produce sufficient T4. Classification is according to:
- *site of abnormality:* primary (thyroid), secondary (pituitary), and tertiary (hypothalamus);
- *onset of abnormality:* congenital (prenatal) or acquired (postnatal);
- *severity:* compensated hypothyroidism (thyroid axis jeopardized but able to produce normal T4 levels); and decompensated hypothyroidism (thyroid axis unable to maintain normal T4 levels).

Hypothyroxinaemia is defined as FT4 levels below the reference range in the absence of an elevated TSH. This biochemical profile is encountered in the preterm infant; severe non-thyroidal illness ('sick euthyroid syndrome', in which T3 is typically low initially but FT4 may eventually decrease as well); malnutrition, anorexia nervosa, diabetic ketoacidosis, and in association with certain drugs. During recovery, thyroid hormone levels spontaneously return to normal but TSH often overshoots transiently.

Hyperthyrotropinaemia is a purely descriptive term which refers to a mild elevation of TSH (e.g. 7–15 mU/L) in the context of normal FT4 (or T4) concentrations.

Hyperthyroidism refers to over-production of T4 and/or T3, and is almost invariably primary with TSH suppression.

Goitre refers to thyroid gland enlargement. It is best inspected with the neck slightly extended, asking the child to swallow to make the gland more obvious; best palpated when standing behind the child; and described clinically in terms of size, texture (e.g. smooth or nodular), consistency, and symmetry. Goitres may be sub-classified according to thyroid function: hypothyroid, hyperthyroid, or euthyroid.

Neonatal hypothyroxinaemia

Preterm babies are susceptible to transient hypothyroxinaemia (TH), the incidence of which increases with decreasing gestational age and increasing neonatal morbidity. The hypothyroxinaemia may be secondary to immaturity of the hypothalamic–pituitary axis and the T4 level may be normal for the infant's gestational age. TSH levels are within the reference range. TFTs should be repeated after two weeks and kept under surveillance. Treatment is only indicated if the T4 level remains low with an elevated TSH.

There is a recognized correlation between the severity of hypothyroxinaemia and neonatal outcome. However, causality has never been established and to date there is no evidence that thyroid hormone replacement therapy improves outcomes in this population. A Cochrane review does not support the use of thyroid hormone supplementation in preterm infants to reduce neonatal mortality, neonatal morbidity or improve neurodevelopmental outcomes (Osborn and Hunt 2007). A United Kingdom randomized controlled trial of L-T4 supplementation in babies below 28 weeks' gestation showed no beneficial effect on brain growth in treated infants (Ng et al. 2013). At present supplementation of preterm babies with thyroid hormones cannot be recommended but there is a need for further research.

Hyperthyrotropinaemia

This non-specific label should only be used once mild compensated primary congenital hypothyroidism (e.g. due to thyroid ectopia) has been excluded by thyroid imaging. Neonatal hyperthyrotropinaemia may reflect the physiological TSH surge or be caused by delayed maturation of the hypothalamic–pituitary–thyroid axis. It is more common in preterm infants. No treatment is required but the infant should be kept under surveillance until the TSH normalizes.

Transient neonatal hypothyroidism

Transient TSH elevation, with or without a low FT4 (or T4), accounts for roughly 25% of cases referred by the screening laboratory if TSH is measured on day 5. It is strongly associated with sick and/or preterm newborns and those suffering from congenital malformations (Table 6.2). More rarely, it is caused by transplacental transfer of maternal medication, transplacental transfer of maternal TSH receptor blocking antibodies, or iodine deficiency or excess. If TSH elevation is >10 mU/L, then treatment should be started (see section 'Congenital hypothyroidism').

Congenital hypothyroidism

Congenital hypothyroidism is one of the most common disorders in paediatric endocrinology with a prevalence of 1 in 6700 live births in countries where newborn screening is not performed, increasing to 1 in 2000–3000 live births when screening is carried out (Grosse and Van Vliet 2011). It is the most common cause of preventable learning difficulties. Worldwide, iodine deficiency is the dominant cause. In areas with

Table 6.2 Causes of permanent and transient, syndromic and non-syndromic neonatal hypothyroidism.

Primary congenital hypothyroidism	Permanent, non-syndromic	Thyroid dysgenesis (75%)	Ectopia (40%)
			Athyreosis (30%) True (thyroglobulin undetectable) Apparent (thyroglobulin detectable)
			Hypoplasia in situ (5%)
		Thyroid dyshormono-genesis (20%)	Autosomal recessively inherited defects within structurally normal thyroid gland due to mutations in genes encoding: Thyroglobulin Thyroid peroxidase Pendrin (Pendred syndrome) Dual oxidase 2;dual oxidase maturation factor 2 Dehalogenase system • Sodium/iodide symporter
		Rare causes (<5%)	Transplacental transfer of thyroid peroxidase or thyrotropin receptor blocking antibody Maternal radio-iodine exposure
	Permanent syndromic	Thyroid dysgenesis	Mutations in: GNAS (Albright's hereditary osteodystropy) PAX8 (with kidney agenesis/other genito-urinary malformations) TTF-1/NKX2–1 (with lung disorders; choreoathetosis) TTF-2/FOXE1 mutation (with cleft palate, spiky hair)
		Thyroid dyshormonogenesis	Mutation in Pendrin gene with goitre and deafness (Pendred's syndrome)
	Transient	Maternal causes	• Iodine deficiency • Excess iodine exposure • Blocking TSHR antibodies
		Foetal abnormalities	Congenital abnormalities Syndromic disorders including Down syndrome
		Postnatal problems	Perinatal illness (e.g. hypoxia, sepsis, exchange transfusion) Iodine exposure
Central congenital hypothyroidism	Permanent	Idiopathic with other pituitary deficiencies isolated	ectopic posterior pituitary +/− septo-optic dysplasia (almost always sporadic) • deficiency in PIT-1 (dominant or recessive). • beta-TSH (recessive) • IGSF1 syndrome (X-linked)

Source: Adapted from Donaldson and Jones (2013), and reproduced with kind permission.

severe iodine deficiency, congenital hypothyroidism is endemic and leads to learning difficulties, short stature, deafness, and neurological abnormalities.

Aetiology

Thyroid dysgenesis

This accounts for approximately 70% of permanent congenital hypothyroidism. The most common form is *thyroid ectopia* when caudal migration is incomplete, resulting in an ectopic (usually sublingual) gland which is always hypoplastic. *Athyreosis*, where no thyroid tissue is detectable on imaging is the second commonest cause. It may be subdivided into apparent athyreosis, in which thyroglobulin is detectable, and true athyreosis when it is not (Gagné et al. 1998). *Hypoplasia in situ* is less common than ectopia and athyreosis. It may result from a TSH receptor mutation which, if severe, causes severe hypoplasia or even apparent athyreosis; and from a PAX8 mutation. Inherited or de novo gene mutations affecting the transcription factors NKX2-1 and FOXE1 genes, sometimes in association with syndromes (see Table 6.2), are responsible for probably <2% of cases of thyroid dysgenesis. Hemiagenesis is not a cause of congenital hypothyroidism since the contralateral lobe compensates.

Thyroid dyshormonogenesis

Autosomal recessive defects in thyroid hormone synthesis account for 15–20% of congenital hypothyroidism in the United Kingdom but occur more commonly in parts of the world where the prevalence of consanguinity is high (e.g. the Middle East, North Africa). The most common genes affected are TPO and thyroglobulin. Pendred's syndrome – sensorineural deafness with or without dyshormonogenetic goitre – is due to a mutation in the Pendrin gene. DUOX2 mutations result in congenital hypothyroidism which may be transient in nature. Mutations in the iodotyrosine dehalogenase gene result in iodine wasting with a goitre, similar to that of dietary iodine deficiency. Sodium iodine symporter gene defects are rare, and show lack of uptake on radioisotope scan.

In contrast to infants with thyroid dysgenesis, in whom thyroid hypoplasia is found, thyroid imaging of infants with biosynthetic defects will show a normal or enlarged thyroid gland in situ, provided that the defect is distal to the TSH receptor.

Other causes of congenital hypothyroidism are rare. TSH or TRH deficiency accounts for hypothyroidism in approximately 1 in 100 000 births and usually occurs in the context of malformations associated with multiple pituitary deficiencies, for example, septo-optic dysplasia.

Thyroid screening in the newborn

Background

Newborn screening for congenital hypothyroidism using dried capillary blood spots was developed in the 1970s, in response to the combination of difficulty in achieving an early clinical diagnosis and the severe neurodevelopmental consequences of a late diagnosis, especially beyond three months of age (Grosse and Van Vliet 2011). By the early 1980s, newborn screening was established in North America and most of Europe, but has yet to be implemented in many parts of the world, including the Maghreb countries of North Africa.

It is important to recognize that no screening programme is perfect and that occasional errors – missed patients, mis-labelling and loss of samples – are inevitable. Thus clinical vigilance is essential, whether newborn screening is in place or not.

Type and timing of sampling

Screening samples are usually collected as capillary blood from the baby's heel but cord blood sampling may be more feasible in resource-limited settings. Guidelines from the European Society for Paediatric Endocrinology (ESPE) recommend that screening should take place 48–72 hours after birth (Léger et al. 2014). In the United Kingdom, screening is normally performed between days 4 and 7. In North America, babies are usually tested between 48 hours and four days, but may be tested before 48 hours of age if they are discharged from the hospital prior to that time. Early sampling may lead to false positive results and it is important that the TSH value is interpreted in the light of age-appropriate reference ranges.

Screening tests

Options include TSH measurement only (the most sensitive method for primary hypothyroidism but which will miss central hypothyroidism), T4 measurement only (which will miss compensated hypothyroidism) and measurement of both T4 and TSH (the ideal but most labour-intensive and costly method). In most of the United Kingdom and North America, TSH-only measurement is used.

Protocol for notification of positive results

Since 2002 in Scotland, a capillary TSH of ≥25 mU/L (measured on whole blood) triggers immediate notification by the laboratory, which should be achieved within a set standard of 14 days (Mansour et al. 2017). When the capillary TSH value ranges between 8 and 24 mU/L, a second sample is requested, and the infant is referred if the repeat value is ≥8 mU/L. Values of <8 mU/L are reported as normal.

Second screening for preterm infants, sick neonates, and in multiple births

The ESPE guidelines recommend repeat sampling at discharge in infants who were born preterm (gestation <37 weeks) or were ill at the time of initial sampling, neonates from multiple births in whom foetal blood mixing may have occurred, infants exposed to iodine, and recipients of blood transfusion, dopamine infusion, etc. The rationale for second testing is that TSH suppression might occur in sick and preterm infants, thus masking true congenital hypothyroidism. While Public Health England also advocates repeat screening at 28 days in preterm infants (NHS guidelines for Newborn Blood Spot Sampling 2016), this approach has not been adopted by all centres, some arguing that the delayed TSH rise in such infants is usually transient in nature.

Point-of-care testing

Devices are being developed for measuring TSH on capillary blood at the time and place of patient care (point-of-care testing). This approach hold promise for screening in areas with restricted resources.

Clinical assessment of infants with suspected congenital hypothyroidism

Awareness of the clinical symptoms and signs is required for the detection of infants missed on the screening programme and for the assessment of infants with high TSH values. Given the increased prevalence (5%) of non-thyroidal malformations (particularly cardiac) in congenital hypothyroidism, and the association with dysmorphic syndromes (e.g. Down, Albright's hereditary osteodystrophy), a thorough examination is indicated.

History

- Sleepiness
- Poor feeding
- Prolonged jaundice
- Constipation
- Hoarse cry
- Parental consanguinity
- Family history of congenital hypothyroidism
- Maternal history of thyroid disease ± treatment

Signs

- Dysmorphic features suggestive of underlying syndrome
- Lethargy
- Jaundice
- Large tongue
- Goitre
- Coarse facies
- Umbilical hernia
- Dry skin
- Large anterior fontanelle, wide sagittal sutures, persistent posterior fontanelle

- Hypothermia
- Cold extremities
- Peripheral cyanosis
- Oedema

Initial investigation of infants with TSH elevation

Biochemical

If hypothyroidism is suspected on neonatal screening, then an urgent venous sample for FT4 (or T4) and TSH measurement should be taken to confirm the diagnosis.

Thyroglobulin measurement is helpful in selected cases, being undetectable (<2 µg/L) in true athyreosis and mutations in the thyroglobulin gene, detectable in apparent athyreosis, often high-normal or elevated (>400 µg/L) in thyroid ectopia, and usually markedly elevated (>1000 µg/L) in dyshormonogenesis (except if due to mutations in Tg). Transplacental transfer of TSH receptor blocking antibodies only accounts for ~1% of cases (Brown et al. 1996).

Imaging
X-ray of knee

Failure of one or both epiphyses to appear on a knee radiograph reflects the severity of intrauterine hypothyroidism and is advocated by some centres as part of the initial assessment.

Thyroid imaging

ESPE guidelines recommend thyroid imaging (Figure 6.5) by radioisotope scanning, ultrasound, or both. If athyreosis or ectopia are confirmed, the diagnosis of permanent congenital hypothyroidism is secure, the parents can be informed that lifelong thyroxine treatment will be required, and reassured that the risk of recurrence is low (<2%). The functional disorders with a thyroid gland in situ, entail a one in four risk in siblings and may be permanent or transient.

While few centres dispute that thyroid imaging in the assessment of newborns with TSH elevation should now be accepted as part of good clinical practice, the optimal mode of imaging remains controversial.

1 *Radioisotope scanning:* ^{99m}Tc-pertechnetate or ^{123}I-labelled sodium iodide scanning will provide information about the presence and site of the thyroid gland and is the gold standard in the diagnosis of thyroid ectopia. Increased size and uptake in a eutopic gland are suggestive of dyshormonogenesis (see

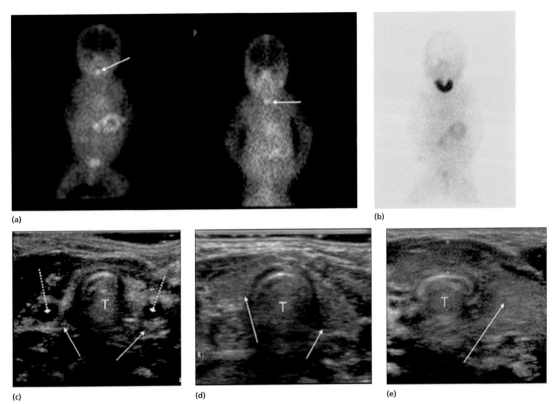

(a)   (b)

(c)   (d)   (e)

Figure 6.5 Isotope (a and b) and ultrasound (c–e) images from infants with thyroid ectopia (a), thyroid hypoplasia due to a TSH receptor defect (d), and dyshormonogenesis (e). The isotope scans show lingual ectopia, a normally sited small gland, and avid uptake into an enlarged gland, respectively. The coronal ultrasound scans show non-thyroidal tissue in the thyroid fossa of the infant with thyroid ectopia, reduced thyroid volume in the infant with thyroid hypoplasia, and a bulky gland in the infant with dyshormonogenesis. Note that the non-thyroidal tissue has a hyperechoic and heterogeneous texture (arrowed), compared with that of the thyroid tissue shown in the two other infants (arrowed), and that it also wraps around the major vessels (broken arrows). T, trachea.

Figure 6.5). There are important caveats with radioisotope scanning: uptake may be decreased or absent in babies with eutopic glands following exposure to iodine in the presence of maternal TSH receptor blocking antibodies, or (more rarely) iodine transport defects. If radioisotope scanning is performed after a few days of thyroxine treatment, TSH should be measured on the same day to help interpret the findings.

2 *Ultrasound scanning:* In skilled hands, thyroid ultrasound is of value in defining thyroid size and morphology. Use of colour Doppler enables vascularity to be assessed. Disadvantages include high observer dependence; inability to detect ectopic thyroid tissue in some cases, even with colour Doppler; and the risk of misinterpreting fatty tissue in the thyroid fossa as dysplastic thyroid. The latter pitfall has been highlighted by a study reporting non-thyroidal tissue in the thyroid fossa of infants with proven thyroid ectopia on radioisotope scanning (Jones et al. 2010, see

Figure 6.5) and may account for a relatively high prevalence of thyroid hypoplasia in some previous studies. Correct interpretation of thyroid ultrasound requires not only subjective evaluation but, in the case of eutopic glands, objective measurement of thyroid volume using normative data from the region/country concerned.

3 *Dual scanning (both radioisotope and ultrasound scanning):* Performing both types of scan on the same day complements their advantages and enables early diagnosis in around 80% of patients (Lucas Herald et al. 2014). However, neither modality satisfactorily predicts transient hypothyroidism.

Treatment of congenital hypothyroidism

Neonatal period
When an infant is found by the screening laboratory to have TSH elevation, she/he should be seen by the

clinician within 24 hours. Most families will be deeply shocked by the discovery of an abnormal result on their apparently well baby, and the disclosure that the child may have a lifelong disorder. *Initial* counselling should therefore be brief and simple, reassuring the parents that the treatment of permanent congenital hypothyroidism is straightforward and the outlook excellent, provided that observance with medication is meticulous.

In centres where same-day venous TFTs are available, the need for treatment with levo-thyroxine (L-T4) can be judged from the venous FT4 and TSH values. Biochemical severity can be graded according to FT4 values of <5 pmol L (severe), 5–10 pmol/L (moderate), and 10–15 pmol L (mild) (Léger et al. 2014). L-T4 should be started immediately, therefore, if TSH elevation is confirmed and FT4 is <15 pmol/L. When same-day venous TFT's are not available, L-T4 should be started if capillary TSH is ≥40 mU/L since decompensated hypothyroidism is likely, but may be deferred for 48–72 hours if TSH is <40 mU/L and the infant clinically euthyroid (Pokrovska et al. 2016).

Treatment should be started within 14 days of age in infants with venous TSH >20 mU/L and/or fT4 < 15 pmol/L. Well infants with normal fT4 and venous TSH 6–20 mU/L may be observed initially, and thyroid imaging should be performed. If, however, TSH elevation >10 mU/L persists, L-T4 treatment followed by discontinuation of L-T4 treatment and retesting at three years is a pragmatic and safe strategy.

L-T4 can be administered as crushed tablets, mixed with a few millilitres of water, breast or formula milk, and given via a spoon or syringe. The smallest tablet is 25 µg, but this can be halved. Liquid forms of thyroxine should only be used if pharmaceutically produced and licensed. The initial dose of T4 should be 10–15 µg/kg per day depending on the severity of the hypothyroidism, equating to 37.5–50 µg daily in most term infants. The aim of treatment is to normalize FT4 and TSH within two weeks if possible, given the evidence of a better neurodevelopmental outcome.

During the early weeks of treatment, once the shock of the diagnosis has settled down, detailed and careful counselling is essential. Information leaflets and visual aids are very useful, as is contact with a similarly affected child and family or a support group.

Infancy

FT4 should be maintained in the upper half of the reference range for age (15–20 pmol/L), with TSH in the lower half (0.5–3 mU/L). Sometimes the initial fall in the TSH with treatment is delayed in which the thyroxine dose should be titrated against FT4, keeping this near the top of the reference range. Parents should be aware of symptoms of over-treatment with thyroxine including crying, irritability, poor sleeping, and diarrhoea.

Beyond infancy

L-T4 dose can be estimated by assuming a full replacement dose (e.g. in athyreosis) of 100 µg (m²/day (3–4 µg/kg/day), calculating body surface area from the formula $\sqrt{[\text{length (cm)} \times \text{weight (kg)}/3600}$. L-T4 requirement depends on the type and severity of hypothyroidism, being lower in children with ectopia, mild dyshormonogenesis and transient congenital hypothyroidism. A suggested dosage schedule, based on the requirement in the absence of thyroid tissue, is given in Table 6.3. L-T4 dosage should be pre-emptively increased to keep pace with body surface area or weight, rather than allowing the TSH levels to rise due to under-treatment. Most children do well when free T4 is kept between 12 and 20 pmol/L and TSH between 0.5 and 5 mU/L.

NB Soya milk formulas, iron medication, calcium, and fibre administered in close time proximity to L-T4 can interfere with L-T4 absorption. Disorders associated with malabsorption, e.g. coeliac disease, may affect T4 levels as may medications which increase T4 degradation, e.g. anticonvulsants. Such patients require more frequent follow-up and higher doses of L-T4.

Follow-up and retesting in selected cases

Follow-up

Table 6.3 gives guidance as to how frequently patients should be seen, with clinic attendance no less than every three months in the first year and yearly after three years. Follow-up should be more frequent if there are concerns about compliance, if TFT's are abnormal or if the dose has been altered. If the TSH is >5 mU/L and the T4 level is in the lower half of the normal range or below the normal range, then the dose should be raised by 12.5–25 µg per day and the TFTs should be repeated in four to six weeks. Conversely, the dose should be reduced by a similar amount if the TSH level is <0.5 mU/L.

The prevalence of sensori-neural hearing loss is increased in congenital hypothyroidism, even after allowing for Pendred's syndrome. Thus audiology

Table 6.3 Suggested schema for follow-up of patients with congenital hypothyroidism. Thyroxine (L-T4) dose is for athyreosis and equivalent to 100 μg/m²/day.

Age	L-T4 dosage guide (μg)	Clinic frequency	Growth monitoring	Assessment/education
Birth–1 mo	See text	Weekly	Length, weight, OFC	Initial investigations including imaging; L-T4 dose titration; counselling
1–6 mo	37.5	2–4 wk	Length, weight, OFC	Consolidation of family education/counselling
6–12 mo	37.5–50	4–8 wk	Length, weight, OFC	Neurodevelopment
1–3 yr	50–75	4–6 mo	Height, weight, OFC	Neurodevelopment Preschool audiology
3–16	75–150	Annually[a]	Height and weight (pubertal staging not normally necessary)	Child and adolescent education including pre-conceptual counselling in girls

[a] More frequent follow-up in the case of problems with compliance/adherence.

should be carried out at three years in all affected children, with repeat testing in patients who had severe hypothyroidism at birth.

Re-evaluation of thyroid status

Retesting should normally take place after the age of three years, by which time neurodevelopment is largely complete so that potential short-term exposure to hypothyroidism carries a low risk of harm. Re-evaluation is unnecessary in infants already known to have an unequivocal cause of congenital hypothyroidism including athyreosis or ectopia, confirmed on scanning during infancy, genetically proven dyshormonogenesis (with the exception of DUOX2 deficiency which may cause transient hypothyroidism) and in children where venous TSH has been >10 mU/L after 12 months of age while on treatment – indicative of underdosage or poor compliance with thyroxine.

However, retesting is required in children who were preterm and/or sick at birth; those with eutopic glands of indeterminate cause; patients in whom thyroid imaging was not performed in infancy; and when the dose of thyroxine has not needed increasing since early childhood. In children requiring re-evaluation, the ESPE guidelines suggest decreasing the thyroxine dose by 30% and checking thyroid function two to three weeks later. If TSH is >10 mU/L, the diagnosis of congenital hypothyroidism is confirmed. Thyroid imaging may then be performed, to establish the aetiology. If thyroid function remains normal, the dose is decreased further before rechecking thyroid function after two to three weeks. If thyroid function is normal

four weeks after stopping treatment, the child can be discharged with a diagnosis of resolved transient hypothyroidism.

Outcome

Neonatal screening programmes have revolutionized the outlook for babies with congenital hypothyroidism and the overall prognosis is now excellent. However, subtle neurocognitive deficits may occur in some children with severe intrauterine hypothyroidism despite adequate postnatal treatment. There is also concern that overtreatment with L-T4 may cause deficit in attention and memory.

Influence of prenatal hypothyroidism on outcome

Lower intelligence quotient (IQ) has been reported in children with serum T4 of <40 nmol/L prior to treatment, superimposed on the effect of a lower socioeconomic status. (Tillotson et al. 1994). Special attention to severely affected children form socially deprived families is therefore essential.

Influence of adequacy of postnatal treatment on outcome

Failure to comply with treatment, especially during the first three years of life, may impair normal brain development. The relationship between intellectual and education outcome, and the quality of postnatal treatment and follow-up has been demonstrated in France (Léger et al. 2011).

Influence of over-treatment on behaviour and attention

Work from Canada and Spain has shown that exposure to high thyroxine levels adversely affects attention (Rovet and Erlich 1995; Rovet and Alvarez 1996; Alvarez et al. 2010). However, although a Norwegian study found more memory and behaviour problems in adults with congenital hypothyroidism compared with sibling controls, a link between high L-T4 dosage in early childhood could not be confirmed (Oerbeck et al. 2005).

Although it is difficult to separate the effects of congenital hypothyroidism itself from the effects of inadequate treatment and/or over-treatment, the available evidence indicates that outcome can be optimized by:

- prompt diagnosis and treatment;
- avoidance of both under- and over-treatment by frequent biochemical monitoring and clinic visits;
- good compliance by family and, in adolescence, the patient;
- continuing family and patient education.

Acquired hypothyroidism

This condition can be difficult to recognize as its onset may be insidious and it has often been present for a number of years prior to diagnosis.

Aetiology

Primary Acquired Hypothyroidism

- Iodine deficiency
- Autoimmune (Hashimoto's) thyroiditis
- Thyroid surgery
- Following irradiation to neck (e.g. craniospinal irradiation, total body irradiation)
- Radioactive iodine therapy
- Antithyroid drugs (e.g. carbimazole)
- Goitrogens

Secondary and Tertiary

- Craniopharyngioma and other tumours impinging on the hypothalamic–pituitary axis
- Neurosurgery
- Cranial irradiation

Iodine deficiency

Although this is the most common worldwide cause of hypothyroidism, it more commonly results in a euthyroid goitre. Clinical iodine deficiency is rare in Europe, but an estimated 11 of 35 countries are iodine-deficient (Lazarus 2014) and there is some evidence that iodine supplementation in mild-to-moderate deficiency improves cognition (Taylor et al. 2013). The condition is suspected in cases of goitre, a family history of iodine deficiency and from a knowledge of the regional iodine status. Measurement of urinary iodine concentration (UIC) is valuable for the assessment of iodine status in populations but of limited use in individual diagnosis. The World Health Organization (WHO) classifies iodine deficiency as mild, moderate, and severe if UIC is 50–99, 20–49, and < 20 µg/L. Iodine deficiency is treated with trace amounts of iodine and prevented by iodization of salt. This is practised widely in North America but inconsistently in Europe.

Autoimmune (hashimoto's) thyroiditis

This is the most common cause of acquired hypothyroidism in the Western world. It is more common in girls, particularly in adolescence, and there is a family history in approximately a one-third of cases. Presentation may be with euthyroid goitre, goitre with compensated hypothyroidism, goitre or an atrophic gland with decompensated hypothyroidism or during screening because of the presence of another autoimmune condition. Autoantibodies are present in 95% of cases. Autoimmune thyroiditis may be associated with other autoimmune diseases, such as diabetes mellitus, coeliac disease, and Addison's disease, as well as with skin disorders, such as alopecia areata and vitiligo.

Hashimoto's thyroiditis is common in Down syndrome, affecting 8.9% of Scottish children (Noble et al. 2000). Regular screening is indicated, one method being annual capillary blood spot TSH screening from one year of age onwards. If the TSH is raised, then venous TFT's and a TPO antibody measurement should be performed. TSH screening will not detect Hashimoto's disease if it goes through a hyperthyroidism phase (see p. 156) but this condition should be clinically obvious.

Autoimmune thyroiditis is also increased in Turner syndrome (especially with isochromosome X), with a 6.6% prevalence in a Polish study (Gawlik et al. 2011).

Miscellaneous causes

These include the hypothalamic–pituitary disorders in which other anterior pituitary hormone deficiencies will almost invariably be present. Dietary goitrogens, such as iodide, cabbage and soya beans, have also been reported to cause hypothyroidism.

The clinician should be wary of diagnosing hypothyroidism in obese children. Obesity results in TSH resistance, causing mild hyperthyrotropinemia (5–7.5 mU/L) but with normal FT4. L-T4 treatment is not indicated in this situation, and weight reduction will lead to normalization of TSH. Occasionally pseudohypoparathyroidism (see Chapter 10) may present as mildly raised TSH, for example, on newborn screening.

Clinical features

History
• Slowing of linear growth ± short stature
• Weight gain
• Tiredness
• Constipation
• Cold intolerance
• Delayed puberty (occasionally sexual precocity)
• Menstrual irregularity
• Presence of other autoimmune disorders
• History of slipped capital femoral epiphysis
• Family history of thyroid or other autoimmune disorders

Signs
• Short stature
• Myxoedematous facies

• Goitre
• Obesity
• Dry skin
• Increase in body hair
• Pallor
• Vitiligo
• Proximal muscle weakness
• Delayed relaxation of ankle reflexes
• Delayed puberty (occasionally precocious puberty)

The principal symptoms of acquired hypothyroidism are tiredness and weight gain, while the key signs are pallor, myxoedematous facies, and short stature relative to the mid-parental height (Figure 6.6). If previous heights are available, it may be possible to pinpoint the start of the hypothyroidism. The goitre is usually diffuse and non-tender with a firm texture but is nodular in some cases and is occasionally tender. Usually puberty is delayed, but, occasionally, with severe hypothyroidism cross-stimulation of FSH receptors by extremely elevated TSH concentrations may lead to incomplete sexual precocity with enlarged ovaries on ultrasound scan in girls and testicular enlargement with low testosterone in boys. Paradoxically, in all but the most severe cases of acquired hypothyroidism, children do well at school, methodically doing their homework until it is completed.

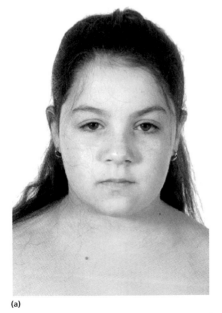
(a)

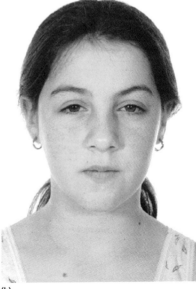
(b)

Figure 6.6 Girl with acquired hypothyroidism caused by Hashimoto's disease (a) before and (b) after treatment.

Investigations

These will depend on the cause of the hypothyroidism. FT4 and TSH are required to confirm the diagnosis and TPO antibodies should be measured to determine the aetiology. In long-standing hypothyroidism, bone maturation is delayed. A thyroid ultrasound should be done if a nodule is palpable or if there is clear asymmetry but is otherwise not essential. If there is no goitre and the autoantibody screen is negative, then an isotope or ultrasound scan should be performed to exclude a late presentation of thyroid dysgenesis. Inappropriately low or normal TSH values in the face of low FT4 suggests pituitary or hypothalamic disease which can be further investigated with further pituitary testing and MRI.

Treatment

Treatment is with T4 100 µg/m² per day given as a single daily dose. Children with clinical hypothyroidism can start on full replacement but some clinicians prefer to prescribe a small dose of T4, 25–50 µg once daily. TFTs should be measured every two to four weeks and the dose adjusted in 25 µg steps as necessary until TFTs have normalized. Regardless of how treatment is initiated, the parents should be warned that treatment for severe hypothyroidism may be associated with short-term adverse symptoms including irritability, poor concentration, emotional lability, and benign intracranial hypertension. School performance may also temporarily deteriorate. Catch-up growth with increased height velocity will occur, often with initial weight loss. In those with compensated hypothyroidism, adverse symptoms are much less likely and treatment can be increased more quickly.

There is controversy as to which euthyroid patients with compensated autoimmune thyroiditis should be treated since a spontaneous return to the euthyroid state is possible. When TSH is as high as 20 mU/L or more, it is wise to treat with L-T4 irrespective of accompanying symptoms or FT4 levels. When TSH is 6–10 mU/L in a well patient with normal FT4, a watch-and-wait approach is advised. In patients who are well with TSH 10–20 mU/L, the choice lies between a period of close observation and elective L-T4 treatment, and should be discussed with the family. There is some evidence that treatment will cause a reduction in thyroid volume in patients with goitre. Occasionally, treatment may be associated with the development of a slipped upper femoral epiphysis or Perthes' disease, both of which cause leg pain and a limp. However, the former is more likely to be seen as a presenting feature of hypothyroidism. Families should be told that in the unlikely event of the child developing leg pain or a limp, they should attend the emergency department that day.

Follow-up

Considerable surveillance and reassurance may be required by some families during the first few months following diagnosis. Thereafter, clinic visits and TFTs should take place 6–12-monthly. The TSH level is a sensitive marker of under- or over-replacement. In the case of non-compliance, FT4 will be normal if L-T4 was taken on the day of the clinic visit but the TSH level will be raised.

Outcome

The prognosis for autoimmune thyroiditis is very good and the outlook partly depends on whether the child will develop other autoimmune diseases. Most patients need treatment for life, but spontaneous remission may occur and should be suspected if L-T4 dose requirement is low. Complete catch-up growth following treatment can be expected in mild to moderate cases but not always in severely affected children with prolonged hypothyroidism, especially when treatment is initiated after puberty has started. Parents of children with severe hypothyroidism should be warned that it may take several months before their child is completely back to normal.

Hyperthyroidism

Aetiology

- Graves' disease
- Autoimmune (Hashimoto's) thyroiditis
- Neonatal thyrotoxicosis
- Syndrome of pituitary T4 resistance
- Autonomous nodules
- TSH-dependent hyperthyroidism (rare):
  - TSH-secreting adenoma
  - activating mutations of the TSH receptor

Hyperthyroidism due to Graves' disease and Hashimoto's thyroiditis

This is caused by the development of antibodies which bind to the TSH receptor and cause inappropriate, unregulated stimulation of T4 production. TPO antibodies are usually also present. The condition is uncommon, with an incidence of 0.8 per 100 000 children per year, but often more severe than in adults when it does occur. Paediatric onset is usually in the second decade. It is six times more common in girls and in up to 60% of cases there is a family history of thyroid disease. It occurs more commonly in children with other autoimmune disorders, including diabetes mellitus, and there may also be a family history of non-thyroidal autoimmune disease. Graves' ophthalmopathy, rarely severe in children, usually takes the form of eye prominence or frank proptosis (exophthalmos) (Figure 6.7). It results from infiltration of the orbit and surrounding structures with lymphocytes, mucopolysaccharides, and oedema.

Hashimoto's thyroiditis

Autoimmune thyroiditis usually causes hypothyroidism but may cause thyrotoxicosis ('Hashitoxicosis') in a small proportion of patients. TPO antibodies are almost always present, TSH receptor antibodies negative, and eye signs absent.

Graves' or Hashimoto's disease?

An absolute distinction between the two conditions may not always be possible, some believing that they represent different ends of a spectrum. However, separating the two disorders was shown to be clinically helpful in a Scottish study of 66 patients with thyrotoxicosis. Of 13 patients with Hashimoto's disease, 10 showed spontaneous remission compared with 10 of

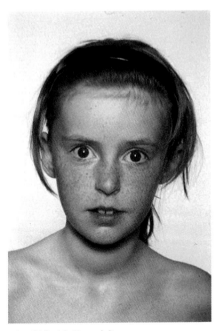

Figure 6.7 Girl with Graves' disease.

53 patients with Graves' disease (Kourime et al. 2017). Thus, while medical treatment of Hashimoto's is as for Graves' disease, neither radioactive iodine nor surgery are usually indicated.

Clinical features of hyperthyroidism in children and adolescents

The onset of both Graves' and Hashimoto's disease is usually insidious but may be acute.

History

- Anxiety
- Irritability and hyperactivity
- Tiredness
- Deteriorating school performance and handwriting
- Weight loss despite increased appetite
- In young children, increased height velocity often with tall stature relative to the parents
- Palpitations
- Heat intolerance
- Sleep disturbance
- Increased stool frequency
- Menstrual irregularities or amenorrhoea
- Family history

Examination

- Goitre (usually diffuse)
- Eye signs (in Graves' disease)
  - mild: lid retraction/slight prominence
  - *moderate:* clinically obvious orbital projection – exophthalmos
  - *severe:* marked exophthalmos ± oedema and injection of the conjunctivae (rare).
- Tachycardia with bounding pulses
- Hypertension with wide pulse pressure
- Hyperdynamic precordium; heart murmur
- Facial flushing
- Tremor
- Tongue fasciculations
- Sweatiness
- Relative tall stature (height centile usually above parental target range centiles)
- Thyroid bruit
- Choreiform movements

   Thyroid crisis or storm is a form of thyrotoxicosis characterized by an acute onset which may be precipitated by surgery, infections, drug withdrawal/non-compliance, and radioactive iodine treatment. The patient develops hyperthermia, severe tachycardia, and restlessness and may become delirious, comatose, or die. It is rare in childhood.

Diagnosis

The diagnosis is usually obvious and is confirmed by finding elevated FT4, FT3, or T3 with TSH suppression. Rarely, FT4 is normal but FT3 or T3 levels are elevated, so-called 'T3 toxicosis'. TSH receptor antibodies are elevated in Graves' disease and TPO antibodies are usually positive in both Graves' and Hashimoto's.

Treatment of hyperthyroidism in children and adolescents

This can be divided into *first line treatment* – medical and *second line treatment* – either with radioactive iodine or surgery.

Initial medical treatment

Symptoms of anxiety, palpitations, and tremor can be distressing, and oral Propranolol treatment 0.5–1 mg/kg/day in divided doses makes the child more comfortable. This should be reduced and stopped when FT4 has normalized and symptoms have resolved. In children with asthma, the selective β-blocker Atenolol may be given. Neither should be used in patients with heart failure.

Antithyroid drugs (ATDs) are given as Methimazole (MMI) or Carbimazole which is the pro-drug of MMI into which it is metabolized. Carbimazole is used in the United Kingdom and is available in 5 and 20 mg tablets. It may be started at 5 mg daily, increasing by 5 mg every two days in two or three divided doses and building up to 0.75 mg/kg/day, maximum dose 30 mg daily, over a two-week period. The rationale of this slow and cautious approach is to minimize the chance of side effects, including nausea.

The patient is seen weekly at this stage and the opportunity taken to counsel the family carefully, particularly when the TSH receptor antibody results are available. After four to eight weeks, FT4 and FT3/T3 will fall to within the reference range but the TSH will remain suppressed for several more weeks. The rapidity of the response is usually proportional to the size of the gland. When the FT4 normalizes at ~ 15 pmol/L the β-blocker may be reduced and stopped, and one of two ATD strategies put into place.

Dose titration regimen

When FT4 is ≤15 pmol/L, the dose of Carbimazole is reduced to 0.5 mg/kg/day, giving this as a single daily dose. Dose is titrated further according to the FT4 and FT3/T3 levels to maintain the hormone levels in the centre of the reference range. It is important *not* to wait for the TSH to normalize before reducing the Carbimazole dose and to titrate against the FT4 levels. Because adverse effects from Carbimazole and MMI are more common in patients receiving high doses, the aim is to use the lowest dose necessary to maintain a euthyroid state.

When FT4 and FT3/T3 are stable on the reduced dose of Carbimazole, the patient is seen monthly and, when good control is achieved, every three months. TSH receptor antibody titre may be repeated annually to give an idea of disease activity.

Block and replace regimen

An alternative is not to reduce Carbimazole when FT4 normalizes but instead to introduce L-T4 in the dose of 50–100 µg daily to counter the hypothyroidism which will occur on 0.75 mg/kg/day of Carbimazole. Carbimazole and FT4 are given as single daily doses.

Dose titration or block and replace?

The American Thyroid Association (ATA) guidelines favour dose titration in adults since the block and replace regimen requires a higher ATD dose with more risk of adverse effects and no proof that remission rates are better (ATD guidelines 2016). Also, it is easier to monitor disease activity and hence the imminence of remission, with dose titration. Advocates of block and replace claim smoother control with avoidance of hypo- or hyperthyroidism, and the need for less frequent monitoring.

Adverse effects of anti-thyroid drugs

Side effects of Carbimazole and MMI include rashes, painful joints (most often wrists and ankles), neutropenia, and liver dysfunction. *Neutropenia* occurs in approximately 0.3% of patients, usually within the first three months. A slightly greater percentage may develop mild to moderate leucopenia. Patients should be asked to report symptoms of infection, especially sore throat, mouth ulcers, fever, and bruising. In such instances, treatment should be stopped and an urgent full blood count performed. Whenever possible, written information should be provided to back up the verbal advice. Stopping the medication nearly always leads to resolution of the problem after one to two weeks. In severe cases, granulocyte colony stimulating factor may be used. Routine measurement of full blood count is unhelpful and not advised.

An itchy erythematous *rash* occurs in 2–5% of patients on Carbimazole and MMI. This side effect is more common with higher doses and these should rarely exceed 30 mg daily, an apparently higher dose requirement suggesting compliance problems. Carbimazole and MMI can cause *liver problems*, characterized by cholestatic dysfunction (rather than hepatocellular inflammation or liver failure) and, rarely, liver failure.

Propylthiouracil (PTU) has also been used to treat thyrotoxicosis. Unfortunately, there is a 1 in 1000 risk of liver failure in children treated with PTU and a percentage of patients may require liver transplantation or die (Rivkees and Mattison 2009). In view of this, PTU should be restricted to the very few patients in whom Carbimazole or MMI have led to a toxic reaction and in whom both radioactive iodine and surgery are not considered an option.

Management of graves' ophthalmopathy

This is usually mild in children and adolescents compared with adults. Dry or painful eyes can be treated with hypromellose eye drops ('artificial tears'), one drop to each eye up to four times a day. In the case of significant symptoms or impaired eye movements, early referral to an ophthalmologist is indicated but treatment with steroids or decompression is rarely required.

Duration of treatment with antithyroid drugs

While hyperthyroidism from Hashimoto's thyroiditis can be expected to remit spontaneously, remission rates for Graves' disease are lower and the family must be counselled that many years of Carbimazole or MMI may be required. Given the relative severity of Graves' disease in children and the spectrum of severity, there is no logic (and no evidence) to support giving ATD treatment for a fixed period, for example, two or three years, and then stopping therapy to see if the patient has remitted spontaneously. Moreover, work from France and Japan suggests that the chance of spontaneous remission in Graves' disease is enhanced by prolonged, low dose ATD therapy (Léger et al. 2012; Ohye et al. 2014).

A logical approach, therefore, is to titrate the dose of ATD to keep serum FT4 between 10 and 20 pmol/L and TSH between 1 and 3 mU/L. In this way, disease activity can be monitored. When the dose requirement falls to, say, 5 mg daily or less of Carbimazole, it may be cautiously lowered further with a view to stopping treatment altogether. If, however, a high or moderate dose of ATD is required to keep the patient euthyroid, then stopping treatment is unlikely to result in remission and should not be attempted. Since the block and replace regimen conceals the patient's hyperthyroid status, it is necessary to stop L-T4 periodically to assess disease activity, and this should be done before attempting to reduce and stop ATD treatment. Monitoring of TSH-receptor antibody may also reflect disease activity.

Some patients and families will struggle with adherence to ATD therapy, resulting in a poorly controlled disease which can cause considerable problems, including educational disruption. In this situation second line treatment should be implemented sooner than later (see sections 'Radioactive iodine' and 'Thyroid surgery'). However, the Scottish study of Kourime et al. showed that long-term compliance with L-T4 was often problematic in adult patients who had received ablative treatment with surgery or radioactive iodine in adolescence. This shows that second line treatment should not be undertaken lightly. It also underlines: (i) the importance of careful and realistic counselling of families from the time of diagnosis onwards; and (ii) the need to encourage a culture of regular and disciplined tablet-taking, given that this will be necessary in the long term in roughly 50% of patients with Graves' disease.

Radioactive iodine

The goal of radioactive iodine therapy is to give a sufficient dose to ablate thyroid tissue. This treatment induces lifelong hypothyroidism, rather than remission of the hyperthyroidism, in almost all cases. High dose ablative treatment minimizes the risk of cancer, and radioactive iodine treatment is now regarded as safe in children from five years onwards.

Radioiodine therapy should be conducted in collaboration with a nuclear medicine specialist or an adult endocrinologist with a special interest in thyroid disorders. Treatment is administered orally as I-131 (or ^{131}I) which is a radioactive isotope of iodine. ^{131}I given as the dose of 450 megabecquerel (MBq) = 12.2 millicurie (mCi) will almost always achieve hypothyroidism within six months. Teenage girls should undergo pregnancy testing prior to ^{131}I administration. ATD medication should be stopped five days prior to treatment and symptoms of hyperthyroidism can be treated with β-blockers if necessary. Analgesia may be needed to treat the neck pain of radiation thyroiditis and rarely nausea may occur. The patient should be closely monitored so that treatment with L-T4 can pre-empt the onset of severe hypothyroidism. In the rare cases when hyperthyroidism persists beyond six months, then patients can be retreated.

In the minority of children with severe eye disease, radioactive iodine should be used with caution as it may exacerbate the ophthalmopathy. Steroid treatment for several weeks may be helpful. Alternatively, surgery may be required.

Thyroid surgery

The main advantage of this treatment is the rapid cure of the thyrotoxicosis. It is particularly useful in young children (under 10 and particularly under 5 years of age) in whom definitive treatment is required and in those with a very large thyroid gland. Euthyroid status must be induced prior to surgery. Ten to fourteen days prior to surgery, iodides (e.g. Lugol's solution, see Table 6.4, 0.1–0.3 ml, three times a day [tds], orally) should be administered to decrease the vascularity of the gland and inhibit release of thyroid hormone.

ATA guidelines stress the importance of thyroidectomy being carried out by a 'high-volume thyroid surgeon' since this will reduce the risk of complications. These include recurrent laryngeal nerve palsy with a

Table 6.4 Early detection and management of neonatal thyrotoxicosis. (after Léger 2017).

Check TSH receptor antibody (TRAB) titre in 3rd trimester of pregnancy in women with a history of Graves' disease, past or present. *This includes mothers in whom ablative treatment has been carried out previously.*

If maternal TRAB titres are undetectable no further action is needed.

If maternal TRAB is above the laboratory reference range neonatal follow up is required

Neonatal thyrotoxicosis is likely if maternal TRAB is x 2–3 above normal

In babies of mothers with detectable TRAB

Check cord blood for TRAB, FT4 and TSH

Check thyroid function days 3, 5, 7, 10, and 15 (keep baby in hospital for first seven days)

Examine for evidence of thyrotoxicosis (tachycardia, excessive crying, goitre)

If biochemical evidence of thyrotoxicosis (FT4 > 30 pmol/l, TSH < 0.1 mU l⁻¹ ± symptoms and signs:

Give Carbimazole or Methimazole 250 μg kg⁻¹ three times daily initially

Propranolol 1 mg kg⁻¹ twice daily for 2 wk (monitor pulse, blood pressure and blood glucose)

Titrate Carbimazole dose to keep FT4 ~15–20 pmol/l

Check TRAB monthly and stop Carbimazole when titres become undetectable (usually within 3 months)

Reproduced with kind permission of author and Karger publications.

resultant hoarse voice, hypoparathyroidism causing hypocalcaemia, unsightly keloid scar formation, and haematoma. Most surgeons favour total or near-total thyroidectomy which will render the patient hypothyroid. Sub-total thyroidectomy carries a risk of recurrence but can be considered in patients with a history of particularly poor tablet-taking in whom compliance with L-T4 replacement is likely to be problematic.

Neonatal thyrotoxicosis

This rare condition is caused by the trans-placental transfer of maternal TSH receptor antibodies which stimulate the foetal and neonatal thyroid. The higher the thyroid stimulating immunoglobulin level in pregnancy, the greater the risk that the infant will develop thyrotoxicosis. This disease may occur in infants of mothers with active hyperthyroidism who are on treatment and in those women previously treated with radioactive iodine ablation or thyroidectomy and are currently euthyroid on L-T4 replacement but who still have high titres of circulating thyroid-stimulating immunoglobulin. Only 2% of infants of mothers with Graves' disease are affected but the condition can be life-threatening. Foetal demise can occur but this should not occur in neonates if they are appropriately treated and monitored. The foetal and neonatal management of the condition is comprehensively covered in a mini-review by Juliane Léger (2017).

Table 6.4 shows how neonatal Graves' disease can be predicted, and thyrotoxicosis pre-empted. Early treatment will prevent severe symptoms occurring and since the half-life of thyroid-stimulating immunoglobulins is approximately 12 days and resolution of the disease corresponds to their degradation, the disorder is self-limiting over a 3–12-week period.

When the risk of neonatal Graves' disease has not been recognized, for example, if antenatal care has been inadequate or if the past history of maternal Graves' disease has not been elicited or its significance appreciated, the baby may present with full-blown features of the condition. These include goitre, tachycardia, arrhythmias, hypertension, cardiac failure, increased appetite, weight loss, increased stool frequency, irritability, and exophthalmos. In these severely affected babies, initial treatment with Lugol's solution (5% iodine, 10% potassium iodide = 130 mg iodine/ml) blocks thyroxine production, exerting an effect within 48 hours. Sedatives may be required, for example, oral chloral hydrate 30 mg/kg given eight hourly as necessary. Prednisolone, which inhibits the conversion of T4 to T3 and inhibits thyroid hormone secretion, can be used in particularly severe cases in the dose of 2 mg/kg/day orally. Heart failure may require treatment with diuretics.

Outcome is usually favourable but babies should be examined for evidence of craniosynostosis and thyroid function monitored for several weeks after discharge. Neurodevelopmental follow-up is indicated in babies in whom severe foetal and neonatal hyperthyroidism has been documented.

Other causes of hyperthyroidism

Thyroid hormone resistance syndrome

This rare disorder has been described in over 1000 people in the world. In approximately 75% of cases there is evidence of a family history. It results from a dominant mutation in the thyroid hormone receptor β (TRβ) gene so that tissues fail to respond to thyroid hormones. This results in the body trying to compensate by the thyroid gland secreting increased amounts of T4 and T3. Blood levels of these hormones are therefore high, although the TSH level is not suppressed. Because the abnormality in the thyroid hormone receptors may vary from one tissue or organ to another, the responsiveness of the cells to the excess thyroid hormones also varies. There may be retardation of growth and a delay in the way the bones mature. Some of the cells in the brain may be relatively unresponsive so that the person has learning difficulties and an attention deficit when concentrating, although the IQ is usually normal. Other tissues continue to respond to the increased amounts of thyroid hormone and this may manifest itself as hyperactivity and tachycardia. A goitre is nearly always present.

Most people with this condition have few symptoms and treatment is not usually required. The diagnosis is important as it allows appropriate family counselling. Symptoms of thyrotoxicosis, particularly tachycardia, can be treated with a β-blocker.

Autonomous nodules

Very rarely an autonomous nodule or nodules, due to an activating somatic TSH receptor mutation, may cause hyperthyroidism. McCune–Albright syndrome is associated with autonomous thyroid adenomas. The nodules, which are follicular adenomas, can be diagnosed clinically and by isotope scanning and are very rarely malignant. Treatment is generally surgical.

TSH-dependent hyperthyroidism

TSH-dependent hyperthyroidism is a very rare condition which is caused by a pituitary TSH-secreting tumour (a 'TSHoma'). Thyroid hormone levels are elevated and the TSH is normal or raised. Neuroradiological (MRI) evaluation is required.

Activating mutations of the TSH receptor

Rarely activating germline mutations of the TSH receptor can be responsible for familial and sporadic cases of nonimmune hyperthyroidism. These patients may present in the neonatal period or in childhood with a goitre and suppressed TSH levels. Hyperthyroidism with a multinodular goitre occasionally occurs in patients with the McCune–Albright syndrome due to an activating mutation of the α subunit of the G protein.

Thyroid neoplasia

Thyroid cancer is rare in childhood and adolescence, accounting for ≤3% of carcinomas. Its epidemiology and management have recently been reviewed (Vaisman et al. 2011; Ross et al. 2016). Table 6.5 shows the different histological types of thyroid neoplasia.

The following points should be borne in mind:
- Papillary carcinoma accounts for 90% of paediatric thyroid cancer.
- The disease tends to be more advanced at diagnosis in children than in adults, with capsular invasion and involvement of regional lymph nodes.
- Paradoxically, the prognosis for survival is better than in adults.
- Thyroid nodules are rare in childhood but carry a higher risk of being malignant than in adults – 22% vs 14% (Gupta et al. 2013).

Presentation

This is usually with painless and diffuse enlargement of the thyroid gland. Alternatively, the family may have noticed one or more nodules. Depending on the

Table 6.5 Classification of thyroid neoplasia.

Follicular tumours
Papillary carcinoma
Follicular adenoma
Follicular carcinoma
Anaplastic carcinoma

Non-follicular tumours
Medullary carcinoma
Lymphoma
Teratoma
Metastatic
Miscellaneous

extent of the spread of disease there may be accompanying hoarseness, dysphagia, cervical lymph node enlargement, and lung metastasis.

Risk factors

These include exposure to low dose irradiation (e.g. as in the 1986 Chernobyl nuclear accident), head and neck irradiation (e.g. for Hodgkin's disease); and a family history of medullary thyroid carcinoma (MTC) (see section 'Medullary thyroid carcinoma').

Investigation

Thyroid function is normal and thyroid antibodies usually negative. Ultrasound will show thyroid texture and confirm the presence of nodules. Radioisotope scan may show areas of absent uptake. Nodules which take up radioisotope are usually benign. If there is *any* doubt, the case should be discussed with a clinician with appropriate experience and training, who will be able to perform fine needle aspiration (FNA).

Treatment

If the clinical picture is suggestive of malignancy, or if FNA result is positive or suspicious, then surgery is indicated. Surgery consists of removal of the affected lobe followed by total thyroidectomy if frozen sections confirm malignancy. Postoperative T4 therapy should lead to complete suppression of TSH so as not to stimulate tumour regrowth. Radioactive iodine treatment is also given if there is evidence of metastatic disease or distant lymph node involvement. Follow-up consists of regular clinical assessment and measurement of thyroid function to ensure TSH suppression. Thyroglobulin is also measured since it indicates the presence or absence of functioning thyroid tissue. Ultrasound is also useful in detecting neck recurrences. The prognosis in the papillary and follicular carcinomas is very good, even in those with metastases, and life expectancy is normal.

Medullary thyroid carcinoma

MTC is an aggressive tumour arising from the parafollicular C cells and usually secretes calcitonin and occasionally other hormones, such as adrenocorticotrophic hormone (ACTH). It is related to de novo or dominantly inherited mutations in the *RET* proto-oncogene which may be isolated or associated with other tumours in one of the multiple endocrine neoplasia (MEN) syndromes. The three phenotypes are:

- *MTC* which may be familial or sporadic (75% of cases);
- *MEN2A*. MTC, pheochromocytoma and hyperparathyroidism. A mutation in codon 634 of the *RET* gene is commonly found.
- *MEN2B*. MTC, pheochromocytoma and multiple mucosal neuromata. A mutation in codon 918 of the *RET* gene is found in 97% of patients.

In children with a family history of MEN2A or MEN2B in whom genetic studies have shown that the child is affected, prophylactic thyroidectomy is now recommended before the age of five years for MEN2A and before one year in MEN2B to pre-empt the inevitable development of medullary thyroid cancer, which has a poor prognosis once it has become clinically evident. Follow-up includes calcitonin monitoring.

Miscellaneous disorders

Colloid (simple) goitre

During adolescence the thyroid gland may become diffusely enlarged. TFTs and an autoantibody screen should be performed and, if both these are normal, the diagnosis – by elimination – is that of a colloid goitre. The goitre usually resolves spontaneously. However, in some cases the goitre can fluctuate in size and in a minority of cases results in a large nodular goitre in later life. There is no evidence that T4 treatment to suppress the TSH is helpful in colloid goitre, but this is sometimes tried if the goitre is large. Rarely, surgery is required for cosmetic reasons.

Subacute thyroiditis

In this condition, the thyroid gland is acutely inflamed because of a viral infection. There is often evidence of a recent or intercurrent upper respiratory tract infection. The patient may be febrile and the gland may be enlarged, tender, and painful. The inflammation results in leakage of preformed thyroid hormones into the circulation. TFTs may be normal but are usually elevated with symptoms and signs of hyperthyroidism. Inflammatory markers such as the ESR are raised while TPO antibody levels may be weakly positive. A radioisotope scan is sometimes performed to confirm the diagnosis and will demonstrate reduced or absent radioiodine uptake (in contrast to abnormally high uptake characteristic of Graves' disease).

Treatment is with analgesics and non-steroidal anti-inflammatory drugs but, in severe cases, steroids may be needed. A beta blocker may also be necessary to manage symptoms. Antithyroid medication is not indicated. Hyperthyroidism usually lasts for one to four weeks and may be followed by a period of hypothyroidism as the gland recovers. The total course of the illness is two to nine months with most patients making a complete recovery but, occasionally, permanent hypothyroidism may occur.

Transition

Transitional clinics specifically for children with thyroid disorders are rare. More commonly the patient may be seen in an adolescent endocrine clinic.

After the age of 16 years, males with congenital and acquired hypothyroidism can be discharged to the care of their general practitioner (family doctor). Most will just require annual reviews with annual TFT's.

In the case of girls with hypothyroidism, in whom periconceptual adherence to L-T4 treatment is important for foetal well-being, there is a case for transfer to adult services and supervision/counselling into early adulthood.

Adolescents with active thyrotoxicosis which is still requiring medical treatment are best transferred from paediatric to adult care at a suitable age (16–18 years). In patients who have undergone second line treatment with radioactive iodine or surgery, it is reasonable to refer back to the general practitioner once the patient has been stabilized on T4 and has normal TFTs. Patients should be informed about the risk of neonatal Graves' disease in the event of a future pregnancy.

Adolescents treated for thyroid cancer should remain under follow-up by an endocrinologist.

When to involve a specialist centre

- Neonatal thyrotoxicosis.
- Investigation of familial and/or goitrous congenital hypothyroidism.
- Graves' disease that is difficult to control or relapses.
- A thyrotoxic crisis.
- Suspected thyroid neoplasia and MTC, MEN2A, and MEN2B.
- Hypothyroidism secondary to pituitary disease.
- Multinodular goitre.

Future developments

- Advances in molecular genetics are likely to lead to a better understanding of the aetiology of congenital hypothyroidism together with clearer guidelines on

the investigation, treatment, and prognosis of congenital hypothyroidism.
- Point of care assessment of capillary TSH or thyroid ultrasound may develop in countries where mass newborn screening is still unavailable.
- Further insight into the effect of maternal thyroid dysfunction on foetal development may lead to thyroid screening in pregnancy.
- Further research should determine whether preterm infants with hypothyroxinaemia should be treated with T4.

Controversial points

- Should preterm neonates <1500 g or acutely ill neonates >1500 g have repeat TFTs and, if so, when?
- Should infants with suspected congenital hypothyroidism undergo imaging with isotope scan, or thyroid ultrasound, or both?
- Should first-degree relatives of children with autoimmune thyroiditis or Graves' disease have their thyroid function checked?
- What initial dosage regimen should be administered to infants with congenital hypothyroidism?
- For how long should patients with Graves' disease receive therapy with anti-thyroid drugs?
- Should all pregnant women have their TFTs measured to avoid possible adverse effects on their infants?
- Should adolescent and young adult females with unremitting Graves' disease undergo ablative therapy (radioactive iodine or thyroidectomy) before the age at which they are likely to become pregnant to avoid the need for MMI during pregnancy?

Common pitfalls

- A normal T4 with a high TSH level may indicate that T4 has been taken on the day of the blood test but irregularly prior to that. Diplomatic questioning should help determine if the problem is non-compliance or if a higher T4 dose is needed.
- Children with congenital hypothyroidism who have been shown to have a eutopic gland and/or at the age of three years are on a small dose of T4 are often found to have transient disease. Failure to re-evaluate these children may result in unnecessarily prolonged treatment with L-T4.
- Children with thyrotoxicosis with a normal FT4 (or T4) and a suppressed TSH level who still have symptoms should have their FT3 (or T3) measured. The

FT3 may be elevated and accounts for their symptoms and the suppressed TSH.

- A low FT4 (or T4) level with a normal or only slightly elevated TSH level (TSH < 10 mU/L) should prompt consideration of the possibility of secondary or tertiary hypothyroidism.
- Mild TSH elevation in obese children usually reflects TSH resistance, which resolves with weight reduction. Such children do not require L-T4 treatment

Case histories

Case 6.1

A 13-year-old girl presented at clinic having been diagnosed as having hypothyroidism by her family doctor who had confirmed the diagnosis with TFTs. She also had a two-year history of a limp in her left leg. On examination, she was short and obese with a goitre and other signs of hypothyroidism. She had limitation of movement of her left hip and a limp.

Questions and Answers

1 What is the most likely diagnosis?

Slipped upper femoral epiphysis and Hashimoto's disease.

2 What investigations should be done?

Frontal and lateral hip X-rays (a frontal X-ray alone may not demonstrate the slipped epiphysis) and thyroid autoantibodies.

3 What is the treatment?

In spite of the long history, urgent referral to an orthopaedic surgeon and urgent surgery are necessary. An acute or chronic slip of the epiphysis may cause avascular necrosis of the femoral head. Prophylactic pinning of the other femoral head is advocated by some surgeons. T4 treatment should also be started.

Case 6.2

An endocrinological opinion was sought about the following series of TFTs. They were taken from a boy with congenital hypothyroidism caused by an ectopic gland who had been treated with T4 from day 15 of life. At five years of age, he was in a mainstream school but had speech delay and behavioural problems (Table 6.6).

Table 6.6 Thyroid function tests.

Age	FT4 (normal 12–26 pmol/l)	TSH (normal 0.5–6.0 mU l^{-1})
10 mo	20.9	2.5
1.5 yr	22.9	3.7
2.1 yr	9.0	53.8
2.2 yr	10.6	79.6
2.3 yr	32.7	0.91
2.6 yr	9.3	44.2
3.1 yr	22.8	32.5
4.7 yr	23.9	34.5
5.1 yr	18.5	29.3

Abbreviations: FT4, free thyroxine; TSH, thyroid-stimulating hormone.

Questions and Answers

1 What is your interpretation of these results?

These results indicate poor compliance. The FT4 values are normal as a result of the tablets having been taken in the few days prior to the blood test. However, the half-life of TSH is longer and the elevated TSH values point to a lack of compliance.

2 Are there any measures you could have taken or would take now to alter the situation?

Earlier recognition and action might well have reduced this boy's poor compliance, developmental delay, and behavioural problems. If, despite full explanations and maximum support, the situation did not improve, then there would be grounds for considering child protection proceedings.

Case 6.3

A 13-year-old boy was referred to the regional endocrine clinic for consideration of growth hormone (GH) treatment. He also had delayed puberty and intermittent headaches. On examination, his height was >– 4.0 SD with evidence of growth failure for at least four years. His weight was –1.0 SD and he was prepubertal (G1P1). A recent GH stimulation test at the referring hospital showed a maximum response to a diethylstilbestrol primed clonidine test of 5 mU/L. He was said to have had normal TFTs two years previously with a FT4 = 9.2 pmol/L (9–24) and a TSH of 1.2 mU/L (0.4–4.0).

Questions and Answers

1 Are these TFTs normal?

They are highly suggestive of secondary or tertiary hypothyroidism.

2 What is the likely overall diagnosis?

Panhypopituitarism secondary to a pituitary tumour.

3 Is there a problem in interpreting his clonidine test?

Yes, one can get a low GH level in any form of untreated hypothyroidism. A growth hormone stimulation test should, ideally, be performed after the patient has received L-T4 and euthyroid state has been restored. However, he is likely to be GH-deficient and in fact had a large cystic craniopharyngioma.

Case 6.4

An 11-year-old girl with Down syndrome is referred with tiredness, mild diarrhoea, and a TSH of 9.2 mU/L (0.4–4.0) and a FT4 of 14.1 pmol/L (9–24). She also has a raised TPO antibody titre.

Questions and Answers

1 Would you treat this child with T4?

The thyroid function is only mildly deranged with a normal FT4 and a slightly raised TSH. This slight abnormality is unlikely to cause any symptoms. Most children with Down syndrome have an atrophic thyroiditis with no goitre. TSH levels sometimes rise transiently and can fluctuate. If the TSH rises to above 10 mU/L, the child should have TFTs six monthly. If the TSH rises above 15 mU/L, the child should have TFTs three monthly and is likely to eventually require T4. In the above situations the family should be told of the symptoms to look out for. If the TSH ≥ 20 mU/L with a normal FT4, the patient should be treated with T4.

2 What other investigations would you consider doing?

A general paediatric approach should be taken, looking for the large number of causes of tiredness and diarrhoea in a child with Down syndrome. The two most important investigations are a full blood count looking for anaemia and a coeliac screen.

3 What is the likely diagnosis?

The likeliest diagnosis is coeliac disease. The anti-transglutaminase antibodies were positive and a jejunal biopsy confirmed coeliac disease. Coeliac disease is an immunological disorder and is more common in Down syndrome. The tiredness and diarrhoea resolved on a gluten-free diet.

References

Alvarez, M., Iglesias Fernández, C., Rodríguez Sánchez, A. et al. (2010). Episodes of over treatment during the first six months in children with congenital hypothyroidism and their relationships with sustained attention and inhibitory control at school age. *Horm. Res. Paediatr.* 74 (2): 114–120.

Brown, R.S., Belisario, R.L., Botero, D. et al. (1996). Incidence of transient congenital hypothyroidism due to maternal thyrotropin receptor-blocking antibodies in over one million babies. *J. Clin. Endocrinol. Metab.* 81: 1147–1151.

Donaldson, M. and Jones, J. (2013). Optimising outcome in congenital hypothyroidism; current opinions on best practice in initial assessment and subsequent management: current opinions on thyroid disease in childhood. *J. Clin. Res. Pediatr. Endocrinol.* 5: 13–22.

Fisher, D.A. and Klein, A.H. (1981). Thyroid development and disorders of thyroid function in the newborn. *N. Engl. J. Med.* 304 (12): 702–712.

Gagné, N., Parma, J., Deal, C. et al. (1998). Apparent congenital athyreosis contrasting with normal plasma thyroglobulin levels and associated with inactivating mutations in the thyrotropin receptor gene: are athyreosis and ectopic thyroid distinct entities? *J. Clin. Endocrinol. Metab.* 83 (5): 1771–1775.

Gawlik, A., Gawlik, T., Januszek-Trzciakowska, A. et al. (2011). Incidence and dynamics of thyroid dysfunction and thyroid autoimmunity in girls with Turner's syndrome: a long-term follow-up study. *Horm. Res. Paediatr.* 76 (5): 314–320. https://doi.org/10.1159/000331050.

Grosse, S.D. and Van Vliet, G. (2011). Prevention of intellectual disability through screening for congenital hypothyroidism: how much and at what level? *Arch. Dis. Child.* 96: 374–379.

Gupta, A., Ly, S., Castroneves, L.A. et al. (2013). A standardized assessment of thyroid nodules in children confirms higher cancer prevalence than in adults. *J. Clin. Endocrinol. Metab.* 98 (8): 3238–3245:https://doi.org/10.1210/jc.2013-1796.

Jones, J.H., Attaie, M., Maroo, S. et al. (2010). Heterogeneous tissue in the thyroid fossa on ultrasound in infants with proven thyroid ectopia on isotope scan – a diagnostic trap. *Pediatr. Radiol.* 40 (5): 725–731.

Kourime, M., McGowan, S., Al Towati, M. et al. (2017). Long-term outcome of thyrotoxicosis in childhood and adolescence in the west of Scotland: the case for long-term antithyroid treatment and the importance of initial counselling. *Arch. Dis. Child.* 103: 637–642. https://doi.org/10.1136/archdischild-2017-313454.

Lazarus, J.H. (2014). Iodine status in Europe in 2014. *Eur. Thyroid. J.* 3 (1): 3–6.

Léger, J. (2017). Management of fetal and neonatal Graves' disease. *Horm. Res. Paediatr.* 87: 1–6. https://doi.org/10.1159/000453065.

Léger, J., Ecosse, E., Roussey, M. et al. (2011). Subtle health impairment and socioeducational attainment in young adult patients with congenital hypothyroidism diagnosed by neonatal screening: a longitudinal population-based cohort study. *J. Clin. Endocrinol. Metab.* 96: 1771–1782.

Léger, J., Gelwane, G., Kaguelidou, F. et al. (2012). Positive impact of long-term antithyroid drug treatment on the outcome of children with Graves' disease: national long-term cohort study. *J. Clin. Endocrinol. Metab.* 97: 110–119.

Léger, J., Olivieri, A., Donaldson, M. et al. (2014). European Society for Paediatric Endocrinology Consensus Guidelines on screening, diagnosis and management of congenital hypothyroidism. *J. Clin. Endocrinol. Metab.* 98 (8): 3238–3245. https://doi.org/10.1210/jc.2013-179621: jc20131891.

Lucas-Herald, A., Jones, J., Attaie, M. et al. (2014). Diagnostic and predictive value of ultrasound and isotope thyroid scanning, alone and in combination, in infants referred with thyroid-stimulating hormone elevation on newborn screening. *J. Pediatr.* 164 (4): 846–854:https://doi.org/10.1016/j.jpeds.2013.11.05.

Mansour, C., Ouarezki, Y., Jones, J. et al. (2017). Trends in Scottish newborn screening programme for congenital hypothyroidism 1980–2014: strategies for reducing age at notification after initial and repeat sampling. *Arch. Dis. Child.* 2016: 312156. https://doi.org/10.1136/archdischild-2016-312156.

Neumann D, Krylová K, Jones JH (2018) Serum thyroglobulin in late pregnancy, cord blood and three-day old neonates born to healthy, iodine-supplemented Czech women; implications for evaluation of suspected congenital hypothyroidism (submitted).

Ng, S.M., Turner, M.A., Gamble, C. et al. (2013). An explanatory randomised placebo controlled trial of levothyroxine supplementation for babies born <28 weeks'gestation: results of the TIPIT trial. *Trials* 14 (211): https://doi.org/1 0.1186/174www.5-6215-14-211.

NHS (2016) Guidelines for Newborn Blood Spot Sampling. https://assets.publishing.service.gov.uk/government/uploads/system/uploads/attachment_data/file/511688/Guidelines_for_Newborn_Blood_Spot_Sampling_January_2016.pdf (accessed 13 October 2018).

Noble, S.E., Leyland, K., Findlay, C.A. et al. (2000). School-based screening for hypothyroidism in Down syndrome by dried blood spot TSH measurement. *Arch. Dis. Child* 82: 27–31.

Oerbeck, B., Sundet, K., Kase, B., and Heyerdahl, S. (2005). Congenital hypothyroidism: no adverse effects of high dose thyroxine treatment on adult memory, attention, and behaviour. *Arch. Dis. Child.* 90: 132–137.

Ohye, H., Minagawa, A., Noh, J.Y. et al. (2014). Antithyroid drug treatment for Graves' disease in children: a long-term retrospective study at a single institution. *Thyroid* 24: 200–207.

Osborn, D.A. and Hunt, R.W. (2007). Prophylactic postnatal thyroid hormones for prevention of morbidity and mortality in preterm infants. *Cochrane Database Syst. Rev.* 24 (1): CD005948. https://doi.org/10.1002/14651858.CD005948.pub2.

Pokrovska, T., Jones, J., Shaikh, G., and Donaldson, M. (2016). How well does the capillary TSH test for newborn thyroid screening predict the venous free thyroxine level? *Arch. Dis. Child.* 101: 539–545. https://doi.org/10.1136/archdischild-2015-309529.

Rivkees, S.A. and Mattison, D.R. (2009). Propylthiouracil (PTU) hepatoxicity in children and recommendations for discontinuation of use. *Int. J. Pediatr. Endocrinol.* 2009: 132041. https://doi.org/10.1155/2009/132041.

Ross, D.S., Burch, H.B., Cooper, D.S. et al. (2016). American Thyroid Association guidelines for diagnosis and management of hyperthyroidism and other causes of thyrotoxicosis. *Thyroid* 26: 1343–1421.

Rovet, J. and Alvarez, M. (1996). Thyroid hormone and attention in congenital hypothyroidism. *J. Pediatr. Endocrinol. Metab.* 9 (1): 63–66.

Rovet, J.F. and Erlich, R.M. (1995). Long-term effects of L-thyroxine therapy for congenital hypothyroidism. *J. Pediatr.* 126: 380–386.

Taylor, P.N., Okosieme, O.E., Dayan, C.M., and Lazarus, J.H. (2013). Therapy of endocrine disease: impact of iodine supplementation in mild-to-moderate iodine deficiency: systematic review and meta-analysis. *Eur. J. Endocrinol.* 170 (1): R1–R15. https://doi.org/10.1530/EJE-13-0651.

Tillotson, S.L., Fuggle, P.W., Smith, I. et al. (1994). Relation between biochemical severity and intelligence in early treated congenital hypothyroidism: a threshold effect. *BMJ* 309: 440–445.

Vaisman, F., Corbo, R., and Vaisman, M. (2011). Thyroid carcinoma in children and adolescents – systematic review of the literature. *J. Thyroid Res.* 2011: 845362. https://doi.org/10.4061/2011/845362.

Further Reading

Francis, G.L., Waguespack, S.G., Bauer, A.J. et al. (2015). Management guidelines for children with thyroid nodules and differentiated thyroid cancer (the American Thyroid Association guidelines task force on paediatric thyroid cancer). *Thyroid* 25 (7): https://doi.org/10.1089/thy.2014.0460.

Useful Information for Patients and Parents

The British Society for Paediatric Endocrinology (BSPED) provides patient information as well as citing other sources of information: www.bsped.org.uk/media/1415/hypothyroidism-in-childhood.pdf

London Institute of Child Health fact sheet on congenital hypothyroidism, https://www.gosh.nhs.uk/conditions-and-treatments/conditions-we-treat/congenital-hypothyroidism deals with the management of congenital hypothyroidism (accessed 10 October 2018).

European Society for Paediatric Endocrinology, http://www.eurospe.org/patient/index.html has booklets on hypothyroidism including congenital and acquired hypothyroidism and hyperthyroidism for parents and patients in easy and average readability formats in English, French, Italian, Spanish, and Turkish (accessed 10 October 2018).

The Thyroid Foundation of Canada, www.thyroid.ca contains educational material on paediatric thyroid disorders in English and French (accessed 10 October 2018).

The British Thyroid Foundation, http://www.btf-thyroid.org/ contains educational information about the thyroid gland mainly relating to adult thyroid disease (accessed 10 October 2018).

7

Differences in Sex Development and Common Genital Anomalies

Introduction

In 2006, the term 'disorders of sex development (DSDs)' was proposed to replace 'intersex', which was felt to be derogatory. Along the same lines, but to keep the same acronym, the term 'differences' can now be used instead of 'disorder', thus, differences in sex development. In the restricted sense, people with DSDs present with external genitalia that are sufficiently ambiguous to cause uncertainty as to which sex should be assigned and this is the major focus of this chapter. However, in the broader sense, DSDs encompass all situations when the karyotype is at partial or complete variance with the primary or secondary sex characteristics. Understanding normal sex differentiation and its genetic and hormonal control is a prerequisite to properly understand and manage people with DSDs. Perhaps even more so than in other fields of paediatrics, a basic understanding of the usefulness and limitations of the various cytogenetic and molecular tools available to the practitioner is important (see Chapter 13). Practitioners also need to be cognizant of the rapidly evolving social norms and values regarding sex and of the cultural differences in the way families react to and deal with a child with a DSD. The vast majority of people with gender incongruence have typical male or female genitalia and are not discussed in this chapter (see Further Reading for recent guidelines). However, having a DSD may increase the probability of a change in gender identity.

Normal sex differentiation and its genetic and hormonal control

Basic concepts of the embryology of sex differentiation

An essential concept is that the human embryo is bipotential until 40 days gestation. Regardless of whether they are derived from a 46,XX or a 46,XY zygote, the gonads and the internal (Müllerian and Wolffian ducts) and external genitalia (genital tubercle and urethral and genital folds) have a similar appearance. After 40 days, the gonads differentiate into either testes, which start producing anti-Müllerian

Practical Endocrinology and Diabetes in Children, Fourth Edition. Malcolm D.C. Donaldson, John W. Gregory, Guy Van Vliet, and Joseph I. Wolfsdorf.
© 2019 John Wiley & Sons Ltd. Published 2019 by John Wiley & Sons Ltd.

hormone (AMH), a glycoprotein, at about six to eight weeks, and then testosterone, or into ovaries. Recent studies have shown that the differentiation of both the ovaries and the testes requires activation of specific gene cascades and that the ovaries actively inhibit Wolffian duct stabilization, thus challenging the long-held concept of 'female development by default'. However, this concept still applies to the differentiation of the external genitalia and of the urogenital sinus (see section 'Urogenital Sinus').

Genetic control of gonadal sex determination

A detailed discussion of this complex process is beyond the scope of this chapter. With few exceptions, the presence of a Y chromosome containing a normal SRY (sex-determining region of the Y chromosome)

gene will result in the differentiation of the bipotential gonad into a testis. However, a number of other genes, acting upstream or downstream of SRY, are required for normal testicular development. As noted above, some genes are also actively involved in the differentiation of the ovary. The list of these genes constantly expanding (see Further Reading).

Internal genitalia

From six to eight weeks, in the presence of a testis, the Müllerian system involutes under the influence of AMH secreted by the Sertoli cells, while the Wolffian system is stabilized by testosterone secreted by the Leydig cells, which are stimulated by placental human chorionic gonadotrophin (hCG), and develop into the epididymis, vas deferens, seminal vesicles, and ejaculatory ducts (Figure 7.1). It is important to note that

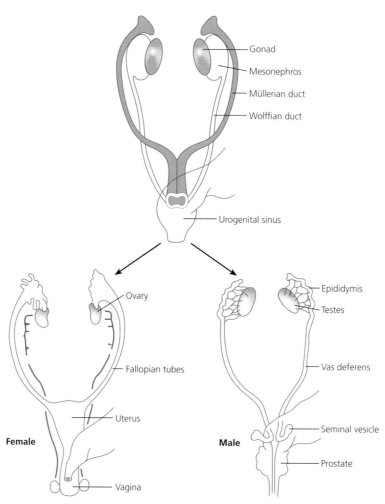

Figure 7.1 Differentiation of the internal genitalia.

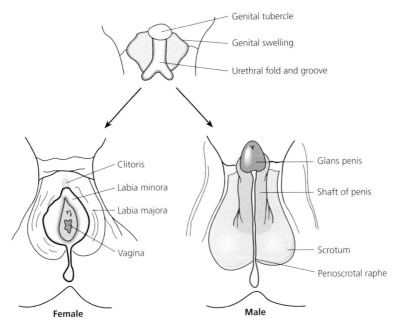

Figure 7.2 Differentiation of the external genitalia from the common anlage.

AMH exerts its effect in a paracrine fashion (i.e. a local effect near its site of production), while testosterone acts both locally (to stabilize the Wolffian ducts) and in a classical endocrine way (to masculinize the urogenital sinus and the external genitalia) after being transported through the bloodstream to its target tissues. In the absence of a testis, the Wolffian system involutes and the Müllerian system develops into the Fallopian tubes, uterus, and the upper third of the vagina.

Urogenital sinus

Under the influence of testosterone, the sinus narrows to form the posterior urethra, and the prostate and the glands of Cowper develop from outgrowths of the sinus. In the absence of testosterone, the sinus forms the lower two-thirds of the vagina and the urethra, and its outgrowths form the para-urethral glands of Skene and the vestibular glands of Bartholin that secrete mucus to lubricate the vagina.

External genitalia

From eight weeks onwards in the male, under the influence of dihydrotestosterone (DHT), converted from testosterone in genital skin by 5-alpha reductase type 2, the genital tubercle will grow to form the penis,

the urethral folds will develop into the corpus spongiosum surrounding the urethra and the genital folds will fuse in the midline to form the scrotum and ventral part of the penis (Figure 7.2). In the female, the same structures will form the clitoris, the labia minora, and the labia majora.

Classification of DSDs

Historically, individuals with ambiguous genitalia had been classified according to the histology of their gonads. Thus, those with both ovarian and testicular tissue were called true hermaphrodites (now ovotesticular DSD), those with only ovarian tissue female pseudohermaphrodites and those with only testicular tissue male pseudohermaphrodites. Since the discovery of the human sex chromosomes in 1956, gonadal biopsies are only required to establish a diagnosis of ovotesticular DSD, a very rare occurrence. Table 7.1 shows the nomenclature proposed in 2006. Of note, mixed gonadal dysgenesis (most often associated with 45,X/46,XY mosaicism), the second most common cause of ambiguous genitalia (after virilizing congenital adrenal hyperplasia [CAH]), occupies a separate niche in both the old and the new nomenclatures.

Table 7.1 Previous and new classification of disorders of sex development.

Previous	New
Intersex	Disorders of sex development (DSD)
Male pseudohermaphrodite	46, XY DSD
Undervirilization of an XY male	
Undermasculinization of an XY male	
Female pseudohermaphrodite	46, XX DSD
Overvirilization of an XX female	
Masculinization of an XX female	
True hermaphrodite	Ovotesticular DSD
XX male or XX sex reversal	46, XX testicular DSD
XY sex reversal	46, XY complete gonadal dysgenesis

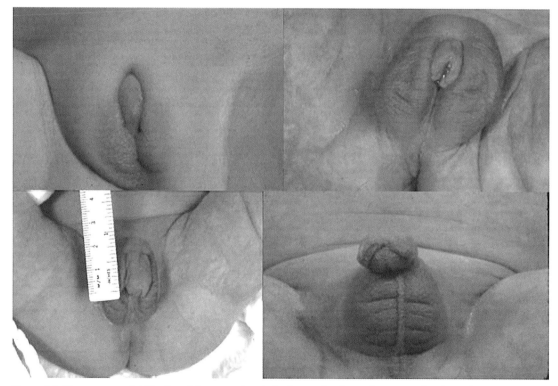

Figure 7.3 The spectrum of virilization of the external genitalia that can be observed in genetic females with CAH due to 21-hydroxylase deficiency.

46,XX DSDs

By far the commonest form of 46,XX DSD is CAH from 21-hydroxylase deficiency. The pathophysiology of this condition and its medical management are described in detail in Chapter 8. In genetic females affected with the severe form of the disease, masculinization of the external genitalia is usually detected at birth. However, virilization can sometimes be relatively mild and may be missed in the neonatal period. At the extreme end of the spectrum, masculinization may be complete, with a penile urethra, and the neonate may be thought to be a boy with bilateral cryptorchidism. Figure 7.3 illustrates the spectrum of virilization of the external genitalia that can be observed in 46,XX infants with CAH due to 21-hydroxylase deficiency.

Much less common enzyme defects that can cause in utero virilization of 46,XX foetuses involve 11-β-hydroxylase and aromatase deficiencies. By contrast, 3-β-ol-dehydrogenase, 17-α-hydroxylase and P450-oxidoreductase (POR) do not typically induce in utero virilization of 46,XX foetuses.

46,XY DSD

Biosynthetic defects

Synthetic defects in the adreno-gonadal enzyme pathways from cholesterol to testosterone (and in its reduction to DHT in genital skin) can cause ambiguous genitalia in 46,XY individuals in spite of the presence of two normally differentiated testes (Figure 7.4). All of these enzyme defects are inherited in an autosomal recessive fashion. Specifically, 3-β-ol-dehydrogenase and 17-β-hydroxysteroid dehydrogenase deficiencies will result in reduced testosterone production during the embryonic period and therefore incomplete virilization. 5-α-reductase deficiency, which results in decreased DHT production in genital skin, should also be considered in incompletely virilized 46,XY neonates. Lastly, a deficiency of the steroidogenic acute regulatory (StAR) protein, which transports cholesterol inside the mitochondria (see Chapter 8 on adrenals), also causes an autosomal recessive form of 46,XY DSD, generally with a completely female external appearance and severe adrenal insufficiency. Likewise, the under-virilization of 46,XY newborns with Smith–Lemli–Opitz syndrome, which is due to a deficiency of 7-dehydrocholesterol reductase and is associated with multiple congenital malformation, can be very severe.

Abnormal testicular development (testicular dysgenesis)

Leydig cell hypoplasia is suggested by severe under-masculinization, occasionally with female external genitalia, in a genetic male with identifiable gonads and raised gonadotrophins. Many individuals with this condition have been shown to have biallelic inactivation of the LH (luteinizing hormone)/hCG receptor. In contrast, because foetal pituitary LH only begins to control testosterone production by Leydig cells after 13 weeks of gestation, congenital gonadotrophin deficiency typically presents with micropenis and cryptorchidism, but not with abnormal sex differentiation. Testicular dysgenesis may also be associated with heterozygous inactivating mutations in steroidogenic factor 1 (SF-1); adrenal insufficiency may be associated. In 46,XX subjects SF-1 mutations are associated with premature ovarian failure. However, a specific diagnosis remains elusive in many under-virilized males with testicular dysgenesis.

Androgen resistance

Complete androgen insensitivity syndrome (CAIS) is an X-linked recessive disorder caused by inactivating androgen receptor (AR) mutations. These mutations can occur de novo or be inherited through the mother who is a healthy carrier. There may be a history of amenorrhea and infertility on the maternal side of the

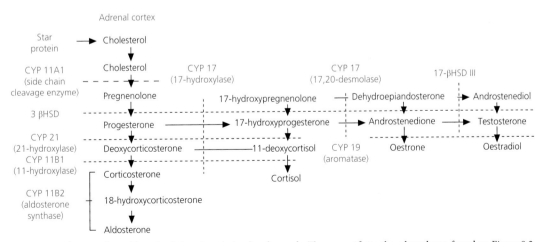

Figure 7.4 Pathways of steroid synthesis in adrenal gland and gonads. Those specific to the adrenals are found on Figure 8.2.

family. Half of the genetically male offspring of carrier mothers will be phenotypic females with absent Müllerian structures, intra-abdominal or inguinal testes, and a short vagina. The diagnosis is usually made in the index case upon the discovery of gonads on palpation or at operation for an inguinal hernia in a female infant. With the increased use of amniocentesis, the diagnosis may also be suspected when a phenotypically female baby is born after a 46,XY karyotype has been found on amniocentesis. The 'classical' presentation with primary amenorrhoea in an adolescent with normal breast development but without sexual hair has become the exception.

Although completely insensitive to androgen, individuals with CAIS are normally sensitive to oestradiol which is aromatized from the high testosterone levels produced at puberty. This accounts for normal breast development and female body habitus, but there is little or no pubic and axillary hair because of the androgen resistance. AMH production by the foetal testes being normal, Müllerian structures are absent, hence the amenorrhea.

Mixed gonadal dysgenesis

Mixed gonadal dysgenesis is the term applied to 45,X/46,XY mosaicism associated with ambiguous genitalia, a streak gonad on one side, and a dysgenetic testis on the other. The external and internal phenotype will depend on the degree of testicular dysgenesis. With severe androgen and AMH deficiency, the external genitalia will be under-masculinized and both vagina and uterus will be present. Regression of the uterine horn and of the Fallopian tube on the side where testicular differentiation occurred may be seen, illustrating the paracrine action of AMH. If testicular dysgenesis is relatively mild, Müllerian regression will have occurred and the external genitalia may be male. Indeed, 45,X/46,XY mosaicism may be found in boys with unexplained short stature and features of Turner syndrome, suggesting that in these subjects the gonads are 46,XY and the growth plates 45,X.

Pure gonadal dysgenesis

In pure gonadal dysgenesis, the gonads are reduced to fibrous streaks, the external genitalia are female, and Müllerian structures (i.e. female internal genitalia) are present. It can occur either sporadically or in familial form. This phenomenon has been found in some cases to be due to deletion or mutation of SRY. The streak gonads should be removed as soon as the diagnosis is established because of the risk of gonadoblastoma.

Pure gonadal dysgenesis can also be seen in association with a 46,XX karyotype; mutations that completely inactivate the follicle-stimulating hormone (FSH) receptor have been found in some cases, although these more commonly lead to premature ovarian failure.

Initial investigation of DSDs

External genitalia that are sufficiently ambiguous to pose the dilemma of sex assignment are observed in 1 in 5000–10 000 newborns. Both parents should be seen as soon as possible. The key points in counselling are the following:

- Initial counselling by attending staff, backed up as quickly as possible by a senior paediatrician and a paediatric endocrinologist.
- Key phrase is: 'There is something the matter with the way that the baby's genitals have been formed, so that we cannot at present say whether the child is a boy or a girl'.
- Infant should be referred to as 'the baby' or 'the child'.
- Mother and baby should be in a single room.
- Registration of name should be postponed.
- Investigations should be undertaken without delay to allow sex assignment.

History

- Consanguinity.
- Pregnancy history:
  - increased body hair and acne (suggests aromatase or POR deficiency);
  - virilization (suggests a tumour).
- Age at menopause in the maternal grandmother (SF-1 mutations).

Examination

- General examination to rule out dysmorphic syndrome ± congenital anomalies (25% of subjects with a DSD have extra-genital malformations).
- Palpation of the abdomen and inguinal regions for gonads.
- Meticulous description ± diagram of abnormal genitalia, using neutral words (see description of the bipotential embryo above) and including labioscrotal folds; genital tubercle; nature and size of opening below genital tubercle; identification where possible of urethral meatus and vaginal opening; and presence and site of gonad(s).
- Examination of anus.
- Measurement of blood pressure (CAH due to 11-β-hydroxylase deficiency may lead to hypertension, but

this is seldom present in neonates; conversely, cortisol and aldosterone deficiency may lead to hypotension and shock).

- Medical photograph with legs spread apart and ruler next to the genital tubercle.

Of note, premature girls, because of the lack of subcutaneous fat, may appear to have clitoral hypertrophy. In these cases, it is useful to estimate the ratio of the distance between the anus and the posterior labial fourchette to the distance between the anus and the base of the clitoris: a ratio less than 0.5, regardless of gestational age, reasonably excludes androgenization during the first trimester.

Further investigations and management

The following professionals should be informed as soon as possible:

- paediatric endocrinologist;
- radiologist, surgeon, and mental health professional with expertise in DSD;
- medical geneticist.

If access to the professionals listed above is difficult, then transfer to a specialist centre for specific tests or for general management may be necessary.

The following investigations should be carried out as quickly as possible:

- *Karyotype:* This takes a minimum of three days. In contrast, fluorescent *in situ* hybridization (FISH) to determine the presence of a Y chromosome or DNA amplification by polymerase chain reaction (PCR) to determine the presence of SRY sequences gives a 'provisional karyotype' within hours.
- *Abdominal ultrasound:* most importantly to determine if a uterus is present; may also be useful for imaging the gonads and adrenals.
- *Plasma 17-hydroxyprogesterone* (17-OHP).

- *Genitography:* This is usually only necessary prior to feminizing genitoplasty to define the point of confluence of the vagina and urethra.

Aetiological diagnosis, sex assignment, and initial management of DSDs

Figure 7.5 shows a simplified flow diagram giving the main diagnostic possibilities. As stated above, the commonest cause of ambiguous genitalia is CAH due to 21-hydroxylase deficiency in a 46,XX newborn. The diagnosis of 21-hydroxylase deficiency is based on the measurement of plasma 17-OHP, with the sample being taken on day 3 (the overlap between affected and normal being too great prior to this) and the result being requested urgently. In addition, the plasma levels of androstenedione, testosterone, and dehydroepiandrosterone-sulfate (DHEAS) will be elevated in CAH. Blood glucose should be measured, although significant hypoglycaemia is seldom present. However, babies with CAH are at risk of salt wasting and plasma electrolytes are often measured early after birth in newborns with genital ambiguity. This may give a false sense of reassurance, because plasma electrolytes are usually normal initially. Due to renal immaturity, the initial salt-wasting episode typically occurs only in the second or third week of life, so that the infant's weight should be carefully monitored even if the plasma electrolytes were normal initially. If there is significant weight loss (up to 10% weight loss is within normal limits in newborns but babies should regain their birth weight by 14 days of age) or if subsequent weight gain is insufficient, plasma electrolytes should be measured again and, if hyponatraemia develops, urine sodium should be measured to document inappropriate natriuresis.

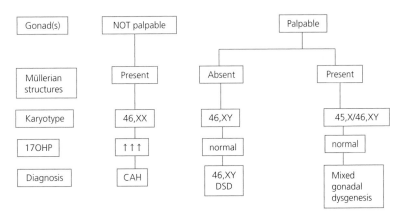

Figure 7.5 Main diagnostic possibilities in neonates with ambiguous genitalia.

Based on their normal female internal genitalia and potential fertility, sex assignment is almost universally female in 46,XX infants with 21 hydroxylase deficiency. Likewise, newborns with ambiguous genitalia due to mixed gonadal dysgenesis are usually assigned female. The presence of a uterus in this condition makes assisted fertility possible. However, the gonads should be removed because of the risk of gonadoblastoma.

Whether in CAH or in mixed gonadal dysgenesis, the psychosexual consequences of clitoral/vulvar surgery in infancy are controversial. Some jurisdictions now allow that no sex be assigned at birth, so that the individual may choose (or not) a male or female assignment after reaching the age of legal autonomy. Most parents are still uncomfortable about this option.

From the point of view of diagnosis and of sex assignment, the most difficult cases are 46,XY infants with partial androgen insensitivity syndrome (PAIS) in whom the growth potential of the phallus at puberty is unpredictable. In contrast, 46,XY individuals with enzyme defects or testicular dysgenesis have normal sensitivity to androgens and can therefore be assigned a male sex if diagnosed early enough. The diagnosis in this group of individuals has classically been based on the measurement of precursor/product ratios of various plasma steroids before and after stimulation with hCG. There are many different protocols for hCG stimulation, the simplest being a single intramuscular (im) injection of $3000\,units\,m^{-2}$ with measurement of plasma steroids five days later. However, several of the enzymes described above are present in various isoforms encoded by different genes (only one of which has deleterious mutations) and expressed in different organs so that these plasma ratios may be misleading. For example, mutations inactivating *SRD5A2* will reduce 5-α reductase activity in genital skin and cause 46,XY DSD; however, *SRD5A1* is not mutated, so that the enzyme activity in the liver is intact and the plasma testosterone/DHT ratio may be normal. Molecular analysis of the relevant genes (targeted exome sequencing) is therefore being increasingly used to establish a diagnosis based on a limited clinical and biochemical phenotype. Another example is 46,XY babies with under-virilization and salt wasting, but normal testes, who are likely to have 3-β-ol-dehydrogenase deficiency until proven otherwise and in whom the diagnosis can be readily confirmed by sequencing *HSD3B2*.

Ultimately, criteria for sex assignment include the specific diagnosis, presence of female internal genitalia (i.e. vagina, uterus), size and androgen sensitivity of the genital tubercle, parental wishes, and cultural considerations. The advice given as to sex assignment should ideally result from a consensus between expert professionals and the parents. In cases where parents and health care providers disagree and psychological support was not able to change the parents' choice, it is probably wise to let the parents' opinion prevail.

Management of CAIS should start with intensive counselling of the individuals, of their parents and of all health professionals involved, to dispel any notion of 'ambiguity'. Because intra-abdominal testes have a high propensity to develop cancer, orchidectomy is recommended. The age at which orchidectomy should be performed is controversial: if the diagnosis of CAIS is certain, some argue that it is preferable for the individual to allow breast development from her endogenous oestrogens. Testicular tumours have been reported as early as at 14 years but remain rare. For this reason, some adult women with CAIS prefer to forego orchidectomy and to undergo ultrasound surveillance.

In contrast to CAIS, PAIS results in a wide phenotypic spectrum ranging from severely ambiguous genitalia to isolated male infertility. The management of these cases is difficult and controversial unless masculinization is relatively mild, in which cases they should be treated as subjects with CAIS; however, orchidectomy should be performed before puberty to avoid the risk of virilization at that time. A greater proportion of infants with PAIS are now assigned male than in the past.

Psychological challenges faced by individuals with DSDs and outcome

Boy or girl? This is usually the first question asked in the delivery room. It is therefore quite understandable that the birth of a child with sufficient ambiguity of the external genitalia as to make immediate sex assignment impossible is associated with great discomfort on the part of the health professionals and with great parental distress. On the other hand, the discovery, perhaps many years after birth, that the child has abnormal gonads and will be unable to have children without assistance, if at all, is also deeply wounding to many parents. Whatever the time when the DSD is discovered, it is essential for the clinician to invest as much time as possible in counselling parents. It is unrealistic to expect that all the information will be assimilated by the family at the first encounter, and several sessions will be required. It is also unrealistic to rely too much on printed information (e.g. parent booklets) in the early stages. Repeated explanations, assisted by hand drawings, and tailored to the parents' psychological state, education, and ability to comprehend require time, patience, and experience.

In addition to hormonal and surgical treatments as appropriate, these individuals and their parents need long-term access to mental health professionals knowledgeable about DSDs. The current thinking is to inform the parents in full, including about the karyotype, at the time of diagnosis. The child should also be informed in a manner appropriate for his or her stage of cognitive and emotional development. Examination of the genitalia by staff and trainees at follow-up visits should be restricted to what is strictly necessary. If the child is properly counselled by the paediatrician and parents during the prepubertal years, it will be possible to give a full and honest account of the problem at adolescence. The classically difficult scenario is explaining the condition to a girl with CAIS. It may be helpful to phrase the explanation as follows:

> The vast majority of girls and women have two X chromosomes and ovaries but some otherwise normal women have XY chromosomes and testes in the abdomen instead of ovaries; yet, they are completely resistant to testosterone, which is converted to oestrogen, resulting in normal breast development. However, there is no uterus and therefore there will be no menses and pregnancy would require a uterine transplant, which is currently experimental.

Communication with women with the same condition is often helpful. Notwithstanding the use of the approach outlined above from diagnosis onwards, feelings of secrecy and shame remain common. These should be addressed so that by the time of transfer to adult care, the person can explain his or her condition and have as little embarrassment about it as possible.

Transition to adult care

At the end of puberty and after full disclosure, people with DSDs should be transferred to an endocrinologist or a gynaecologist with expertise in these disorders. How this is organized in practice will vary according to local circumstances, but ensuring that the transfer has actually happened is important. Especially in individuals who do not need chronic medication, it is not unusual that they do not show up at the appointment made with the physician in charge of overseeing their evolution and management in adult life. Even individuals on chronic replacement therapy may stop taking their glucocorticoids and present with acute adrenal insufficiency, while gonadectomized or hypogonadal individuals who stop their sex hormones are at risk of developing osteoporosis at an early age.

Studies of subjects with DSD in adulthood are few. The best studied, most numerous and relatively homogeneous group is that of women with CAH. Clearly, the surgical techniques used in the past for feminizing genitoplasty have led to sexual difficulties in many women. When adherence to treatment is good, the clitoral hypertrophy should not progress after birth and clitoral surgery can be avoided. Separating the urethral and vaginal orifices is still performed based on the rationale that a urogenital sinus is a risk factor for ascending urinary infections but even that rationale is questionable.

People with 46,XY DSDs born with ambiguous genitalia are much more heterogeneous. Reports of female-to-male self-reassignment at adolescence of 46,XY subjects with 5-α reductase deficiency whose testes had not been removed in infancy are not generalizable. Importantly, almost half of 46,XY DSD subjects (mostly PAIS), reared male or female, reported that they were neither well informed about their medical and surgical history nor satisfied with their knowledge. This emphasizes the importance of the philosophy of full disclosure that is outlined above and that should now be adopted by all interdisciplinary teams following individuals with DSD.

Sexual orientation and gender identity in subjects with DSD

Gender non-conformity in individuals with typical male of female genitalia has received considerable attention in recent years, both among health professionals and in society at large. This complex and rapidly moving field cannot be reviewed here. We think DSD, sexual orientation, and gender non-conformity are best conceptualized as distinct entities. However, being born with atypical genitalia (and/or androgen exposure of the brain in 46,XX foetuses with CAH) has long-lasting consequences. In girls with CAH, stereotypical male toy preference has been well documented in childhood; homosexual orientation and gender non-conformity in adulthood appear to be substantially increased.

Common genital anomalies with no ambiguity

Fused labia

This benign problem in infant girls is likely due to their low oestrogen milieu. Indeed, twice daily application of oestrogen-containing creams for one to two weeks usually relieves the problem. Longer periods of application of oestrogen creams may lead to breast budding. Referral to a paediatric gynaecologist is only exceptionally needed. If the vaginal opening remains completely obstructed in spite of treatment with topical oestrogen, a pelvic ultrasound will rule out the Mayer-Rokitansky-Küster-Hauser syndrome (congenital absence of the vagina and uterus). However, to avoid undue anxiety, this should be performed by a radiologist with paediatric expertise, given the small size of the normal prepubertal uterus.

Isolated clitoromegaly

As described above, this is a common finding in premature infants and tends to become less obvious with the development of subcutaneous fat. On the other hand, if it is first noted after birth but is isolated (i.e. not associated with accelerated linear growth), the probability that the girl has a 'simple virilizing' form of CAH (i.e. without salt wasting) is low. A short period of watchful waiting may be in order, but if clitoromegaly increases, an androgen-producing tumour of the adrenals or ovaries should be considered.

Micropenis

The length of the penis should be evaluated by pressing firmly on the prepubic fat and should be compared with the existing growth curves. These show that the 10th centile for penile length in term newborns is 2.5 cm. In otherwise normal newborns with true micropenis, the presence of testes should be ascertained. If normal testes are felt with certainty, isolated gonadotrophin deficiency remains possible but can be easily ruled out by measuring plasma testosterone at about two months of age; indeed, the 'minipuberty of infancy' creates a critical window of opportunity to assess the integrity of the hypothalamo–pituitary–testicular axis. If no testes are felt, bilateral anorchia (which results from bilateral testicular torsion some time after sex differentiation is complete) can be ruled out by measuring plasma AMH levels as early as three days after birth (when FSH may still be normal due to inhibition by maternal oestrogens). In infant boys with micropenis due to either gonadotrophin deficiency or anorchia, sensitivity to androgens is normal and treatment with testosterone enanthate (25 mg im monthly for three months) will result in a doubling of penile size.

Penile length increases until about four years of age and then remains stable until puberty. Therefore, by far the most common reason for referral for 'micropenis' at school age is for obese boys with a penis that is buried in prepubic fat. Anosmia may suggest an associated gonadotrophin deficiency, but in its absence these boys can be reassured by a simple physical examination as described above.

Cryptorchidism

The best time to accurately assess the presence and position of the testes is the first year of life, before the cremasteric reflex sets in. Although testicular descent may not be complete at birth in some normal term newborns (in which case one may take advantage of the 'minipuberty' to exclude gonadotrophin deficiency as outlined above), the testes should have reached a scrotal position by the end of the first year. Parents should be informed that their son has two normally descended testes and this should be noted in the health record.

If this is not done, undue concern will arise at a later age and sometimes lead to superfluous investigations and even unnecessary surgeries. Indeed, even by careful examination with warm hands, many school-aged boys will have testicles that are difficult to palpate. The vast majority of these boys have retractile testes and their testes will descend permanently in the scrotum at the beginning of puberty.

If true cryptorchidism is established after repeated examinations, the extent of investigations will depend on its unilateral or bilateral nature and on whether the testes are palpable or not. In the latter case, plasma AMH will establish whether there are intra-abdominal testes (in mid-childhood, plasma FSH may be normal even in the absence of functional gonads). How these intra-abdominal testes can be located by imaging is beyond the scope of this chapter; suffice it to say that ultrasound examinations are useless except if the testes are in the inguinal canal. Otherwise normal boys with incompletely descended but palpable testes, either unilaterally or bilaterally, can be referred for surgery without investigation.

Hypospadias

Hypospadias is defined as incomplete fusion of the urethra with the meatus on the ventral aspect of the penis – the glans, corona, shaft of penis, and (most severe) the perineum. This abnormality is commonly accompanied by chordee – curvature of the penis – caused by fibrosis of the corpus spongiosum.

Isolated hypospadias (hypospadias without micropenis and with normally descended testes in a normal scrotum) is rarely associated with an endocrine disorder.

Surgeons should be asked to refer the following conditions for further investigation, including karyotype:

- perineal hypospadias;
- hypospadias with micropenis;
- hypospadias with cryptorchidism ± scrotal abnormality.

However, even extensive investigation of such individuals does not always lead to a specific diagnosis.

Future developments

- DSDs are relatively uncommon and affected children require help from a variety of specialized health professionals (paediatricians, endocrinologists, surgeons, gynaecologists, geneticists, psychologists, radiologists, and possibly others), who are usually only available at large academic centres. Communication between these health professionals is as important as communication of each professional with the individual and with the family. Designating a primary contact person for the individual is important and this role is often assumed by the paediatric endocrinologist.
- Increased understanding of the genetic basis of DSDs and greater availability of clinical laboratories providing molecular diagnostic services permits the cause of the DSD in more and more individuals to be identified.
- Long-term follow-up data are needed, in particular to help determine the optimal surgical management of the virilized genitalia in females with CAH. Multicentre studies organized jointly by paediatric endocrinologists, surgeons, and psychologist are required.
- The medical, surgical, and psychological management of parents, children, adolescents, and adults affected by DSDs, including those born with ambiguous genitalia, has progressed greatly in part from the feedback given by affected adults but still requires considerable refinement based on continuing this dialogue.
- In countries with low resources, education of local professionals coupled with confidential teleconsultation services will result in improved management of DSDs.

Potential pitfalls

- Incorrect assignment of male sex to masculinized females with 21-hydroxlase deficiency. The absence of palpable gonads in an apparently male infant with hypospadias (or even with a penile urethra) should always arouse suspicion.

- Fusion of the labia minora, a common problem, may give the false impression of an absent vagina.
- Most school-aged boys referred for micropenis have exogenous obesity and a normal prepubertal phallus buried in surrounding fat.

Controversial points

- When should clitoroplasty and vaginoplasty be performed, if at all, in girls with CAH?
- What are the long-term effects of exposure of the foetal brain to androgen levels that are discordant with the genetic and gonadal sex?
- Should the testes of individuals with CAIS be removed and, if so, when?

When to involve a specialist centre

- When a baby is born with ambiguous genitalia.
- Severe hypospadias ± cryptorchidism.
- Complete androgen insensitivity syndrome.
- Mixed or pure gonadal dysgenesis.

Case histories

Case 7.1

A 3.5 kg term newborn is of indeterminate sex, with a genital tubercle measuring 3 × 1 cm, labioscrotal folds, a single urogenital orifice and no gonad palpable. Pelvic ultrasound shows a uterus.

Question and Answer

1 What is the most likely diagnosis and what immediate investigations should be performed?

The most likely diagnosis is congenital adrenal hyperplasia in a genetic female. Essential investigations are the karyotype, which was 46,XX, and the 17-OHP level, which was 110 nmol/L [3663 ng/dL] on day 1 rising to above 300 nmol/L [10,000 ng/dL] on day 3. Although 17-OHP measurement should officially be deferred until day 3, a distinctly elevated level on day 1 in the context of a genital anomaly is highly suggestive.

Case 7.2

A 2.5 kg term newborn has abnormal genitalia with a gonad palpable in one labioscrotal fold and no gonad palpable on the other side. Pelvic ultrasound and genitography show a vagina and uterus. Karyotype is 45,X/46,XY. 17-OHP levels are normal.

Question and Answer

1 What is the diagnosis and what advice would you give regarding sex assignment?

The diagnosis is mixed gonadal dysgenesis with a dysgenetic testis on one side and probably a streak gonad on the other. The presence of Müllerian structures suggests that it is probably appropriate to raise this child as a female. The gonads should be removed.

Case 7.3

A 3.0 kg term newborn has a small genital tubercle (1.5×0.8 cm) and gonads palpable in partially fused labioscrotal folds. Pelvic ultrasound shows no uterus and genitogram shows a blind vaginal pouch. Karyotype is 46,XY; 17-OHP levels are normal.

Question and Answer

1 What is the most likely diagnosis and how should the child be managed?

The absence of female internal genitalia indicates that the gonads are testes which have produced AMH normally. The differential diagnosis is between a biosynthetic defect in testosterone production (rare) or, more likely, PAIS. A family history suggestive of autosomal recessive or X-linked inheritance orients to the former and latter possibility, respectively. LH, FSH and androgens should be measured in plasma before and following stimulation with hCG and, with PAIS, may show normal or high levels. Newborns with such types of DSD have been increasingly assigned a male sex over the past 10 years.

Case 7.4

A baby is born to a 24-year-old G1P1A0 mother at 36 and 5/7 weeks of gestation, weighing 2100 g. The external genitalia are ambiguous, with a genital tubercle measuring 2×1 cm and partial posterior fusion of the genital folds. There are no palpable gonads. There is a posterior cleft palate, postaxial polydactyly and syndactyly of the 2nd, 3rd, and 4th toes. Pelvic ultrasound shows no uterus. Karyotype is 46,XY.

Question and Answer

1 What is the most likely diagnosis and how should the child be managed?

The associated malformations point to a diagnosis of Smith-Lemli-Opitz syndrome. Total plasma cholesterol is low at 0.75 nmol/L and 7-dehydrocholesterol is 147 μmol/L (normally undetectable), pointing to a deficiency of 7-dehydrocholesterol reductase. This can be confirmed by DNA analysis. The prognosis should be guarded.

Further Reading

Délot, E.C., Papp, J.C., DSD-TRN Genetics Workgroup et al. (2017). Genetics of disorders of sex development: the DSD-TRN experience. *Endocrinol. Metab. Clin. North Am* 46 (2): 519–537.

Hembree, W.C., Cohen-Kettenis, P.T., Gooren, L. et al. (2017). Endocrine treatment of gender-dysphoric/gender-incongruent persons: an Endocrine Society Clinical Practice Guideline. *J. Clin. Endocrinol. Metab.* 102 (11): 3869–3903.

Lee, P.A., Nordenström, A., Houk, C.P. et al., Global DSD Update Consortium(2016). Global disorders of sex development update since 2006: perceptions, approach and care. *Horm. Res. Paediatr.* 85 (3): 158–180.

Useful Information for Individuals and Parents

The Androgen Insensitivity Support Group. Website: http://www.aissg.org. It is an international consortium with good information and links to local resources (accessed 13 October 2018).

The Accord Alliance. Website: http://www.accordalliance.org. Provides similar services for DSDs in the broader sense (accessed 13 October 2018).

The following professional associations of paediatric endocrinologists also have useful links for individuals presenting a DSD and their parents:

- British Society for Paediatric Endocrinology and Diabetes. Website: www.bsped.org.uk (accessed 13 October 2018).
- European Society for Paediatric Endocrinology. Website: http://www.eurospe.org (accessed 13 October 2018).
- Pediatric Endocrine Society (North American). Website: http://www.lwpes.org (accessed 13 October 2018).

8 Adrenal Disorders

Physiology

Adrenal anatomy and physiology

The adrenal glands are pyramidal structures which lie adjacent to the upper poles of the kidneys. The adrenal cortex is divided into three zones: the outer zona glomerulosa, the middle zona fasciculata, and the inner zona reticularis. The main types of steroids produced by the adrenal cortex are mineralocorticoids (principally aldosterone), glucocorticoids (principally cortisol), and androgens. Steroidogenesis in the zona fasciculata (primarily cortisol) and reticularis (mainly androgen) is under hypothalamic–pituitary control (Figure 8.1); secretion of aldosterone from the zona glomerulosa is under the control of the renin–angiotensin system.

Hypothalamic–pituitary axis

Corticotrophin-releasing hormone (CRH) is synthesized in the hypothalamus and acts on the corticotrophs of the anterior pituitary to secrete the peptide proopiomelanocortin (POMC). POMC is the precursor of adrenocorticotrophic hormone (ACTH). ACTH binds to its melanocortin-2 receptor (MC-2R), a cell surface receptor in the cells of the adrenal cortex. ACTH also has affinity for the melanocortin-1 receptor (MC-1R) in the skin, so that ACTH excess results in hyperpigmentation. The MC-2R is G-protein coupled, and its activation results in increased adenylate cyclase activity, which in turn increases intracellular cyclic adenosine monophosphate (cAMP). Increased cAMP activity enhances the transport of cholesterol across the mitochondrial membrane by the steroidogenic acute regulatory (StAR) protein.

Cholesterol is metabolized into three types of steroids: (i) glucocorticoid; (ii) mineralocorticoid; and (iii) androgen.

Cortisol, the principal glucocorticoid, is vital for maintaining normal glucose and blood pressure and for combating stress. It follows a circadian rhythm, with high levels on waking and a nadir at midnight. Between 80% and 90% of cortisol is bound to cortisol binding globulin (CBG), and most plasma assays measure total rather than free cortisol. Cortisol exerts a negative feedback at the hypothalamic and pituitary levels. Thus, plasma ACTH concentrations will be elevated in primary adrenal insufficiency and suppressed when cortisol excess is caused by autonomous adrenal lesions or exogenous glucocorticoids. In primary adrenal insufficiency, cortisol levels will depend on the severity of the defect. In severe deficiency, cortisol is low despite massively raised ACTH, but in

Practical Endocrinology and Diabetes in Children, Fourth Edition. Malcolm D.C. Donaldson, John W. Gregory, Guy Van Vliet, and Joseph I. Wolfsdorf.
© 2019 John Wiley & Sons Ltd. Published 2019 by John Wiley & Sons Ltd.

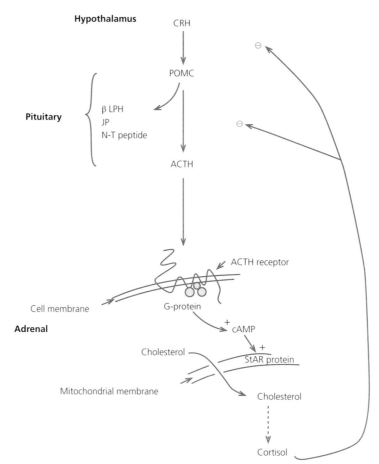

Hypothalamus   CRH

POMC

Pituitary
β LPH
JP
N-T peptide

ACTH

ACTH receptor

Cell membrane   G-protein

Adrenal

⊕
⊖

+
cAMP

Cholesterol
+
StAR protein

Mitochondrial membrane
Cholesterol

Cortisol

Figure 8.1 Schematic diagram of hypothalamic–pituitary–adrenal axis. b LPH, b lipotrophic hormone; CRH, corticotrophin-releasing hormone; JP, joining peptide; N-T peptide, N-terminal peptide; POMC, pro-opiomelanocortin; StAR protein, steroidogenic acute regulatory protein; +, positive effect; −, negative effect.

partial deficiency, basal cortisol may be normal. However, since basal cortisol output is already maximal in this situation, there will be no further increase should a major physical stress occur and signs of acute adrenal insufficiency may then develop.

Steroid pathways

Adrenal steroidogenesis is under the control of the cytochrome P450 (CYP) and the hydroxysteroid dehydrogenase (HSD) enzymes. Pregnenolone is converted along the mineralocorticoid pathway to aldosterone, along the glucocorticoid pathway to cortisol, or along the androgen pathway to testosterone (Figure 8.2). Impairment of cortisol synthesis results from disorders affecting the StAR protein and 3-β-hydroxysteroid dehydrogenase (3-βHSD), CYP

21A2 (21-hydroxylase), CYP 11B1 (11-hydroxylase), and the CYP 17 (17-hydroxylase) enzymes. These enzyme disorders are collectively known as 'congenital adrenal hyperplasia (CAH)', as cortisol deficiency causes increased ACTH secretion and thus enlargement of the adrenal glands. Mineralocorticoid deficiency results from StAR protein, 3-βHSD and CYP 21 deficiencies, while CYP deficiency in 11B1 or 17-hydroxylase deficiency results in mineralocorticoid excess. Finally, deficiency in the enzymes proximal to testosterone – StAR protein, CYP 17 (17,20-desmolase), 17-βHSD and 3- βHSD – results in under-masculinization of males. Lastly, 3-βHSD deficiency does not typically cause in utero virilization in females, because the steroid immediately above the enzyme block is dehydroepiandrosterone, a relatively weak androgen; however, mild postnatal signs of

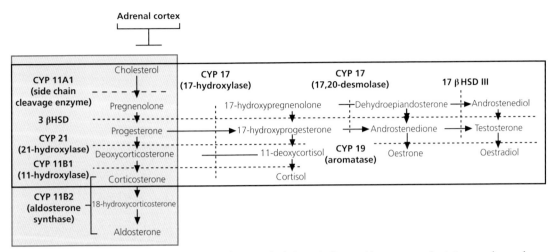

Figure 8.2 Pathways of steroid synthesis in adrenal cortex. Shaded area indicates aldosterone synthesis in zona glomerulosa. Cortisol and androgen are synthesized in the zona fasciculata and zona reticularis, respectively. bHSD, b hydroxysteroid dehydrogenase.

hypersecretion of this weak androgen, such as precocious pubarche, may be observed.

Mineralocorticoid synthesis

Aldosterone synthase, encoded by the *CYP 11B2* gene, converts deoxycorticosterone (DOC) to aldosterone (Figure 8.3). Renin, secreted from the juxtaglomerular apparatus (JGA) in the kidney, causes cleavage of angiotensinogen into angiotensin 1, which is in turn cleaved by angiotensin-converting enzyme (ACE) into angiotensin 2, a potent stimulator of *CYP 11B2* activity, promoting aldosterone secretion from the zona glomerulosa. Renin will therefore be elevated when aldosterone synthesis is impaired, and suppressed with aldosterone excess. Aldosterone enters the distal renal tubular cells, binds to its receptor and enters the nucleus, causing enhanced activity of the $Na^+ K^+$ ATPase ('the sodium pump') and of the amiloride-sensitive epithelial sodium channel (ENaC), resulting in sodium reabsorption.

The following points should be noted:
- Cortisol has a similar affinity for the mineralocorticoid receptor (MR) as aldosterone, but is prevented from competing for this receptor by the enzyme 11-βHSD 2 which converts cortisol to cortisone. 11-βHSD 2 deficiency causes apparent mineralocorticoid excess (AME).
- Mutations inactivating ENaC or the mineralocorticoid receptor result in aldosterone resistance and elevated aldosterone levels – pseudohypoaldosteronism (PHA).

- Mutations activating ENaC result in apparent aldosterone excess despite low levels – Liddle's syndrome.
- Aldosterone excess causes sodium retention with hypernatraemia, hypokalaemia, a metabolic alkalosis and hypertension.

Investigations of adrenocortical function

Biochemical

Glucocorticoid secretion

Glucocorticoid excess and deficiency states are often difficult to diagnose because cortisol levels normally fluctuate widely according to the time of day and degree of stress (Table 8.1). Glucocorticoid excess results in normal or high random cortisol levels, loss of the normal circadian rhythm, an increase in urinary free cortisol and failure of plasma cortisol to suppress with low-dose dexamethasone.

Glucocorticoid deficiency is easy to diagnose if the defect is in the adrenal gland itself (primary adrenal insufficiency) because this will result in elevated ACTH levels and low cortisol levels with absent or impaired rise following synthetic ACTH (Cortrosyn® or Synacthen®) stimulation. The diagnosis is more difficult when the defect lies in the hypothalamus or pituitary gland (central adrenal insufficiency, CAI). In suspected secondary adrenal insufficiency, the low-dose synthetic ACTH test may be helpful. The rationale for this test is

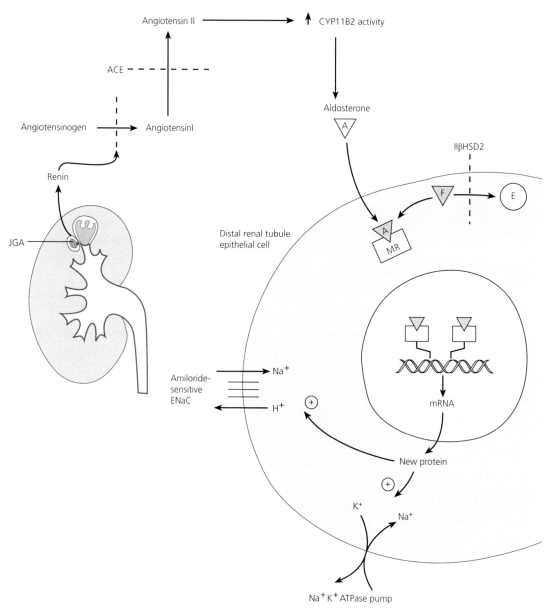

Figure 8.3 Schematic diagram of aldosterone stimulation and action. A, aldosterone; ACE, angiotensin converting enzyme; E, cortisone; ENaC, epithelial sodium channel; F, cortisol; JGA, juxtaglomerular apparatus; MR, mineralocorticoid receptor; 11βHSD2, 11-betahydroxysteroid dehydrogenase 2.

that the adrenal glands, if under-stimulated for months or years, will respond subnormally to quasi-physiological stimulation. A peak stimulated cortisol greater than 550 nmol/L is considered normal, while a peak of less than 400 nmol l^{-1} is considered too low, and a great many patients fall in the grey zone in between. We regard a peak-stimulated cortisol level of >500 nmol l^{-1} as 'normal' (see Table 8.1) while recognizing that any

chosen cut-off level will be somewhat arbitrary and that the biochemical data must be interpreted in the clinical context.

Mineralocorticoid secretion

Mineralocorticoid deficiency is assessed by the measurement of plasma and urinary electrolytes, and of plasma renin and aldosterone (Table 8.2).

Table 8.1 Investigation of glucocorticoid secretion.

Basal samples	Reference values
Plasma	
Fasting glucose	4–7 mmol/L
0800 h ACTH	<20 mU/L
2400 h (sleeping) cortisol	<50 nmol/L
0800 h cortisol	200–700 nmol/L
Saliva	
8 a.m. cortisol	6.5–28 nmol/L (usually 9–16) median 14.5
6 p.m. cortisol	≤10 (mean 1.4)
Urine	
Urinary-free cortisol (random)	<25 µmol /mmol/L creatinine
Suppression tests	
Low-dose dexamethasone (1 mg at 11 p.m.)	Plasma cortisol <50 nmol/L at 8 a.m. the next day
High-dose dexamethasone (2 mg 6-h × 8)	Plasma cortisol <50% basal value 48 h after last dose
Stimulation tests	
CRH (1 µg/kg IV)	Doubling of ACTH (usually to 8–25 mU/L)
	Cortisol peak ≥600 nmol/L with >20% increase over basal value
Standard short Synacthen (250 µg m^{-2} IV)	Peak cortisol >500 nmol/L± doubling of basal value
Low-dose short Synacthen (500 ng m^{-2} IV)	Peak cortisol >500 nmol/L± doubling of basal value
Insulin hypoglycaemia (min blood glucose <2.2 mmol/L)	Peak cortisol >500 nmol/L
Metyrapone test	Doubling of plasma 11 deoxycortisol and urinary tetrahydrodeoxycortisol

ACTH, adrenocorticotrophic hormone; CRH, corticotrophin-releasing hormone.
Source: Reference values are taken from the Institute of Biochemistry, Glasgow Royal Infirmary. Salivary cortisol data kindly provided by Dr J. Schulga are derived from 147 healthy children aged 5–15 years.

Adrenal androgen secretion

Adrenal androgen status is assessed by plasma steroid analysis under basal and stimulated conditions (Table 8.3). Monitoring of patients with 21 hydroxylase deficiency is routinely based on the measurement of plasma 17-hydroxyprogesterone (17-OHP) and androstenedione at the time of clinic visits. If available, salivary or capillary profiles collected at home may add information about adherence to treatment.

Glucocorticoid excess

Cushing's syndrome

Cushing's syndrome, unless iatrogenic, is very rare in childhood (Figure 8.4). However, its principal feature, obesity, is extremely common, so that the possibility of Cushing's syndrome is often raised.

Imaging

If a central cause for glucocorticoid excess or deficiency is discovered, imaging of the hypothalamic–pituitary area by magnetic resonance imaging (MRI) will be required. Adrenal ultrasound to detect adrenal enlargement is very operator-dependent and computed tomography (CT) or MRI are needed to identify discrete lesions.

Causes

The causes of Cushing's syndrome in childhood are the following:
- Iatrogenic: glucocorticoids by mouth, inhalation, skin preparations or nose drops
- Cushing's disease (ACTH-secreting pituitary tumour)
- Adrenal tumour (cortical adenoma or carcinoma)
- Primary adrenal hyperplasia: bilateral micronodular dysplasia (± Carney complex) and McCune–Albright syndrome
- Ectopic ACTH syndrome (exceedingly rare in children).

Table 8.2 Investigation of mineralocorticoid secretion.

Electrolytes	Normal values	Mineralocorticoid excess	Mineralocorticoid deficiency
Sodium	Na 135–145 mmol/L	Normal or ↑	↓
Potassium	K 3.5–4.5 mmol/L	Normal or ↓	↑
Aldosterone (pmol l^{-1})[a]			
Infants <1 mo	1000–5500	↑ in hyperaldosteronism	↓ in hypoaldosteronism
Infants 1–6 mo	500–4500	↓ in AME and Liddle's syndrome	↑↑ in PHA
Infants 6–12 mo	160–3000		
Children 1–4 yr	70–1000		
Children 5–15 yr	30–600		
Adults	30–420		
Plasma renin activity (ng (ml/h)[b] (supine for 30 min)			
Infants (<1 yr)	<31	Suppressed	↑
Children 1–4 yr	<26		
Children 5–15 yr	<9		
Adults	<2.6		

AME, apparent mineralocorticoid excess; PHA, pseudohypoaldosteronism.
[a] Aldosterone data obtained using Diagnostic Products Corporation Coat-A-Count Aldosterone Kit.
[b] Plasma renin activity data obtained using BioChem ImmunoSystems Renin Maia Kit (Code 129640).

Clinical diagnosis

Symptoms
- Obesity
- Slow growth (overtaken by siblings and peers)
- Fatigue
- Emotional lability

Signs
- Cushingoid habitus with moon face, central obesity, and buffalo hump
- Facial plethora
- Acne
- Hirsutism
- Striae
- Hypertension

Growth
- Height below mid-parental centile
- Height velocity subnormal
- Bone age usually delayed

The crucial difference between obesity, as a result of Cushing's syndrome/disease, and exogenous obesity is in the growth pattern. Cushing's syndrome/disease is almost always associated with a slower, and exogenous obesity with a faster, rate of linear growth. Appreciation of this difference in growth will largely protect children with simple obesity from being investigated for Cushing's syndrome, although the occasional child with familial short stature and exogenous obesity may cause confusion. It is important not to subject children with simple obesity to investigation of Cushing's syndrome since plasma and urine cortisol levels may be elevated in these subjects. Steroid biochemistry should also be interpreted with care in adolescent girls who may be on the oral contraceptive pill since this treatment increases CBG levels and hence plasma cortisol.

Investigations

Where exogenous steroid excess (by a steroid other than cortisol) is suspected, a low or undetectable 0800 hours plasma cortisol will usually confirm suppression of the pituitary–adrenal axis (see Table 8.1) and a low-dose ACTH test is seldom necessary. If the features of Cushing's syndrome are accompanied by virilization, then an adrenal tumour is likely and an adrenal CT scan should be performed promptly.

Diagnosis of Cushing's syndrome or disease

The following can be carried out in a non-specialist centre (from most to least practical):
- plasma cortisol levels at 8 a.m. after taking dexamethasone 1 mg orally at 23 p.m. the night before: if cortisol <50 nmol/L, Cushing's syndrome or disease is reasonably excluded. If the patient is very obese (>100 kg), use 2 mg of dexamethasone. Timing of dexamethasone administration and blood draw is critical.

Table 8.3 Investigation of adrenal steroid precursors and androgens.

17-hydroxyprogesterone

Plasma (nmol l⁻¹)

Normal neonates	<13	
Stressed/preterm neonates	<40	
Neonates with CAH	>100	
Adults		
Basal	<13	
60 min after 250 μm iv Synacthen	<20	

Blood spot (nmol/L)	*Extraction assay*	*Direct assay*
Stressed/preterm neonates	<70	<140
Neonates with CAH	>180	>350

Saliva (nmol/L of saliva)

Children 5–15 yr 09.00 h	0.16–0.66 (median range 0.22–0.4)	

Androstenedione (mean ± SD)	Male	Female
Plasma (nmol/L)		
1–2 mo	1.5 ± 0.45	0.66 ± 0.24
>6 mo–adrenarche	<0.4	<0.4
Adult male	3.7 ± 0.9	
Adult female		
follicular phase		2.7 ± 1.0
luteal phase		5.2 ± 1.5
Saliva (nmol/L)		
5–15 yr 09.00 h	0.04–0.96 (median range 0.2–0.7)	

Testosterone (mean ± SD)	Male	Female
Plasma (nmol/L)		
First wk	1.15 ± 0.15	0.45 ± 0.3
1–2 mo	8.8 ± 2.7	0.28 ± 0.13
>6 mo–prepubertal	<0.3	<0.3
Adult male	19.8 ± 4.7	
Adult female		
follicular phase		0.75 ± 0.2
luteal phase		1.28 ± 0.3

Dehydroepiandrosterone sulfate (μmol/L of plasma)	Male	Female
Infancy, pre-adrenarche	<2	<2
Adult	2–9	2–11

Source: Blood spot 17-hydroxyprogesterone data are from A.M. Wallace et al. (1986). Salivary data are from Dr Schulga (see Table 8.1). Plasma androstenedione and testosterone data are from M.G. Forest (1979).

- Measurement of plasma cortisol levels at 8 a.m. and 4 p.m., looking for loss of the normal circadian rhythm.
- Measurement of three consecutive 24-hour urinary free cortisol estimations, looking for elevated cortisol excretion.
- Plasma or salivary cortisol at midnight <50 nmol/L).

Aetiological diagnosis of hypercortisolism

This can be difficult. Referral to a specialist centre is recommended.

- *ACTH measurement at 8 a.m..* Undetectable values suggest a primary adrenal lesion, detectable levels pituitary Cushing's and elevated levels ectopic ACTH syndrome.
- *High-dose dexamethasone suppression test,* measuring at 9 a.m. plasma cortisol, then giving dexamethasone 2 mg at 9 a.m., 3 p.m., 9 p.m., and 3 a.m. × 2, i.e. eight doses over 48 hours, then re-measuring plasma cortisol at 9 a.m. A fall in cortisol to below more than 50% of the basal value is suggestive of pituitary Cushing's (Cushing's disease), while failure to suppress suggests ectopic ACTH syndrome.

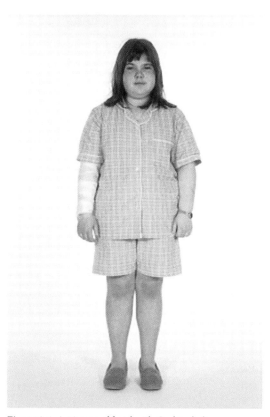

Figure 8.4 A 10-year-old girl with Cushing's disease causing growth failure and obesity.

- According to the ACTH level, imaging of either adrenal (CT or MRI) or pituitary (high-resolution MRI) should be carried out.
- The final step in the investigation of Cushing's disease is a stimulation test with desmopressin, or CRH if ACTH does not respond to the former. The selected stimulus is then administered with bilateral inferior petrosal sinus sampling. This should only be carried out in a specialist centre and is helpful in confirming the pituitary origin of the ACTH secretion and the side of the microadenoma.

Treatment

Iatrogenic Cushing's syndrome must be managed by withdrawal of the glucocorticoid preparation or, if this is not possible, by minimizing the dosage given, or converting to an alternate day regimen. If severe adrenal suppression has occurred, hydrocortisone replacement may be required for months, or even years, following treatment. Treatment of an adrenal or pituitary tumour is by surgical resection, followed by hydrocortisone replacement if the other adrenal gland

is suppressed. After bilateral adrenalectomy, mineralocorticoids should be given as well.

Cushing's disease is treated by trans-sphenoidal surgical exploration with removal of the microadenoma. If none is identified, but petrosal sinus sampling has suggested lateralization of ACTH secretion, then a hemihypophysectomy can be carried out. A post-operative cortisol level of <50 nmol/L [<1.4 µg/dL] indicates that the adenoma has been completely removed and the patient is cured. The treatment of choice for Cushing's disease following failed pituitary exploration is direct pituitary irradiation. The alternative, bilateral adrenalectomy, carries a long-term risk of Nelson's syndrome (growth of the corticotroph adenoma).

The ectopic ACTH syndrome may be seen as part of an established malignancy. Occasionally, small carcinoid lesions (e.g. lungs, pancreas) may be responsible, requiring location by CT scanning with selective venous sampling where necessary, and surgical removal.

Cushing's syndrome caused by bilateral micronodular dysplasia with or without primary pigmentation (Carney's syndrome), or the McCune–Albright syndrome, should be treated medically if features are mild to moderate, otherwise by bilateral adrenalectomy. When surgical resection is impossible (e.g. with infiltrating carcinoma), or in pituitary Cushing's disease when there may be a delay of several months before remission occurs (e.g. following radiotherapy), then medical therapy must be given. Useful agents include metyrapone and ketoconazole. In adrenal carcinoma, the adrenal cytotoxic o,p'-dichlorodiphenyl-dichloroethane (o,p'-DDD) (mitotane) is of temporary benefit.

Follow-up

After definitive treatment of Cushing's syndrome, patients should be seen three-monthly to monitor growth rate, body composition, and signs of recurrence.

Glucocorticoid deficiency

Adrenal insufficiency caused by hypothalamic–pituitary disease – central adrenal insufficiency (CAI)

Causes

The causes of CAI are as follows:
- *Congenital:*
  - idiopathic congenital hypopituitarism;
  - septo-optic dysplasia;

- other mid-line central nervous system (CNS) disorders;
- isolated ACTH deficiency (mutations in TPit, POMC, or NFKB2).
- *Acquired*
  - craniopharyngioma;
  - cranial irradiation (e.g. for head and neck tumours);
  - surgery to hypothalamic–pituitary area;
  - steroid therapy
  - vascular insult, trauma, meningitis.

Clinical features

ACTH deficiency is usually seen in association with several other anterior pituitary hormone deficiencies. Severe ACTH deficiency at birth causes hypoglycaemia, poor feeding, convulsions and jaundice. The jaundice is of the cholestatic type and resolves once hydrocortisone is started.

In older children, the symptoms of CAI are non-specific. Cortisol deficiency is responsible for tiredness and lack of energy, with increased susceptibility to and a longer recovery period from minor illnesses. Children with POMC deficiency also have severe obesity and red hair. Some POMC mutations lead to high, not low, plasma ACTH. NFKB2 mutations are also associated with common variable immunodeficiency.

Investigations

In the newborn infant, dynamic studies are difficult to perform. If congenital hypopituitarism is strongly suspected (hypoglycaemia, jaundice, micropenis, low plasma free thyroxine (FT4) and random plasma cortisol levels less than 50 nmol/L [1.4 μg dL]), then replacement should be instituted without delay. In more doubtful cases where the child is reasonably stable, 1 μg ACTH can be given intravenously and the cortisol response assessed at 30 minutes. Peak values of <550 nmol/L [<19 μg/dL] are suggestive of prenatal hypostimulation of the adrenal glands.

In children with suspected CAI, especially survivors of cancer, investigation depends on the severity of symptoms and the clinical context. Children who have received doses of >3000 cGy are particularly at risk. Cortisol secretion can be assessed by carrying out a low-dose ACTH test, or a salivary cortisol profile. An undetectable plasma dehydroepiandrosterone sulphate (DHEAS) level at an age when adrenarche should have occurred (>8 years) is indirect evidence of at least partial ACTH deficiency.

Treatment

Hydrocortisone, 10 mg/m² per day should be given divided in two or three doses per day. Treatment during an intercurrent illness or during surgery is as for 21-hydroxylase deficiency (see section 'Treatment'). Once the child is on glucocorticoid replacement, biochemical monitoring is not usually necessary.

Primary adrenal insufficiency

Causes

- *Congenital:*
  - adrenal hypoplasia – X-linked (DAX-1 mutation) or autosomal recessive;
  - CAH;
  - familial glucocorticoid deficiency (FGD) (autosomal recessive) or resistance.
- *Acquired:*
  - isolated autoimmune adrenalitis (Addison's disease);
  - adrenalitis associated with other autoimmune endocrinopathies;
  - adrenoleukodystrophy (ALD);
  - tuberculosis;
  - bilateral adrenalectomy;
  - drugs (e.g. cyproterone).

Congenital adrenal hypoplasia

In the newborn period, cortisol deficiency will cause hypoglycaemia and jaundice, while aldosterone deficiency will result in hyponatraemia, hyperkalaemia, poor feeding, vomiting, and failure to thrive. Investigations will show elevated renin and ACTH, but low or normal 17-OHP. Symptoms usually start from day 10 onwards. Boys with a DAX-1 (dosage-sensitive sex reversal, adrenal hypoplasia critical region, on chromosome X, gene 1) mutation may have bilateral cryptorchidism in infancy and gonadotrophin deficiency in adolescence.

Familial glucocorticoid deficiency

Familial glucocorticoid deficiency (FGD, also known as 'hereditary unresponsiveness to ACTH') is an autosomal recessive disorder in which the adrenal cortex is unable to respond to ACTH. In about 25% of cases, a mutation on the ACTH receptor MC2-R can be identified. These children, who tend to be tall, are classified as having FGD type 1. FGD without an MC2-R mutation is termed FGD type 2. Recently, mutations in a new gene encoding a protein called melanocortin 2 receptor accessory protein (MRAP) have been identified in some cases of FGD type 2.

MRAP is required for the expression of MC2-R at the cell membrane. More recently identified causes include mutations in *NNT* (some with associated mineralocorticoid deficiency and insulin-dependent diabetes) or in *TXNRD2*.

Patients present with jaundice, poor feeding, failure to thrive, and hypoglycaemia in infancy. Older children may present with collapse and coma, sometimes with fatal consequences so that the diagnosis is only made post mortem. Investigations show elevated ACTH, low cortisol with poor or no response to ACTH and normal renin levels. Plasma potassium is usually normal but a degree of hyponatraemia may be present. This is attributable to cortisol deficiency causing impaired water secretion at the renal tubule.

Treatment

Congenital adrenal hypoplasia should be treated similarly to 21-hydroxylase deficiency (see section 'Treatment'), although the dose of hydrocortisone used can be somewhat lower (as there is no need to suppress ACTH to prevent hyperandrogenism). FGD should be treated with hydrocortisone but not fludrocortisone or salt.

Acquired adrenal insufficiency

Causes

Autoimmune adrenalitis (Addison's disease) is the most common cause of acquired primary adrenal deficiency. Although seen in isolation, it may also be associated with other autoimmune disorders, such as diabetes mellitus and Hashimoto's thyroiditis, and with the polyglandular autoimmune (PGA) syndromes. PGA 1, also known as autoimmune polyendocrinopathy with endocrinopathy, muco-cutaneous candidiasis and ectodermal dystrophy (APECED), is a recessive condition caused by mutations in the AIRE (autoimmune regulator) gene on chromosome 21 and has its onset in childhood and adolescence. Components of APECED syndrome include the following:

- *Endocrine:*
  - Addison's disease;
  - hypoparathyroidism;
  - primary ovarian failure;
  - diabetes mellitus;
  - hypophysitis.
- *Non-endocrine:*
  - vitiligo;
  - alopecia;
  - malabsorption;

- hepatitis;
- keratitis;
- immune deficiency – increased prevalence of infections, particularly mucocutaneous candidiasis.

ALD is an X-linked recessive disorder affecting both the CNS and the adrenal cortex. Onset may be in childhood or early adulthood. The phenotype is highly variable, even within families, so that the presence and severity of neurological impairment and adrenal failure vary from case to case. Severely affected individuals suffer progressive neurological disability, and ultimately death. The neurological symptoms may precede those of adrenal insufficiency, or vice versa. Therefore, in all males with primary adrenal insufficiency other than CAH, plasma very long chain fatty acids must be measured.

Clinical features of primary adrenal insufficiency

Symptoms include tiredness, weight loss, and, in the final stages, vomiting, drowsiness, and coma. Examination shows increased pigmentation (Figure 8.5), especially in the skin creases, old scars and buccal mucosa, with signs of recent weight loss, and low or normal blood pressure.

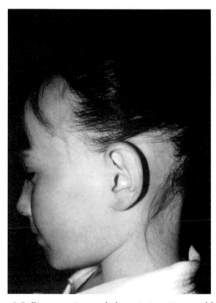

Figure 8.5 Pigmentation and alopecia in a 10 year-old-girl who also had nail dystrophy caused by *Candida*. Investigations showed both Addison's disease and hypoparathyroidism. Genetic studies showed a homozygous 13-bp deletion in exon 8 of the autoimmune regulator gene on chromosome 21q22.3.

Investigations

Fasting glucose is normal or low. In acute adrenal insufficiency, sodium is low, potassium is high, and there may be severe hypoglycaemia. Basal cortisol is low or normal with no rise following ACTH administration. Plasma ACTH and renin activity are high. Given the association between Addison's disease and other autoimmune diseases and ALD, the following is recommended at diagnosis and yearly thereafter:
- autoantibody screen (adrenal, thyroid, islet cell, parietal cell);
- calcium, phosphate, complete blood count (CBC), vitamin B_{12}, folate, thyroid-stimulating hormone (TSH), and alanine amino transferase (ALT).

Treatment

Acute adrenal insufficiency is managed by intravenous (IV) fluids with 0.9% saline and added 5% glucose, IV hydrocortisone (see p. 182) and conversion to oral hydrocortisone and fludrocortisone once recovery has occurred (Table 8.4).

Follow-up

Once a patient is on established treatment with hydrocortisone and fludrocortisone, clinical monitoring and adjusting the dosage as body surface area increases are usually sufficient and there is no need for laboratory investigations.

Mineralocorticoid excess

Apart from the secondary hyperaldosteronism seen in cardiac and renal patients and in chronic volume depletion (leading to activation of the renin–angiotensin system), mineralocorticoid excess is very rare.

Table 8.4 Dosage schedules for mineralocorticoid, glucocorticoid and salt therapy in adrenal disorders.

Disorder	Mineralocorticoid	Glucocorticoid	Salt
Hypothalamo–pituitary-adrenal insufficiency	Not required	Hydrocortisone 8–10 mg m²/day	
Primary adrenal insufficiency (Addison's disease)	Fludrocortisone 100–200 µg/day: • Not related to body size • Decrease if high BP and suppressed renin	Hydrocortisone 10–12 mg/m²/day	
Congenital adrenal hypoplasia	As for primary adrenal insufficiency	For first 6 mo consider treatments as for CAH. (see p. 190), then hydrocortisone 10–12 mg/m²/day	
FGD	Not required	As for primary adrenal insufficiency (Addison's disease)	
CAH (21-hydroxylase deficiency)			
Salt-wasting	As in Addison's	For first 6 mo of life, see pp. 195. Oral hydrocortisone 10–15 mg mg/m²/day thereafter. Dexamethasone 0.25 mg hs after epiphyseal fusion (check for iatrogenic Cushing's)	5 mmol/L/kg/day in three divided doses for first yr
Simple virilizing	As above if renin ↑ at diagnosis	As above	Not required
Pseudohypoaldosteronism	Not usually effective		Sodium chloride 10–40 mmol kg/day + calcium or sodium resonium

ACTH, adrenocorticotrophic hormone; CAH, congenital adrenal hyperplasia; FGD, familial glucocorticoid deficiency.

Causes

- *Iatrogenic*
- fludrocortisone overdosage, carbenoxolone or liquorice ingestion.
- aldosterone-secreting adrenal adenoma/hyperplasia (Conn's syndrome).
- *Enzyme blocks.* 11-hydroxylase, 17-hydroxylase, 11-βHSD 2 deficiencies;
- CYP11B2/CYP11B1 chimeric rearrangements;
- activating mutation of ENaC (Liddle's syndrome).

Secondary hyperaldosteronism does not normally present to the endocrinologist. Fludrocortisone overdosage may result in hypertension with or without hypokalaemia. Carbenoxolone is rarely used, but liquorice addiction can cause the syndrome of AME, brought about by 11-βHSD 2 inhibition (see below). Aldosterone-secreting adrenal adenomas are rare in childhood, and other causes of hyperaldosteronism must be ruled out before invasive procedures, such as selective adrenal vein sampling, are performed.

Two of the enzyme disorders causing CAH, 11-hydroxylase and 17-hydroxylase deficiencies, cause hypertension with hypokalaemia. 11-hydroxylase deficiency causes virilization in girls and sexual precocity in boys from infancy, but affected children are hypertensive because of the high levels of DOC, rather than salt-losing as in 21-hydroxylase deficiency. 17-hydroxylase deficiency causes cortisol and androgen deficiency but mineralocorticoid excess, so that affected 46,XY individuals are phenotypically female and may present with pubertal failure in association with hypertension and hypokalaemia. Deficiency of the enzyme 11-βHSD 2 results in failure to metabolize cortisol to cortisone, with consequent occupation of mineralocorticoid receptors by cortisol (Figure 8.3). The clinical features are those of mineralocorticoid excess but aldosterone levels are suppressed, hence the term AME.

Mutations of the *CYP 11B2* gene may lead to a chimeric enzyme which is under ACTH control, resulting in glucocorticoid-suppressible hyperaldosteronism. This condition should be suspected in the hypertensive adolescent, with or without hypokalaemia, in whom there is a family history of hypertension and cerebral haemorrhage. Treatment is with dexamethasone or amiloride.

Liddle's syndrome is autosomal dominant and caused by an activating mutation of the ENaC, leading to increased sodium absorption with aldosterone and renin suppression. Treatment is with amiloride.

Mineralocorticoid deficiency

Causes

Aldosterone deficiency
- Congenital adrenal hypoplasia.
- Addison's disease.
- *Enzyme disorders:*
  - StAR protein deficiency;
  - 3-βHSD deficiency;
  - CYP 21 (21-hydroxylase) deficiency; or
  - CYP 11B2 (aldosterone synthase) deficiency.

Aldosterone resistance (pseudohypoaldosteronism)
- Autosomal dominant or sporadic – affects renal tubule.
- Recessive – affects kidneys, colon, and sweat and salivary glands.

Clinical features and investigation

Mineralocorticoid deficiency causes salt-wasting with polyuria, vomiting, dehydration, and hyperkalaemia which, if severe and untreated, leads to cardiac arrest. In older children, the salt-wasting tendency is partially offset by an instinctive increase in salt intake. Congenital adrenal hypoplasia and Addison's disease are discussed above; the three types of CAH causing salt-wasting are discussed below.

PHA may be associated with salt-wasting and dangerous hyperkalaemia in the newborn period. Affected infants do not respond to large doses of fludrocortisone, and treatment consists of generous sodium replacement (Table 8.4) and resins to combat hyperkalaemia. The dominant and sporadic forms are milder and resolve with age. The autosomal recessive variety, caused by inactivating mutations in the ENaC, is severe and runs a protracted course.

Sex steroid excess

Androgen excess

Adrenal causes of androgen excess
- Adrenocortical adenoma and carcinoma.
- *CAH:*
  - CYP 21 (21-hydroxylase) deficiency and CYP 11β1 (11-hydroxylase) deficiency;
  - 3-βHSD deficiency in females;
  - 11-βHSD 1 deficiency.

Isolated premature pubarche is common (see Chapter 5) but virilization in girls or prepubertal boys suggests an androgen-secreting tumour or an enzyme defect.

Adrenocortical tumour

Clinical features
Virilization develops over a period of weeks or months and accelerated linear growth and bone maturation then become apparent. In boys, the testes are prepubertal (Figure 8.6).

Investigations
These show a marked elevation of one or more of the adrenal androgens, androstenedione, and DHEAS. Abdominal ultrasound, followed by CT or MRI scanning, should be obtained without delay.

Treatment
Treatment is by surgical removal wherever possible. If the tumour is well circumscribed and <5 cm in diameter, the prognosis is good. Pathological features are usually not helpful in predicting the risk of recurrence or of metastases.

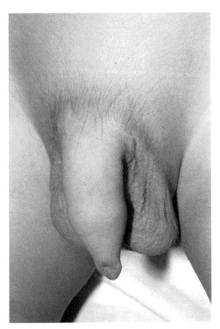

Figure 8.6 Penile enlargement, pubic hair development and scrotal laxity with prepubertal (2 ml) testes in a two-year-old boy. Investigation showed a small tumour in the right adrenal cortex.

Adrenal enzyme defects

21-hydroxylase deficiency is by far the most common adrenal enzyme disorder and will be discussed in detail. 11- and 17-hydroxylase deficiencies are discussed above (see p. 182). 3-βHSD deficiency in females causes mild postnatal androgenization because of high DHEAS levels. Deficiency in P450 oxidoreductase, the electron donor for 21- and 17-hydroxylases and aromatase, may be associated with bone abnormalities.

21-hydroxylase deficiency

Incidence
In most populations, the incidence is about one in 15 000 births.

Pathogenesis and classification
21-hydroxylase deficiency results from mutations in the *CYP21B* gene, which is situated on chromosome 6. The phenotype of 21-hydroxylase deficiency correlates reasonably well with the following genotype:
- Salt-wasting 21-hydroxylase deficiency (SW 21-OHD) results from a child inheriting two severe mutations, leading to complete or near-complete loss of 21-B function, with <1% of normal 21-hydroxylase activity.
- Simple virilizing 21-hydroxylase deficiency (SV 21-OHD) occurs if one of the two mutations (e.g. point mutation Ile172Asn) is relatively mild with 1–5% preservation of 21-hydroxylase activity. Significant salt loss does not occur, although plasma renin activity is often elevated.
- Non-classical or late onset 21-hydroxylase deficiency (NC 21-OHD) results if one mutation is mild (e.g. Val 281Leu). Likely an ascertainment bias, it is diagnosed more often in females.

Clinical features
SW 21-OHD females present with virilization at birth. The clitoris is enlarged and there generally is posterior fusion of the labia majora (Figure 8.7). The vagina and urethra usually enter a common urogenital sinus, with the distal end of the vagina becoming increasingly more distant from the pelvic floor with the severity of virilization. Virilization can be graded in severity according to the Prader classification (Figure 8.8).

Males with SW 21-OHD usually present in the second week of life, with a salt-losing crisis heralded by poor feeding, vomiting, poor weight gain, and listlessness. Examination shows dehydration with pigmentation of the scrotum. Biochemistry reveals hyponatraemia and hyperkalaemia. Death may occur before the diagnosis is considered. For this reason, neonatal screening for SW 21-OHD is being implemented in an increasing number of countries. However, this is not yet universal because the positive predictive value of a high 17-OHP is very low, especially in premature or stressed neonates.

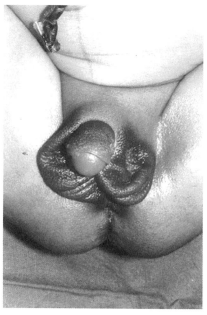

Figure 8.7 Severe virilization with fusion of labia majora and gross clitoral enlargement in a female infant with 21-hydroxylase deficiency.

Boys with SV 21-OHD, and girls with SV 21-OHD in whom virilization at birth has been mild and/or missed, will present later in childhood (usually two to four years) with signs of androgen excess – long-standing growth acceleration and advanced bone age, enlarged penis or clitoris, and pubic hair. Both girls and boys with SV 21-OHD enter true puberty early when treated with glucocorticoids because of priming of the hypothalamic–pituitary axis. This leads to premature closure of the epiphyses and an adult height below target.

NC 21-OHD is a rare cause of hyperandrogenism in adolescent and adult females and should be considered in the differential diagnosis of the polycystic ovary syndrome.

Diagnosis

SW 21-OHD is diagnosed in females with ambiguous genitalia, no palpable gonads, hyperpigmentation of the labia majora and a uterus on ultrasound, and in boys with a salt-wasting crisis. Biochemical confirmation is based on high plasma androgens and 17-OHP (values usually >100 nmol l^{-1} [>3300 ng dl^{-1}]).

In SV and NC 21-OHD, 17-OHP elevation is milder. Levels are higher between 8.00 a.m. and 9.00 a.m. In this context, 17-OHP at 0 and 60 minutes after standard ACTH stimulation (250 µg), can be compared to the nomogram published by New et al. in 1983.

Prenatal management

After the birth of a child affected with 21-OHD, the genotype of parents, affected child, and healthy siblings can be determined. The main purpose of prenatal testing is to assist with maternal dexamethasone treatment. Pre-pregnancy counselling as to the pros and cons of this intervention is important. If the

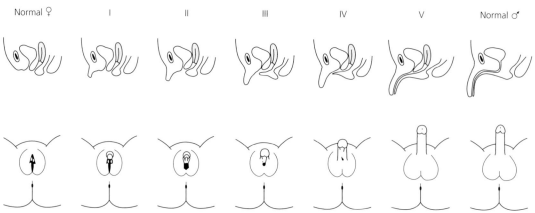

Figure 8.8 Prader classification of five stages of virilization in the female infant.

mother chooses to be treated, dexamethasone 20 µg/kg per day should be started by four to six weeks' gestation. This should be continued throughout pregnancy if the foetus is an affected female, but stopped if the foetus is male or an unaffected female. Determining the sex of the embryo and *CYP21B* genotyping based on free embryonic DNA in maternal blood will allow shortening unnecessary treatments. The demonstrated benefit of reducing or preventing virilization in girls must be offset against hypertension, weight gain, striæ, and mood changes in the mother. The possible long-term physical and psychological deleterious consequences of in utero dexamethasone exposure have led to this treatment no longer being even suggested to the couple by some clinicians.

Neonatal management

Diagnosis and management of 21-OHD in newborn females are part of disorders of sex development (DSD) management (see Chapter 7).

Once the diagnosis has been confirmed, treatment must be started as follows:

1 Fludrocortisone 0.05–0.100 mg per day.
2 Sodium chloride 5 mmol kg per day in three divided doses given as either 6% (1 mmol/ml), 15% (2.5 mmol/ml), or 30% (5 mmol/ml) solution. The solution may be added to milk feeds or given separately (e.g. if mother is breast-feeding).
3 Hydrocortisone 20 mg/m^2 per day in three divided doses.

If clinical evidence of salt-wasting is present (weight loss >10%), manage as follows:

1 Measure electrolytes and 17-OHP. Hyperkalaemia usually precedes hyponatremia and hypoglycaemia.
2 Give 10–30 ml/kg of 0.9% saline over one to three hours depending on the degree of dehydration, then 0.9% saline at a rate sufficient to provide maintenance, and correct any deficit over 24 hours. Monitor capillary glucose.
3 Give hydrocortisone 25 mg intravenously immediately, then 12.5 mg six hourly until enteral administration can be started.
4 When plasma sodium is normal and the infant is stable, start fludrocortisone, sodium chloride and hydrocortisone as above.

Management in infancy

Glucocorticoid Therapy

Treatment consists of oral hydrocortisone, approximately 15 mg/m^2 per day in three divided doses.

Suspensions are unreliable and 10 mg hydrocortisone tablets should be given halved or quartered, asking the pharmacy to prepare powder if needed.

Fludrocortisone Therapy

Fludrocortisone 0.05–0.100 mg per day, with blood pressure monitoring.

Salt Therapy

The dosage of 5 mmol /kg per day should be maintained for the first 12 months of life and is usually discontinued at, or shortly before, the first birthday.

Education and Surveillance

A great deal of time must be invested in counselling the parents at diagnosis. Parent information leaflets are very useful. Contact with a family with an affected child of similar sex can also be very helpful. Management of acute illness should be carefully discussed, and the parents instructed in the administration of intramuscular hydrocortisone in an emergency.

The infant should be reviewed weekly until the parents are comfortable with management, thereafter one- to three-monthly during infancy. Weight and length are measured on each occasion with blood pressure, plasma steroids, and renin at least three-monthly. Routine measurement of electrolytes is not indicated if the child is thriving.

Management of Acute Illness

Infancy is a prime time for acute illness, including gastroenteritis. The key to successful management is correct parental instruction (see Table 8.5), facilitated by provision of a CAH therapy card (similar to the asthma card). A CAH therapy card is shown in Appendix 2. In North America, it is common practice to prescribe a Medic-Alert® bracelet to all patients who are glucocorticoid-dependent. If the following procedure is followed, children with CAH rarely need admission to hospital and duration of hospital stay will be minimized:

1 If the child has an intercurrent illness but is well, feeding and playing normally, and is not febrile, then no change in dosage is required.
2 If the child is unwell with fever, reduced activity, etc., then the oral total daily dosage of hydrocortisone is doubled and given in three divided doses.

Table 8.5 Preoperative and emergency intramuscular (im), bolus, and infusion rate for hydrocortisone dosage (mg) according to body weight and age in months (m) and years (yr) in infants and children with adrenal insufficiency, including congenital adrenal hyperplasia.

Age	Weight (kg)	im dose	Bolus dose	Subsequent 6h infusion rate mg h^{-1}
<6 m	3–7	12.5	6.25	0.5
6 m–5 yr	7–20	25	12.5	1
5–10 yr	20–30	50	25	2
10 yr	30	100	50	3

12.5 mg for infants up to 6 mo, 25 mg from 6 mo to 5 yr, 50 mg from 5 to 10 yr, and 100 mg thereafter. Note that, should the iv line become obstructed or disconnected, cortisol deficiency will immediately ensue, making some centres prefer q6h hydrocortisone injections.

3 If the child is particularly unwell, especially if there is vomiting, drowsiness, or diarrhoea – in which case oral hydrocortisone will not be reliably absorbed – give hydrocortisone intramuscularly in a dose of 12.5 mg for infants up to 6 months, 25 mg from 6 months to 5 years, 50 mg from 5 to 10 years, and 100 mg thereafter (see Table 8.5). If the parents are unable or unwilling to give intramuscular hydrocortisone, then the child should be taken to hospital immediately.
4 If the child does not respond to the intramuscular injection, parents should take the child immediately to hospital. Under these circumstances:
• Take blood for electrolytes, glucose and full blood count.
• Give hydrocortisone intravenously if not given intramuscularly by parents (dosage as above).
• Give 10–30 ml kg^{-1} 0.9% saline over one to three hours depending on the degree of dehydration, followed by 0.9% saline and 5% dextrose to provide maintenance and correct any deficit.
• Give hydrocortisone injections six hourly (dosage given in Table 8.5) until the child is able to tolerate oral medications.
• Genital surgery is discussed in Chapter 7 on DSD.

Medical Management of Children Undergoing Surgery

On the day of surgery, hydrocortisone should be given intravenously at the doses stated in Table 8.5 as soon as an IV line is established. Thereafter, half of this initial dose should be given six hourly (see Table 8.5). This high dose hydrocortisone treatment also covers the mineralocorticoid needs of these patients.

Management of Linear Growth

Chronic treatment consists of daily or twice-daily fludrocortisone therapy to replace aldosterone, and twice- or thrice-daily hydrocortisone to suppress ACTH secretion and thus prevent acceleration of bone maturation and virilization. The limitation of this approach is that the glucocorticoid regimen fails to mimic normal cortisol secretion. Moreover, even if ACTH secretion is normalized, the presence of the enzyme block will still cause androgen excess. Therefore, to achieve satisfactory adrenal suppression, a slightly supraphysiological dose of glucocorticoid is needed. Conversely, insufficient glucocorticoid dosage will result in androgen excess, early epiphyseal fusion, and decreased adult height. Central precocious puberty resulting from priming of the hypothalamus (see Chapter 5 on puberty) can be treated with gonadotrophin-releasing hormone (GnRH) agonists but is not always easy to document with a GnRH stimulation test in children with CAH.

It is also evident that frankly excessive glucocorticoid administration will result in Cushingoid features, obesity, and slow growth with decreased adult height. What is less obvious is that lesser degrees of glucocorticoid overdosage will cause hyperphagia resulting in obesity with normal or increased height velocity and advancing bone age, tempting the clinician to make a further increase in hydrocortisone dosage.

With these considerations in mind, the clinician needs to make a careful judgement as to the optimal glucocorticoid dose, taking the clinical assessment, height velocity, bone age, and biochemical profile into account, and being mindful that adherence problems are common, especially during adolescence.

Hydrocortisone – 10–15 mg/m^2 per day –is usually given in two to three doses, titrating the dosage so that the height velocity is 4–7 cm per year. The manner in which the daily glucocorticoid dose should be administered is controversial. Some favour giving a thrice-daily dose, equally divided, in pre-school children, then a twice-daily dose from school age (when adherence with a thrice-daily regime becomes problematic). Fludrocortisone should be given at 0.150 mg/m^2 per day to bring plasma renin into the reference range.

At clinic visits (no less than every six months), the following should be done:

• Measurement of height, weight, height velocity, and body mass index (BMI) and (in older children) pubertal stage.

• Examination for features of over-treatment (Cushing's syndrome) and under-treatment (including pigmentation and signs of androgen excess).

• Measurement of blood pressure (to monitor fludrocortisone dosage).

• Bone age should be evaluated yearly.

• Most practitioners also measure plasma 17-OHP, androgens and renin activity biannually; this should ideally be done in the morning before taking the tablets. Some centres also measure 17-OHP and androstenedione on capillary samples taken by the patient throughout the day. Normalization of 17-OHP and androstenedione may reflect over-treatment with glucocorticoid and suppression of renin may reflect over-treatment with mineralocorticoid. However, there is great individual variation in biochemical profiles, and surveillance is based primarily on clinical parameters (growth in height and weight, bone age, pubertal progression, and blood pressure).

Morbidity

The sources of morbidity for parents and individuals with CAH are as follows:

A *Parents:*
  1 Shock of initial diagnosis.
  2 In female infants, distress at the genital anomaly and uncertainty about sex at birth.
  3 Anxiety over possible genital surgery and sequellae.

B *Patients:*
  1 Acute illness.
  2 Learning disability in some salt-wasting patients.
  3 *Growth:*
    • poor growth 0–2 years;
    • overgrowth 2–10 years;
    • early puberty;
    • decreased adult height;
    • obesity.
  4 *Urogenital problems:*
    • In males: testicular adrenal rest tumours reducing fertility
    • In females:
    • urinary tract infection;
    • incontinence;
    • vaginal stenosis (haematocolpos, difficulty with tampon insertion and later with penovaginal intercourse).

5 *Psychosexual:*
  • self-esteem/confidence;
  • sexual activity;
  • sexual orientation;
  • gender identity development;
  • fertility.

The principal causes of morbidity are the complications of surgery in girls, and of obesity in both sexes. Strategies to minimize these problems include the use of prenatal dexamethasone, bilateral adrenalectomy during infancy in those with SW 21-OHD associated with severe genotype, adding growth hormone, anti-androgens and aromatase inhibitors, or using sustained-release hydrocortisone. However, none of these options has become standard, despite having been under discussion for many years.

Oestrogen excess

Feminizing adrenal adenomas are exceedingly rare. The clue that the source of sexual precocity lies outside the hypothalamic–pituitary axis is that luteinizing hormone (LH) and follicle stimulating hormone (FSH) are undetectable and do not respond to GnRH.

Sex steroid deficiency

Adrenal androgen deficiency

Causes
• Adrenal hypoplasia.
• *Enzyme disorders:*
  • StAR protein deficiency;
  • 3-βHSD deficiency;
  • 17-hydroxylase deficiency;
  • 17,20-desmolase deficiency;
  • 17-βHSD deficiency.

The androgen deficiency in boys with adrenal hypoplasia is insignificant because gonadal androgen synthesis is intact. However, severe enzyme deficiency affecting both adrenal and gonadal androgen synthesis results in under-masculinization with complete sex reversal in the more severe cases, and ambiguous genitalia in less severe cases. Management is discussed in Chapter 7.

Oestrogen deficiency

Oestrogens are responsible for closure of the epiphyses at adolescence. Gene mutations inactivating the aromatase enzyme or of the oestrogen receptor are associated with tall adult stature.

Adrenal medullary disorder

Phaeochromocytoma and paraganglioma (PPGL)

Chromaffin cell tumours within the adrenal are called phaeochromocytomas while if extra-adrenal they are called paragangliomas. Phaeochromocytoma and paragangliomas (PPGLs) may also occur in association with neurofibromatosis type 1 or as part of the multiple endocrine neoplasia (MEN) syndromes: MEN type 2A (hyperparathyroidism, phaeochromocytoma, medullary thyroid carcinoma), MEN type 2B (phaeochromocytoma, medullary thyroid carcinoma, and tongue and lip neuromas), von Hippel–Lindau syndrome or renal and gastrointestinal tumours in succinate dehydrogenase deficiency. All these may occur sporadically or as dominantly inherited disorders.

Although extremely uncommon in childhood, PPGLs are an important cause of hypertension. It is suggested by the combination of episodic pallor, sweating, and headaches, with either sustained hypertension or raised blood pressure during a symptomatic episode. The diagnosis is made by examining plasma metanephrines in children with hypertension and in children with symptoms suggestive of a PPGLs, even in the absence of hypertension.

Neuroblastoma

Neuroblastoma usually presents to the general paediatrician or oncologist. The diagnosis is suggested by hypertension in the context of malaise, sweating, pallor, and an abdominal mass. There is an increase in catecholamine metabolites in the urine.

Future developments

- Monogenic causes of primary or secondary adrenal disorders are increasingly recognized.
- New strategies to reduce adrenal androgen production in 21-hydroxylase deficiency need further study.
- Determining the risk/benefit ratio of prenatal dexamethasone in all exposed children requires careful long-term surveillance.

Potential pitfalls

- Missing the diagnosis of CAH in fully masculinized female infants.
- Incorrectly diagnosing 21-hydroxylase deficiency in infants with aldosterone resistance (due to obstructive uropathy or to mutations inactivating the ENaC of the mineralocorticoid receptor) or to isolated aldosterone deficiency.
- Misinterpreting non-specific symptoms revealing adrenal insufficiency, such as vomiting and hypoglycaemia, in a patient with another endocrine disorder (such as diabetes).

Controversial points

- Should pituitary surgery for Cushing's disease be performed in one or two designated national centres?
- What is the optimal treatment regimen for infants with 21-hydroxylase deficiency?
- Is prenatal dexamethasone given to prevent virilization in foetuses at risk of 21-hydroxylase deficiency standard of care or investigational?

When to involve a specialist centre

- When Cushing's disease is either seriously suspected or confirmed.
- Endogenous primary and secondary adrenal insufficiency states.
- Conditions causing mineralocorticoid excess.
- CAH.

NB: Involvement of a specialist centre does not preclude a shared care arrangement.

Transition

- Ensuring that adolescents with CAH are seamlessly transferred to an endocrinologist who treats adults is of great importance. The practical aspects of this transition vary greatly depending on local circumstances (e.g. independent children's hospital vs paediatric department within a general hospital).
- Adolescent females with genitourinary problems related to CAH and its surgery may need joint assessment, sometimes involving joint examination under anaesthesia by a paediatric surgeon, plastic surgeon, and gynaecologist with expertise in feminizing genitoplasty.

Emergency management

Correct emergency management depends on: (i) recognizing adrenal insufficiency in an acute situation; and (ii) giving appropriate glucocorticoid, glucose, electrolyte and fluid treatment to known or suspected cases.

Recognizing adrenal insufficiency

The cardinal symptoms include vomiting, diarrhoea (often mistakenly thought to be infectious in nature) and altered consciousness, and with/without a background history of poor feeding, poor weight gain/weight loss.

Signs of adrenal insufficiency include dehydration, shock, hyperpigmentation (in primary adrenal insufficiency), and genital anomaly (in genetic females with 21-hydroxylase deficiency).

Investigation suggesting adrenal insufficiency includes hypoglycaemia, hyponatraemia (due to salt-wasting from aldosterone deficiency or to impaired free water clearance due to cortisol deficiency), hyperkalaemia, and acidosis.

In the newborn, adrenal insufficiency causes hypoglycaemia, prolonged jaundice and, sometimes, a neonatal hepatitis-like syndrome with conjugated bilirubinaemia and raised liver transaminases. There may be associated features such as roving nystagmus (in septo-optic dysplasia) and low T_4 with low or inappropriately normal TSH in hypopituitarism.

It is particularly important to consider adrenal insufficiency in a newborn infant with unexpected hypoglycaemia, for example, when neither the gestation nor birth weight explains this problem, and especially if there is concurrent jaundice.

Appropriate management of adrenal insufficiency

Hospital admission is almost always required in a patient with known adrenal insufficiency who develops vomiting (see Table 8.1). Such patients should always be seen at the hospital, and only allowed to leave the emergency department after a senior member of staff has been consulted.

- Families should be encouraged to show their adrenal insufficiency or CAH card to the emergency staff.
- Vital signs and capillary glucose should be recorded on arrival by the nursing staff. After the medical history and examination have been completed, a cannula should be inserted and blood taken for glucose, electrolytes, and (if intercurrent infection is a possibility) CBC, and inflammatory markers. Blood, urine, and stool cultures may also be indicated.
- A bolus injection of hydrocortisone should be given (unless an intramuscular injection has already been given recently), and fluid management should be as set out in the section on emergency management of 21-hydroxylase deficiency. Next, hydrocortisone may be given as six-hourly injections (see Table 8.5).

- Before discharge, the glucocorticoid and mineralocorticoid dosages, together with the family situation regarding education and adherence, should be reviewed.

Case histories

Case 8.1
A four-year-old boy with known asthma is admitted acutely with a convulsion, and is found to be hypoglycaemic (blood glucose 0.8 mmol/L [14 mg/dL]). For the past year, his asthma has been well controlled on fluticasone propionate 500 µg twice daily, but recently he has been lethargic and has had more than his fair share of intercurrent illnesses. On examination (after glucose administration), his consciousness level is normal. He looks slightly Cushingoid with some hypertrichosis, especially over the back. Height is on the 3rd centile (mid-parental height 25th centile), weight on the 50th centile, and blood pressure is 120/50. Random plasma cortisol is <24 nmol/L [<1 mg/dL].

Question and Answer
1 How can this boy's Cushingoid features be reconciled with his gross adrenal impairment?

This boy has an iatrogenic combination of Cushing's syndrome (causing the facial appearance, hypertrichosis, a degree of growth failure, and an increased tendency to infections), together with adrenal suppression (lethargy, hypoglycaemia). He is receiving over twice the licensed paediatric dose of fluticasone (400 µg daily). He will require hydrocortisone replacement while the respiratory team modifies his therapy, and his adrenal status should be re-evaluated if and when the dose of inhaled steroid is reduced.

Case 8.2
Four hours after delivery at 41 weeks' gestation with birth weight 3740 g, a baby boy becomes dusky while breast-feeding. True blood glucose is 1.1 mmol/L [<20 mg/dL]. On examination, the baby is noted to have a very small penis. He is started on a glucose infusion. Plasma cortisol is <30 nmol/L and LH and FSH are unmeasurable (<0.5 units/L).

Question and Answer

1 What is the diagnosis, and what other system should be examined in detail?

This baby has hypopituitarism with gonadotrophin deficiency leading to micropenis and ACTH deficiency resulting in hypoglycaemia. Associated central hypothyroidism is documented by a very low plasma free T4 level (2.9 pmol/L), contrasting with an inappropriately normal plasma TSH (3.5 mU/L). On day 6, a head MRI shows an ectopic posterior pituitary.

Case 8.3

A 14-year-old boy is found to be hypertensive (blood pressure 170/130) when he consults his family practitioner with headache. Investigations show normal electrolytes and renal imaging, but plasma aldosterone is elevated at 990 pmol/L [36 ng/dL] and renin completely suppressed. There is a family history of hypertension, with his maternal uncle and grandmother dying young of stroke and the mother being hypertensive during pregnancy.

Question and Answer

1 What diagnostic possibilities should be considered and what further investigations should be performed?

The family history of hypertension in a boy with high aldosterone levels strongly suggests glucocorticoid-suppressible hyperaldosteronism. Molecular genetic studies confirmed a chimeric $C_YP_{11}B_1/2$ gene in both mother and son, and the boy's aldosterone suppressed quickly with dexamethasone. Detailed adrenal imaging in search of adenoma or hyperplasia was unnecessary in this case.

Case 8.4

A boy was admitted, aged 4.7 years, with a short history of vomiting and acidosis. On arrival at the hospital he was comatose; investigations showed plasma sodium 132 mmol/L, cortisol 228 nmol/L (inappropriately low for such a sick child) and ACTH 41 mU/L (normal <20 mU/L). Despite intensive care, he died of cerebral oedema. He was found at post-mortem examination to be hyperpigmented with small adrenal glands. Nasopharyngeal aspirate was positive for influenza A.

His two surviving brothers underwent stimulation testing with synthetic ACTH (Synacthen). Aged 1.6 years, the second brother showed adrenal insufficiency with no response to Synacthen, basal/peak cortisol 321/343 nmol/L, but ACTH (7 mU/L), renin and electrolytes normal. He was treated with hydrocortisone but not fludrocortisone. The youngest brother showed a normal peak cortisol of 680 nmol/L at the age of three months and was not treated.

Aged 1.9 years, the second brother became drowsy and began vomiting after his oral hydrocortisone at 8 a.m. His mother gave him intramuscular hydrocortisone and brought him to hospital where biochemistry showed true blood glucose 1.8 mmol/L, sodium low at 127 mmol/L, but potassium normal at 4.3 mmol/L. He was given 25 mg of hydrocortisone intramuscularly, together with IV 0.45% saline and 5% dextrose, and he made a good recovery.

Questions and Answers

1 What is the differential diagnosis of this family's adrenal disorder?

Congenital adrenal hyperplasia is unlikely, given the small adrenal glands in the oldest brother at post mortem. By contrast, X-linked congenital adrenal hypoplasia is a possibility, although these children commonly present in infancy with salt wasting. Autosomal recessive familial glucocorticoid deficiency is another possibility and would be in keeping with intact mineralocorticoid function. Triple A (or Allgrove) syndrome, another autosomal recessive disorder, can present with adrenal insufficiency prior to the development of alacrima and achalasia. Finally, X-linked ALD can present with adrenal insufficiency rather than neurological signs.

2 What investigations should be carried out to try and ascertain the diagnosis?

Molecular genetic analysis was negative for DAX-1 and ACTH-receptor mutations, but very long-chain fatty acids were elevated in both surviving siblings and mutational analysis indicated that all three brothers shared the common mutation for

ALD (*c.1415 1416delAG*). MRI scan of brain was normal in both surviving brothers initially but when subtle white matter changes were found on surveillance scanning in the second brother at 10 years of age, he underwent a successful pre-emptive bone marrow transplant.

3 How can the low sodium on admission be explained, given that recent renin measurement was normal?

The low plasma sodium on admission at 1.9 years is attributable to impaired water clearance secondary to cortisol deficiency. Cortisol deficiency could partly explain the development of cerebral oedema seen in the deceased brother.

Comment
This family's case history shows the potentially rapid and devastating nature of acute adrenal decompensation, especially in infants and preschool children. Meticulous education of the parents, best given by the endocrine specialist nurse, is the cornerstone of management.

References

New, M.I., Lorenznev, F., Lerner, A.J. et al. (1983). Genotyping steroid 21-hydroxylase deficiency hormonal reference data. *J. Clin. Endocrinol. Metab.* 57 (2): 320–326.

Forest, M.G. (1979). Plasma androgens (testosterone and 4-androstenedione) and 17-hydroxyprogesterone in the neonatal, prepubertal and peripubertal periods in the human and the rat: differences between species. *J. Ster. Biochem* 11: 543–548.

Wallace, A.M., Beastall, G.H., and Cook, B. (1986). Neonatal screening for congenital adrenal hyperplasia: a programme based on a novel direct radioimmunoassay for 17-hydroxyprogesterone in blood spots. *J. Endocrinol.* 108: 299–308.

Further Reading

Crona, J., Taïeb, D., and Pacak, K. (2017). New perspectives on pheochromocytoma and paraganglioma: towards a molecular classification. *Endocr. Rev.* 38 (6): 489–515.

Flück, C.E. (2017). Update on pathogenesis of primary adrenal insufficiency: beyond steroid enzyme deficiency and autoimmune adrenal destruction. *Eur. J. Endocrinol.* 177 (3): R99–R111.

Perry, R., Kecha, O., Paquette, J. et al. (2005). Primary adrenal insufficiency in children: twenty years experience at the Sainte-Justine Hospital, Montreal. *J. Clin. Endocrinol. Metab.* 90 (6): 3243–3250.

Stratakis, C.A. (2016). Diagnosis and clinical genetics of Cushing syndrome in pediatrics. *Endocrinol. Metab. Clin. North Am.* 45 (2): 311–328.

Useful Information for Patients and Parents

- The Congenital Adrenal Hyperplasia Support Group: This group, which was formed in 1991 to assist families affected by congenital adrenal hyperplasia, offers support to families and patients, aims to increase awareness of the condition to the public and to the medical profession, and to raise funds to support research. Website: www.livingwithcah.com (accessed 11 October 2018).
- Child Growth Foundation: CGF offers support to patients and families with CAH; CGF and & Serono publish 'Congenital Adrenal Hyperplasia'; Series No: 6. Website: www.childgrowthfoundation.org (accessed 11 October 2018).
- Warne GL (2009) Your Child with Congenital Adrenal Hyperplasia. Royal Children's Hospital, Victoria (accessed 11 October 2018).
- Kelton S (2009) *Congenital Adrenal Hyperplasia (CAH)*. Family Researched Library. British Columbia's Children's Hospital, Vancouver: famreslib@cw.bc.ca (accessed 11 October 2018).

CARES Foundation: This USA-based organization offers support to families and individuals with CAH. Website: www.caresfoundation.org (accessed 11 October 2018).

9

Salt and Water Balance

Physiology and pathophysiology

Control of salt balance

Regulation of salt balance is achieved primarily through activation of the renin–angiotensin–aldosterone system and the release of atrial natriuretic peptide. Renin is secreted by the juxtaglomerular cells of the kidney in response to sodium depletion or extracellular fluid volume restriction. Renin converts angiotensinogen to angiotensin I which, in turn, is converted by angiotensin-converting enzyme to angiotensin II. Angiotensin II stimulates the production of aldosterone from the zona glomerulosa of the adrenal cortex. Adrenocorticotrophic hormone (ACTH) does not play a role in the *physiological* regulation of aldosterone secretion although serum aldosterone increases upon acute intravenous (IV) ACTH administration. Potassium ions also facilitate the secretion of aldosterone. By contrast, the secretion of both renin and aldosterone may be inhibited by atrial natriuretic peptide.

Aldosterone binds to the mineralocorticoid receptor, resulting in increased reabsorption of sodium in the kidney, sweat and salivary glands. Sodium ions are exchanged for potassium and hydrogen ions in the distal tubule. Cortisol also has a strong binding affinity for the mineralocorticoid receptor but is prevented from doing so as a result of metabolism to inactive cortisone by 11-β-hydroxysteroid dehydrogenase-2 in aldosterone-sensitive tissues.

Control of water balance

Water balance is maintained by the interrelation between thirst, renal function, and the antidiuretic hormone arginine vasopressin (AVP). Vasopressin is synthesized in the supraoptic and paraventricular nuclei of the hypothalamus in a pre-pro-hormone form consisting of vasopressin, neurophysin II, and copeptin. These peptides are then cleaved during transport along the supraoptic–hypophyseal tract to be stored in the posterior pituitary. Vasopressin release is regulated by osmoreceptors in the hypothalamus which detect changes in plasma osmolality from 280 to 295 mOsm/kg as may occur with loss of extracellular water. High concentrations of vasopressin may also be secreted following baroreceptor-detected reductions in blood volume or blood pressure of 5–10%. Baroreceptors are located in the carotid arch, aortic sinus, and left atrium and modulate vasopressinergic neuronal function via vagal and glossopharyngeal stimulation of the brainstem.

Vasopressin binds to a V2 receptor in the renal collecting tubule which regulates the insertion of water channel proteins (aquaporin 2) into the cell membrane. These allow water to flow along an osmotic gradient from the tubular lumen into the cells lining the collecting duct. Other aquaporins (aquaporin 4) allow

Practical Endocrinology and Diabetes in Children, Fourth Edition. Malcolm D.C. Donaldson, John W. Gregory, Guy Van Vliet, and Joseph I. Wolfsdorf.
© 2019 John Wiley & Sons Ltd. Published 2019 by John Wiley & Sons Ltd.

this water to pass to the renal interstitium and circulation. This regulatory mechanism maintains plasma osmolality between 282 and 295 mOsm/kg. When the plasma osmolality exceeds 295 mOsm/kg, vasopressin secretion cannot be increased further and fluid balance is maintained by increased thirst leading to increased fluid intake. The vasopressin effect is under negative feedback modulation by locally generated prostaglandins in the medullary collecting duct cells. Glucocorticoids are also required for free water excretion so that initiation of glucocorticoid replacement in hypopituitary patients may unmask diabetes insipidus (DI).

Hyponatraemia

Aetiology

Hyponatraemia may occur either as a result of salt and water depletion in which salt loss exceeds water loss or following fluid overload resulting in relatively more water than salt. The general mechanisms for the development of hyponatraemia are shown in Table 9.1.

Hyponatraemia associated with extracellular fluid loss is not always a direct consequence of the fluid loss

per se, which is frequently hypotonic or isotonic by comparison with plasma, but may be caused by replacement of these fluid losses with hypotonic fluid (e.g. drinking water alone or use of hypotonic IV fluids).

History and examination

When a child presents with hyponatraemia for which the cause is not immediately apparent, the following points should be highlighted in the history:

1 *Features suggestive of salt loss:*
   - The presence of symptoms causing excess fluid and sodium loss (e.g. weight loss, vomiting, diarrhoea, polyuria) or a compensatory decrease in urine production which may occur when sodium loss has occurred from the skin or gut.
   - Evidence that hyponatraemia is precipitated by intercurrent illness and associated with hyperkalaemia and hypoglycaemia which might suggest adrenal failure.
   - Symptoms of malabsorption or recurrent chest infections or a tendency for hyponatraemia to develop during hot weather which may be indicative of cystic fibrosis.

Table 9.1 Causes of hyponatraemia.

Mechanism	Examples
Salt loss	
Renal disease	Renal tubular defects (e.g. Fanconi, Bartter syndromes)
	Chronic renal failure
	Interstitial nephritis
	Renovascular hypertension
	Diuretic treatment
	Cisplatin toxicity
Aldosterone deficiency	Inherited enzyme disorders (e.g. 21-hydroxylase deficiency), Addison's disease
Aldosterone resistance	Pseudohypoaldosteronism
Cutaneous loss	Excess sweat sodium loss in cystic fibrosis, fluid loss in burns
Gastrointestinal	Vomiting and diarrhoea (e.g. in gastroenteritis)
	Intestinal obstruction (e.g. intussusception)
Water excess	
Renal disease	Acute nephritic syndrome, acute and chronic renal failure
Hypovolaemia or decreases in renal perfusion causing increased proximal renal tubular reabsorption	Cirrhosis, congestive heart failure, nephrotic syndrome
Excessive water intake	Iatrogenic – excessive intravenous fluid replacement
	Primary polydipsia
ADH excess	Syndrome of inappropriate ADH secretion (e.g. in meningitis, pneumonia)
	Over-treatment with DDAVP

- The use of medication (e.g. diuretics) which predispose to hyponatraemia.
- Family history of consanguinity and of specific disorders such as cystic fibrosis, congenital adrenal hyperplasia or hypoplasia, and pseudo-hypoaldosteronism.

2 *Features suggestive of water retention:*
- Excess daily fluid intake.
- Symptoms suggestive of an underlying central nervous system (CNS) or respiratory disorder (e.g. meningitis, raised intracranial pressure, pneumonia) associated with the syndrome of inappropriate antidiuretic hormone secretion (SIADH).
- Symptoms suggestive of heart failure, renal, liver or thyroid disease.

The following points should be highlighted in the clinical examination:

1 The patient should always be weighed.

2 If sodium loss has occurred, clinical signs of volume depletion may be present as shown in Table 9.2. Evidence of growth impairment may suggest a long-standing cause of hyponatraemia resulting from sodium loss. Careful clinical examination should be undertaken of all systems for signs suggestive of intracranial or respiratory disease, cardiac, hepatic, renal or adrenal failure, or hypothyroidism.

3 If signs of volume depletion are absent, this may imply either previous fluid replacement with hypotonic fluids or the presence of water retention. In the latter circumstances, there may be evidence of oedema or rapid recent weight gain. The clinical signs of volume overload are shown in Table 9.2. The rapid onset of a hypo-osmolar state may be associated with neurological manifestations including anorexia, apathy, confusion, headaches, weakness, and muscle cramps. More severe symptoms may include vomiting, depressed deep tendon reflexes, bulbar or pseudobulbar palsy, Cheyne–Stokes breathing, psychotic behaviour, seizures, coma, and death.

Investigations

- Serum and urine electrolytes and creatinine to calculate urinary sodium losses.
- Serum and urinary osmolalities.
- Plasma renin activity, aldosterone, 17-hydroxy progesterone and cortisol.
- Thyroid function tests (TFT).
- Other investigations as indicated for cardiac, respiratory, hepatic, renal, or intracranial disease.
- If the patient is normo-osmolar, plasma proteins, lipids, and glucose.

Differential diagnosis

Hyponatraemia can be spurious either as a result of contamination of the blood sample taken from an IV cannula with hypotonic IV fluids or because of interference with the flame photometer assay by excess serum lipids or proteins.

The key requirement in the assessment of a patient with hyponatraemia is to distinguish between causes associated with excess sodium loss and those associated with water retention, for example, in SIADH.

Table 9.2 Clinical signs of volume depletion and overload.

Volume depletion	Volume overload
1 Weight loss	1 Weight gain
2 Intravenous compartment depletion with • ↓ tissue perfusion • fast, low volume pulse • blood pressure typically low (but may be normal/high due to vasoconstriction) • slow capillary refill (>2 s) • impaired consciousness • pallor due to vasoconstriction	2 Intravenous compartment expansion • fast, high volume (bounding) pulse • high blood pressure • raised jugular venous pressure • gallop rhythm • liver engorgement
3 Interstitial compartment depletion • ↓ skin turgor, sunken eyes • dry mucous membranes	3 Interstitial compartment expansion • peripheral oedema with puffy eyes, ankle and sacral oedema, ascites
4 Increased urine osmolality • Urine sodium low or high depending on aetiology	4 Urine osmolality increased or decreased depending on aetiology

The clinical distinction between these two states is summarized in Table 9.2.

If the cause of the hypo-osmolar state is not clear at presentation, urine osmolalities >100 mOsm/kg associated with urinary sodium concentrations >20 mmol/L suggest acute SIADH or renal, adrenal, or cerebral salt wasting. Urine osmolalities >100 mOsm/kg associated with urinary sodium concentrations <20 mmol/L suggest hypovolaemia or longer-standing SIADH. Plasma renin is usually suppressed in SIADH but elevated in hypovolaemia.

Diagnosis

The causes of hyponatraemia are summarized in Table 9.1. Mineralocorticoid deficiency may be a consequence of idiopathic congenital adrenal hypoplasia or aplasia, biosynthetic defects of aldosterone synthesis (e.g. congenital adrenal hyperplasia) or acquired primary adrenal failure (e.g. Waterhouse–Friderichsen syndrome, autoimmune disease, or following surgical removal). While combined mineralocorticoid and glucocorticoid deficiency will cause hyponatraemia through salt loss, glucocorticoid deficiency (e.g. in hypopituitarism) will cause hyponatraemia due to impaired water excretion. Resistance to aldosterone may occur as a result of inactivation of the mineralocorticoid receptor or of the epithelial sodium channel. Abnormalities of mineralocorticoid physiology are discussed in more detail in Chapter 8.

The various causes of SIADH are summarized in Table 9.3.

Treatment

Where hyponatraemia is a consequence of sodium loss and in the context of clinical signs of significant hypovolaemia, IV colloid or 0.9% saline should be given until there is clinical evidence of circulatory improvement. Adrenal insufficiency should be treated with fludrocortisone and glucocorticoids (see Chapter 8).

SIADH should be anticipated in individuals who have experienced significant head trauma or intracranial surgery and careful postoperative supervision of fluid balance is required. SIADH should be treated by fluid restriction which may range from only 40% to two-thirds of normal intake. Where severe or symptomatic hyponatraemia or excessive thirst makes this approach impractical, then treatment to either increase water excretion or to raise the plasma sodium should be used. Water excretion will be enhanced by the tetracycline antibiotic demeclocycline which impairs the renal response to vasopressin and has been used in adults, giving 3–5 mg /kg eight-hourly. An alternative is the relatively newly available V2 receptor antagonist tolvaptan, though trials of its efficacy in children are ongoing. Plasma sodium can be raised using hypertonic (3%) saline (0.1 ml/kg/min for two hours), aiming to increase plasma sodium concentration by about 10 mmol/L. In this context, it may be necessary to give furosemide with replacement of excreted urinary electrolytes to prevent hypervolaemia. This treatment should be reserved for those with significant neurological symptoms following the relatively acute onset of SIADH, as there is a risk of lethal pontine myelinolysis if serum sodium concentrations rise too rapidly (>10 mmol/L per day).

Endocrine hypertension

Aetiology

Hypertension in childhood as a result of endocrine pathology is usually a consequence of either glucocorticoid or catecholamine excess, as shown in Table 9.4.

Table 9.3 Causes of syndrome of inappropriate antidiuretic hormone secretion (SIADH).

Cause	Examples
Central nervous system disorders	Meningitis, encephalitis, trauma (including surgery), hypoxia, haemorrhage, ventriculo-peritoneal shunt obstruction, Guillain–Barré syndrome
Respiratory disorders	Pneumonia, tuberculosis
Tumours	Thymoma, lymphoma, Ewing's sarcoma
Drugs • AVP stimulants • AVP potentiators • Other	Phenothiazines, tricyclic antidepressants, vincristine, narcotics DDAVP, prostaglandin synthetase inhibitors Chlorpropamide, cyclophosphamide, carbamazepine

Table 9.4 Causes of endocrine hypertension.

Mechanism	Examples
Steroid-mediated	
Glucocorticoid excess	Iatrogenic (pharmacological doses, or over-replacement in deficiency states)
	Cushing's syndrome
	Apparent mineralocorticoid excess (AME)
Mineralocorticoid excess	11β-hydroxylase deficiency, 17α-hydroxylase deficiency
	Liddle's syndrome
	Dexamethasone-suppressible hyperaldosteronism
Catecholamine-mediated	Phaeochromocytoma, paraganglioma, neuroblastoma

History and examination

Key points to highlight in the history and on clinical examination include the following:

- A history of intermittent headaches, sweating, flushes, nausea or vomiting is suggestive of a phaeochromocytoma.
- *Other affected family members.* An autosomal recessive inheritance suggests congenital adrenal hyperplasia caused by 11β-hydroxylase or 17α-hydroxylase deficiency whereas an autosomal dominant pattern might suggest a phaeochromocytoma associated with a multiple endocrine neoplasia syndrome or hereditary phaeochromocytoma-paraganglioma syndrome.
- Virilization in a girl might suggest congenital adrenal hyperplasia.
- Clinical signs of Cushing's syndrome (see Chapter 8).
- The presence of cutaneous signs suggestive of neurofibromatosis, or of mucosal neuromas, which are associated with von Hippel–Lindau disease, may suggest the presence of an associated phaeochromocytoma.

Investigations

The following preliminary investigations should be considered if an endocrine cause of hypertension is suspected:

- serum electrolytes and creatinine;
- three 24-hour urinary-free cortisol (and creatinine) collections;
- urinary steroid metabolite profiling;
- plasma free metanephrine and urinary catecholamine metabolites;
- abdominal ultrasound.

If Cushing's syndrome seems likely, additional investigations to confirm the diagnosis and treatment are described (see Chapter 8). If the urinary excretion of catecholamine metabolites is increased, then a blood sample should be taken for the measurement of free metanephrine. Two-thirds of phaeochromocytomas are located in the adrenal medulla but they may also be found anywhere in the sympathetic chain, most commonly close to the renal hilum or aortic bifurcation. Abdominal imaging, preferably with computerized tomography (CT), magnetic resonance imaging (MRI), ^{123}I-metaiodobenzylguanidine (MIBG) scanning and, possibly, selective venous catecholamine sampling by catheterization may be necessary to locate the site(s).

Diagnosis

The various causes of endocrine hypertension are shown in Table 9.4. Hypertension in 11β-hydroxylase- and 17α-hydroxylase-deficient congenital adrenal hyperplasia results from accumulation of the potent mineralocorticoid deoxycorticosterone, resulting in sodium and water retention with suppression of renin and aldosterone. 11β-hydroxylase deficiency is also associated with excess androgen production and virilization, whereas 17α-hydroxylase deficiency leads to female external genitalia in 46,XY subjects and lack of development of secondary sexual characteristics in both sexes.

Primary aldosteronism is associated with hypernatraemia, increased plasma volume, hyporeninaemia, and hypokalaemia. Hypertension is common in childhood Cushing's syndrome. The syndrome of apparent mineralocorticoid excess (AME) is characterized by low plasma renin and aldosterone concentrations and is associated with a deficiency of 11β-hydroxysteroid dehydrogenase 2 which is responsible for metabolizing cortisol to cortisone to prevent high concentrations of cortisol from binding to the mineralocorticoid receptor.

Liddle's syndrome arises from an abnormality of renal tubular transport caused by an activating mutation of the amiloride-sensitive sodium channel, resulting in increased sodium reabsorption and potassium loss with a biochemical and clinical picture similar to that of AME. Glucocorticoid-suppressible hyperaldosteronism is a rare disorder in which primary aldosteronism is regulated by ACTH rather than renin–angiotensin because of the fusion of regulatory sequences of the 11β-hydroxylase gene to coding sequences of the aldosterone synthase gene.

Treatment

In 11β-hydroxylase- and 17α-hydroxylase-deficient congenital adrenal hyperplasia, hypertension responds to glucocorticoid therapy which suppresses ACTH secretion and thus deoxycorticosterone production. The treatment of Cushing's syndrome is discussed in detail in Chapter 8.

A phaeochromocytoma requires surgical removal in an experienced specialist centre with skilled anaesthetic support. Pre- and perioperative control of blood pressure must be achieved by the initial use of an adequate alpha blockade such as phenoxybenzamine. As this is achieved, supplemental salt intake is needed to expand the extracellular fluid volume. Beta blockers are also necessary to treat alpha-blocker-induced tachycardia. When a neuroblastoma causes catecholamine-induced hypertension, similar medical management will be necessary in the pre-operative period.

Hypernatraemia

The mechanisms of hypernatraemia are shown in Table 9.5 and include gastrointestinal fluid loss in which relatively more water is lost than salt, excessive salt intake (e.g. due to deliberate poisoning as in Munchausen-by-proxy), decreased water intake through impaired thirst, and excessive renal water losses, including diabetes insipidus. It is important to recognize that some patients with neurological disability may have a combination of impaired thirst and

Table 9.5 Causes of hypernatraemia.

Mechanism	Examples
Gastrointestinal fluid loss with relatively more water loss than salt loss	Gastroenteritis with hypertonic dehydration
Decreased water intake	Water deprivation
	Impaired thirst
	• Congenital adipsia and hypodipsia
	• Acquired osmoreceptor damage
Excessive salt intake	Salt poisoning
Vasopressin deficiency (central diabetes insipidus)	
1 Congenital causes	
• Brain malformation	Septo-optic dysplasia, holoprosencephaly
• Familial gene disorder	Autosomal dominant vasopressin deficiency
2 Acquired causes	
• Tumours and infiltrations	Craniopharyngioma, germinoma, Langerhans cell histiocytosis, sarcoidosis
• Inflammatory	Autoimmune
• Trauma	Head injury, neurosurgery
• Other	Narcotic agonists
Vasopressin resistance (nephrogenic diabetes insipidus)	
1 Primary defect in vasopressin/aquaporin responsiveness	*V2 receptor* or *aquaporin 2* gene defect
2 Secondary causes	
• Renal parenchymal disease	Nephrocalcinosis, nephronophthisis, polycystic kidney disease
• Obstructive uropathy	Urethral valves
• Electrolyte disturbances	Hypercalcaemia, hypokalaemia
• Drugs	Lithium, demeclocycline, tolvaptan
• Other	

central diabetes insipidus. Rarely, congenital adipsia/hypodipsia may be seen in the context of a mid-line defect with single central incisor. Unexplained episodic hypernatraemia should raise the possibility of factitious illness caused by the deliberate administration of salt by the child's parent or carer.

Diabetes insipidus

Aetiology

Diabetes insipidus may occur either as a result of inadequate secretion of AVP (cranial or central diabetes insipidus) or when there is resistance to the antidiuretic effect of AVP (nephrogenic diabetes insipidus). Cranial diabetes insipidus may be congenital due to a gene defect or to a cerebral malformation (e.g. septo-optic dysplasia (SOD), holoprosencephaly); or caused by acquired disease (e.g. craniopharyngioma, Langerhans cell histiocytosis, or surgery) of the hypothalamo–pituitary axis (Table 9.5). Autosomal dominant cranial diabetes insipidus may be caused by a mutation of the AVP–neurophysin II gene which leads to impaired processing of the AVP hormone precursor, causing progressive damage to the neurosecretory neurones of the hypothalamus and the development of increasingly severe symptoms of diabetes insipidus with advancing age. In the much less common autosomal recessive form, the symptoms occur earlier. Nephrogenic diabetes insipidus may occur as a consequence of mutations affecting the V2 receptor gene (X-linked) or aquaporin 2 gene (autosomal recessive) or because of disorders of the kidney which impair the function of other components of the urinary concentrating mechanism (Table 9.5).

History and examination

The cardinal symptoms of diabetes insipidus are polyuria and polydipsia. Other causes of these symptoms must be considered – osmotic diuresis from glycosuria in diabetes mellitus and reduced nephron mass in chronic renal failure; excessive intake in habit drinking (psychogenic polydipsia); and impaired renal tubular function in hypercalcaemia and hypokalaemia. Additional clinical features of diabetes insipidus include constipation, fever, vomiting, loss of weight, failure to thrive, and dehydration.

The following points should be highlighted in the history and clinical examination:

- The nature and severity of the polyuria and polydipsia. Excess consumption of flavoured liquids only as opposed to water suggests habitual excess drinking. Drinking from unusual places, such as from the toilet or bath, or unusual fluids, such as shampoo, suggests severe thirst due to an underlying organic disorder.
- Whether the symptoms were present from birth, suggesting a congenital abnormality, or developed later in life, suggesting an acquired disorder.
- Associated neurological symptoms (e.g. blindness, neurodevelopmental delay, headache) and signs (e.g. optic atrophy) or history of a recent neurological disorder suggesting risk factors for hypothalamo–pituitary dysfunction.
- Past medical history of renal disease.
- Symptoms suggestive of diabetes mellitus (weight loss and hyperphagia within the past six weeks) or hypercalcaemia (anorexia, abdominal pain, constipation).
- Medication (e.g. lithium treatment).
- Family history of similarly affected cases.
- Congenital abnormalities especially in the mid-line of the brain and face.
- Blood pressure or presence of enlarged kidneys.
- Growth status – short stature suggestive of associated growth hormone (GH) deficiency in hypopituitarism.

Investigations

Habitual excess drinking is common in toddlers and preschool children, and if often part of a wider management problem including a poor sleeping pattern. The child is otherwise healthy and the problem can usually be both diagnosed and cured by asking parents to stop flavoured fluids but allow the child unrestricted access to water. If symptoms persist, the child should be admitted for observation and the severity of the polyuria and polydipsia be confirmed by measurement of the 24-hour fluid intake and urinary losses. A fasting blood sample should be taken for the measurement of plasma glucose and serum sodium, potassium, calcium, and creatinine concentrations. Urine should be tested for glycosuria and proteinuria.

In a significantly symptomatic individual, simultaneous early morning blood and urine samples should be taken for the measurement of serum electrolytes and osmolality and urinary osmolality. Diabetes insipidus may be confirmed by the presence of a hyperosmolar state (i.e. serum osmolality >295 mOsm/kg) with inappropriately dilute urine (urine osmolarity around <750 mOsm /kg). The plasma or urine sample should then be sent for the measurement of AVP or plasma copeptin concentrations to confirm whether the cause is cranial or nephrogenic (Figure 9.1). In these circumstances, a water deprivation test would be dangerous and is contraindicated. Furthermore, a water deprivation test is not required when there is a clear history of polydipsia and polyuria in the context of underlying disease or treatment (e.g. craniopharyngioma, histiocytosis, and postoperative phase of craniopharyngioma) which is known to cause cranial diabetes insipidus.

Water deprivation test

This test is time-consuming for staff and unpleasant for the child and family. It can usually be avoided, being either unnecessary (young child with habit drinking), unsafe (e.g. postoperative craniopharyngioma) or both. It should only be carried out after consultation with an experienced physician and must be undertaken with particular care in young children. The following protocol can be used:

1 Allow the child to consume their normal overnight fluid intake.

2 Weigh child at 8.00 a.m. at start of the fluid deprivation and measure plasma and urinary osmolalities.

3 Repeat weight, blood and urine samples every two hours and monitor the child carefully to prevent fluid intake.

4 For most children, an eight-hour fast is adequate and the test should be discontinued before then if more than 5% of body weight is lost or the thirst cannot be tolerated longer.

5 At the end of the fluid deprivation, administer desmopressin (DDAVP) either as an injection of 0.3 mg (subcutaneously, intramuscularly, or intravenously) or 5 μg by the intranasal route and collect simultaneous urine and blood samples for osmolality measurements about four hours later. During the four hours following DDAVP, the child can be allowed to drink up to 1.5 times the volume of any urine voided.

Central nervous system testing and other investigations

If a diagnosis of cranial diabetes insipidus is made, an MRI of the hypothalamo–pituitary axis should be performed as there may be a pituitary tumour or stalk abnormality. The serum tumour markers β-human chorionic gonadotrophin (β-hCG) and α-foetoprotein should also be measured. If the MRI demonstrates thickening of the pituitary stalk, repeat scans should

be performed over the next several years to monitor the development of infiltrative disorders, such as Langerhans cell histiocytosis or a germinoma, especially if symptoms, such as headache or additional pituitary hormone deficiencies develop.

Tests of wider anterior pituitary function may also be indicated. Diabetes insipidus may be masked by concurrent glucocorticoid insufficiency so that glucocorticoid replacement should be instituted before diagnostic tests for diabetes insipidus are performed.

Diagnosis

If during the water deprivation test, the plasma osmolality remains between 282 and 295 mOsm/kg and the urine osmolality increases to >750 mOsm/kg, the patient does not have diabetes insipidus and the possibility of primary polydipsia because of abnormal drinking habits should be considered.

A diagnosis of cranial diabetes insipidus is suggested by the development of increased plasma osmolality >295 mOsm/kg in the presence of a urine osmolality <300 mOsm/kg which is then increased to >750 mOsm/kg following the administration of DDAVP. Failure of the urine to respond to DDAVP is indicative of nephrogenic diabetes insipidus. A partial urinary response (300–750 mOsm/kg) to water deprivation or DDAVP suggests partial cranial or nephrogenic diabetes insipidus.

Treatment

Cranial diabetes insipidus

This should be treated with the long-acting AVP analogue DDAVP and the following preparations are available:

- DDAVP subcutaneous injection containing 4 μg/ml. This should only be given in hospital and is not administered on a regular basis.
- DDAVP nasal solution containing 100 μg/ml and given via an intranasal catheter. This preparation is suitable for giving doses of 0.05 ml = 5 μg. For very young children, the pharmacy may need to dilute the solution to 25 μg/ml so that doses of 1.25 μg can be given.
- DDAVP nasal spray (Desmospray) delivering a fixed dose of 10 μg/spray. A low dose DDAVP delivers 2.5 μg/spray.
- DDAVP tablets (Desmotabs) 100 or 200 μg which are scored.
- DDAVP sublingual tablets (Desmomelt) 60, 120 or 240 μg.

Widely varying dose regimens may be required, usually in two or three divided doses. The complete replacement dose of intranasal DDAVP is around 15 μg/m² per day, and 10 μg of nasal DDAVP is roughly equivalent to 100 μg of oral DDAVP and to 60 μg of sublingual DDAVP. In those individuals taking DDAVP by the nasal route, an increase in the dosage of medication may be required during upper respiratory tract illnesses which may cause congestion of the nasal mucosa and impaired drug absorption. For this reason there has been a shift from nasal to oral DDAVP and, in recent years, a further move towards the sublingual preparation.

Patients with cranial diabetes insipidus fall into three broad categories: postoperative craniopharyngioma patients who require very careful monitoring; cranial diabetes insipidus with intact thirst; and cranial diabetes insipidus with impaired thirst.

1 *Postoperative craniopharyngioma patients:* These patients show a triphasic pattern with initial diabetes insipidus for up to 24 hours, followed by a period of vasopressin excess for 2–4 days as the necrosing posterior pituitary gland releases this hormone, followed by permanent diabetes insipidus. DDAVP should not be given regularly during the first phase, will not be required during the second phase, but will be needed regularly thereafter.

2 *Cranial diabetes insipidus with intact thirst:* Since patients may be very sensitive to DDAVP, treatment should start with small doses and gradually increase according to the clinical and biochemical responses. The initial response to therapy should be monitored closely by measurement of fluid intake and output and serum electrolytes and osmolality every few days at the start of therapy. Over-treatment may be recognized by an abnormally low serum sodium concentration and osmolality. Once stabilized on treatment, patients should be reviewed in clinic at least three-monthly as seasonal changes in temperature may alter their requirements for DDAVP. Patients who are experienced in the management of their diabetes insipidus may be allowed to adjust their own doses if they detect recurrence of polyuria. However, patients must be instructed to allow a short period (1–2 hours) of diuresis at a convenient time during the day to allow the excretion of any excess water, which may have occurred during the day and before taking the next dose of DDAVP.

3 *Cranial diabetes insipidus with impaired thirst:* This is seen in some children with neurodisability who have impaired osmoreceptor but normal baroreceptor responses so that they will produce inadequate vasopressin until they become hypovolaemic. It is also seen in some craniopharyngioma patients who have sustained hypothalamic osmoreceptor damage either from the tumour or from surgery. Correction of any hypernatraemia, which may be of long standing, should be gradual in these patients to avoid seizures. A small dose of DDAVP is given initially together with a fixed daily volume of water, for example, 1500 ml/1.73 m².

Nephrogenic diabetes insipidus

This should be managed by treatment of any underlying metabolic cause. In the absence of this, treatment with indomethacin (0.5–1.0 mg/kg twice daily) and/or a thiazide diuretic (e.g. hydrochlorothiazide 0.5–1.0 mg/kg twice daily from birth to 12 years of age, or 12.5–25 mg twice daily in older children) together with a potassium-sparing diuretic such as amiloride (5–10 mg/1.73 m² twice daily) can be tried. Unfortunately, patients with nephrogenic diabetes insipidus often respond poorly to treatment and must be allowed adequate access to liberal amounts of water intake as required.

When to involve a specialist centre

- If the investigation and diagnosis of individuals with disturbances of their salt and water balance are proving difficult (e.g. in determining whether hyponatraemia is caused by salt loss or water retention, whether diabetes insipidus is cranial or nephrogenic, or in cases of suspected diabetes insipidus in infants).
- When a water deprivation test is contemplated.
- Endocrine causes of hypertension which usually require specialist investigations and expertise (e.g. endocrine surgeons).
- Diabetes insipidus, particularly when associated with impaired thirst sensation which can be difficult to manage.
- If patients fail to thrive following the introduction of apparently appropriate treatment for salt or water loss.
- Patients with oncological causes of their salt and water imbalance.
- Multiple hormone dysfunction.

Future developments

- The management of nephrogenic diabetes insipidus remains difficult and further research is required to understand the mechanisms more clearly so that more effective treatments can be developed.

• Excessive urine output and natriuresis leading to hyponatraemia is a recognized complication of a serious CNS insult (so-called 'cerebral salt wasting') which is distinct from SIADH. Clarification of whether this is a consequence of inappropriate atrial natriuretic peptide secretion and appropriate treatment options are required.

• Recent research has suggested that the endocrine control of blood pressure in foetal and early postnatal life may be responsible for the 'programming' of blood pressure in adult life. This hypothesis requires further examination.

Controversial points

• Should intranasal DDAVP be replaced by oral or sublingual DDAVP in most patients?

• What is the most appropriate treatment for nephrogenic diabetes insipidus?

Potential pitfalls

• Failure to recognize the tri-phasic pattern of vasopressin problems following craniopharyngioma surgery, resulting in hypernatraemia in the initial post-operative phase followed by hyponatraemia two to four days later due to the syndrome of inappropriate antidiuretic hormone (ADH) secretion.

• Inappropriate and potentially life-threatening management of hyponatraemia due to failure to undertake a sufficiently careful history and clinical examination to distinguish between causes due to salt loss and those due to water retention.

• An inconclusive water deprivation test result due to inadequate supervision of the patient who surreptitiously obtained water to drink (e.g. from the tap in the toilet while producing a urine sample for measurement of osmolality) or failure to extend the test for a sufficient length of time.

• Symptomatic hyponatraemia following administration of DDAVP at the end of the water deprivation test due to failure to prevent the thirsty child consuming excess water.

• Symptomatic hyponatraemia in a child with cranial diabetes insipidus receiving regular DDAVP due to failure to allow a short period of diuresis each day to excrete any excess fluid intake or due to inadequately frequent outpatient review and adjustment of DDAVP dose to take into account changing fluid requirements through the seasons.

• Failure to plan and frequently adjust the fluid intake in a child with cranial diabetes insipidus and adipsia.

• Inadequately aggressive management of nephrogenic diabetes insipidus leading to failure to thrive.

• Inadequate cortisol replacement in hypopituitary states resulting in poor control of DI; this relates to the role of cortisol in facilitating free water excretion.

Emergencies

• Hypernatraemic dehydration with impairment of consciousness, particularly if accompanied by convulsions, is an indication for admission to a high dependency unit for careful fluid input and output balance, twice daily weight, and cardiovascular monitoring. Shock (capillary refill >2 seconds ± hypotension) is treated with 20 ml/kg boluses of 0.9% saline, otherwise the estimated fluid deficit is replaced slowly (over 48–72 hours), checking the plasma sodium at least 6-hourly in the first instance. NB: If severe hypernatraemia is long-standing, as seen in adipsic and hypodipsic patients, slow oral rehydration over several days is carried out in preference to IV fluids.

• Severe hyponatraemia due to sodium loss is managed with 20 ml/kg boluses of 0.9% saline to correct shock, and replacement of the remaining deficit over 24–36 hours.

• Salt and water management can be particularly difficult in patients with hypopituitarism and diabetes insipidus who are on hormone replacement. Such patients may present to the emergency department with illnesses accompanied by vomiting and/or diarrhoea. In this situation, there may be uncertainty as to their cortisol status. In the context of cortisol deficiency, DDAVP may be ineffective, resulting in dehydration, while the cortisol deficiency itself may cause water retention since cortisol is required to enable water excretion. In the latter situation, a relative excess of DDAVP may lead to water intoxication, dilutional hyponatraemia and possible convulsions, and neurological injury. Where doubt exists about the patient's cortisol status, it is safer to provide the correct dose of cortisol, stop the DDAVP and monitor the input/output balance with regular paired plasma and urine electrolytes and osmolality, which may need to be done hourly initially. High fluid volumes may be required but, provided that water and salt balance are monitored meticulously, this will be safe.

Case histories

Case 9.1

A two-week-old boy was admitted with hyponatraemia following an 11-day history of vomiting, constipation, and failure to regain his birth weight. On examination, he appeared underweight, with no other abnormal signs. The mother's brother was known to have developed a similar problem in infancy and was receiving long-term treatment for this. Initial investigations demonstrated the following:

sodium 114 mmol/L
potassium 8.1 mmol/L
cortisol 241 nmol/L [8.7 μg/dL]
17-hydroxy progesterone 5.4 nmol/L [179 ng/dL]

Questions and Answers

1 What is the most likely diagnosis?

In the context of severe hyponatraemia, the cortisol is inappropriately low. The normal 17-hydroxy progesterone excludes 21-hydroxylase-deficient congenital adrenal hyperplasia and the family history suggests a likely diagnosis of X-linked congenital adrenal hypoplasia.

2 What additional investigations are indicated?

A blood sample for the measurement of plasma glucose, renin, aldosterone, ACTH, luteinizing hormone (LH), follicle stimulating hormone (FSH), testosterone and glycerol (gonadotrophin and glycerol kinase deficiencies are associated with X-linked congenital adrenal hypoplasia). A urine sample for the measurement of steroid metabolites or an ACTH stimulation test will help confirm the diagnosis if there is any doubt.

3 What treatment should the baby be given?

Once the initial blood sample for investigations has been taken, the baby should be treated with IV fluids containing 0.9% saline with additional dextrose to provide a concentration of 10% dextrose. He requires IV hydrocortisone at a dosage of approximately 60 mg/m^2 per day subdivided 8-hourly which can be reduced to 10–15 mg/m^2 per day orally once the patient has recovered from the presenting illness (see Chapter 8). Once the vomiting has ceased, oral fludrocortisone can be added at a dosage of 150 mg/m^2 per day.

Case 9.2

An 11-year-old boy presented with an 8-week history of polyuria and polydipsia. He was otherwise well apart from recent headaches. Investigations in clinic demonstrated the following:

serum sodium 142 mmol/L
serum potassium 3.7 mmol/L
serum urea 2.3 mmol/L [6.5 mg/dL]
serum creatinine 52 μmol/L [0.6 mg/dL]
plasma osmolality 305 mOsm/kg
plasma glucose 6.2 mmol/L
urine sodium 16 mmol/L [112 mg/dL]
urine osmolality 78 mOsm/kg

Questions and Answers

1 What further investigation is required to clarify the diagnosis?

Given that a hyperosmolar state has spontaneously developed in this child, a formal water deprivation test is contraindicated. However, it is not clear whether this child has cranial or nephrogenic diabetes insipidus and the response to DDAVP needs to be evaluated. His urinary osmolality increased from 75 to 530 mOsm/kg and there was a dramatic reduction in his urine output, suggesting that he has cranial diabetes insipidus.

2 What additional investigations are then required?

Given a diagnosis of cranial diabetes insipidus and a history of headaches, a full assessment of pituitary function and cranial imaging are indicated. His hypothalamo–pituitary axis was normal on MRI. A basal blood sample demonstrated normal thyroid function and cortisol concentrations. However, after six months he demonstrated poor growth despite a dramatic resolution of his symptoms with regular DDAVP. Peak serum growth hormone concentration after a stimulation test was 4.7 mU/L (normal >20). Repeat MRI demonstrated the presence of a tumour which was shown to be a germinoma.

Case 9.3

A 13-week-old baby girl is admitted for assessment with poor feeding. She was born at

41 weeks' gestation weighing 3.4 kg to a mother aged 29 years. She became hypoglycaemic during the first 24 hours, and required phototherapy for jaundice. She was not fixing or following by 6 weeks and was found at 10 weeks to have small optic discs and absent electroretinogram response to light by the ophthalmology department. On examination she is a pale, lethargic infant weighing 5.36 kg (−1.05 SD), length 60.5 cm (0.12 SD), head circumference 40.7 cm (0.17 SD). She is hypotonic and has roving nystagmus.

Serum sodium is 163 mmol/L, chloride 124 mmol/L, urea 3.3 mmol/L, creatinine 50 μmol/L. Urine osmolality is low at 132 mOsm/kg. Random cortisol is 220 nmol/L, peak cortisol response to a standard dose of synthetic ACTH (125 μg) is 1269 nmol/L (46 mcg/dL). Free T4 is 13.9 pmol/L with TSH 3.8mU/L. Peak GH after arginine stimulation is low/normal at 8 μg/L (24 mU/L).

Questions and Answers

1 What is the most likely diagnosis?

The finding of roving nystagmus and failure to fix and follow with small optic discs in the context of neonatal hypoglycaemia and jaundice is strongly suggestive of septo-optic dysplasia (SOD) with optic nerve hypoplasia and hypopituitarism (including cortisol and thyroxine deficiency).

2 What further assessment is indicated?

Cranial magnetic resonance imaging to look for absence of the septum pellucidum.

3 What do these results indicate?

The baby is one of the unfortunate minority of subjects with SOD who have diabetes insipidus. She has incipient hypothalamic hypothyroidism but, surprisingly, no evidence of cortisol deficiency on a standard Synacthen test.

4 What treatment should be given?

She clearly requires treatment with DDAVP, given as 25 μg daily initially, adding in T4 25 μg daily when the free T4 falls to 8.9 pmol/L at five months of age.

At seven months the infant is admitted, acutely unwell with poor perfusion, mottled and cold peripheries and capillary glucose only 1.3 mmol/L. Sodium is elevated at 167 mmol/L and glucose 2.2 mmol/L. She is given IV fluids and her DDAVP dose is adjusted, but her diabetes insipidus is very hard to control, with sodium fluctuating between 130 and 156 mmol/L.

5 How can the unsatisfactory progress of this infant be explained?

Clinically the child is ACTH-deficient, and diabetes insipidus cannot be properly controlled in the context of cortisol deficiency since the latter is required for water excretion. The peak cortisol level after Synacthen stimulation was achieved using a standard rather than low dose. Random cortisol levels during illness were 200–300 nmol/L (7.2- 10.9 mcg/dL), and never >500 nmol/L (18 mcg/dL), and the child was accordingly started on hydrocortisone. Only when a full replacement dose of hydrocortisone was given did her diabetes insipidus stabilize. The height remained on the 10th centile until five years of age when it fell to the 3rd centile, with IGF-I low at 35 μg/L after which GH therapy was started.

Comment

This case demonstrates the difficulty of diagnosing central adrenal insufficiency, the important role of cortisol in water balance, and the evolving pattern of GHD in SOD, with normal GH levels often found during infancy.

Case 9.4

A male infant is referred to the ophthalmology department because it was noted at the 12-week check that he was not visually fixing and following. He was born at 38 weeks' gestation weighing 2.95 kg and smiled late, with delayed gross motor development. Ophthalmic assessment showed visual inattention with nystagmus, normal optic discs and electroretinogram but reduced visual-evoked potentials consistent with a visual pathway abnormality. In the course of investigations for developmental delay aged

10 months, he was found to have a very high serum sodium of 160 mmol/L, chloride also high at 120 mmol/L, bicarbonate high/normal at 26 mmol/L, urea 5.9 mmol/L and creatinine 41 μmol/L. Urine specific gravity is 1010, confirming a urine concentration defect. On direct questioning his parents say that he does not appear particularly thirsty but that his nappies are quite wet. The infant is referred to the endocrine team for further assessment.

Questions and Answers

1 What is the most likely diagnosis, based on the information given so far?

It appears that this child has a central nervous system (CNS) disorder affecting neurodevelopment including vision and the hypothalamus with a combination of reduced thirst and diabetes insipidus – hypodipsic DI. In this situation, osmoreceptor function is impaired so that vasopressin response to hypernatraemia is reduced, but baroreceptor function is preserved so that vasopressin will be produced in response to low blood pressure. The high/normal bicarbonate probably reflects volume contraction, with enhanced bicarbonate absorption at the proximal tubule, while the normal urea and creatinine show that the baby is not markedly dehydrated.

2 How should the child be managed initially?

The hypernatraemia will be long-standing in nature, and attempts to abruptly correct it will result in convulsions. The child is thoroughly examined and found to have dysmorphic features including mid-line crease in the nose, sloping forehead, low set posteriorly rotated ears and prominent metopic suture. He is hypotonic, visually inattentive, and has poor peripheral perfusion with doughy texture to the subcutaneous tissues, heart rate 120/min and blood pressure 115/75 (crying). Weight is 14.2 kg (>99.6th centile), length 74 cm (50th centile), head circumference 47.2 cm (50th centile).

Hypodipsic DI in a child with an unclassified dysmorphic syndrome is diagnosed on the basis of the clinical and biochemical findings. A nasogastric tube is passed initially and 1000 ml per day of diluted milk (800 ml milk and 200 ml water) is given together with oral DDAVP 25 μg daily. The sodium normalizes on this regimen and is 144 mmol/L 18 days after it was started, by which time the child has been at home for 2 weeks and managing to take the target volume of fluid orally.

3 What further investigations are indicated?

Further hypothalamic assessment is required, together with a genetic consultation and DNA analysis. The MRI of brain shows absence of the pituitary bright spot but is otherwise unremarkable. Pituitary function testing aged 13 months shows a peak GH of 1.9 μg/L (5.7 mU/L) in response to arginine stimulation but IGF-I is normal for age at 33 μg/L; free T4 is 10 pmol/L with a TSH of 6 mU/L. Peak cortisol response to low dose Synacthen (500 ng/1.73 m^2) is borderline low at 411 nmol/L (14.9 mcg/dL). FSH and LH responses to luteinizing hormone releasing hormone (LHRH) are normal for age. These results indicated hypopituitarism with GH and ACTH deficiency, and incipient hypothyroidism.

The child is started on thyroxine 25 μg daily, and hydrocortisone 2.5 mg twice daily in addition to oral DDAVP. Genetic studies show normal chromosomes and multiplex ligation-dependent probe amplification (MLPA) screening is negative. A further DNA sample is sent for array comparative genomic hybridization (CGH).

4 What approach to management should be adopted?

The management approach towards this severely disabled child must be multidisciplinary, involving ophthalmology, audiology, neurodevelopmental, community, and social work professionals. A case discussion is held to ensure good communication between the various disciplines and to devise an integrated care plan.

Further Reading

Baylis, P.H. and Cheetham, T. (1998). Diabetes insipidus. *Arch. Dis. Child.* 79: 84–89.

Bholah, R. and Bunchman, T.E. (2017). Review of pediatric pheochromocytoma and paraganglioma. *Front. Pediatr.* 5 (155): https://doi.org/10.3389/fped.2017.00155.

Cerdà-Esteve, M., Cuadrado-Godia, E., Chillaron, J.J. et al. (2008). Cerebral salt wasting syndrome: review. *Eur. J. Intern. Med.* 19 (4): 249–254.

Ishikawa, S. and Schrier, R.W. (2003). Pathophysiological roles of arginine vasopressin and aquaporin-2 in impaired water excretion. *Clin. Endocrinol.* 58: 1–17.

Maghnie, M., Cosi, G., Genovese, E. et al. (2003). Central diabetes insipidus in children and young adults. *N. Engl. J. Med.* 343: 998–1007.

Schrier, R.W., Gross, P., Gheorghiade, M. et al. (2006). Tolvaptan, a selective oral vasopressin V2-receptor antagonist, for hyponatremia. *N. Engl. J. Med.* 355 (20): 2099–2112.

Timper, K., Fenske, W., Kühn, F. et al. (2015). Diagnostic accuracy of copeptin in the differential diagnosis of the polyuria-polydipsia syndrome: a prospective multicenter study. *J. Clin. Endocrinol. Metab.* 100 (6): 2268–2274.

Werny, D., Elfers, C., Perez, F.A. et al. (2015). Pediatric central diabetes insipidus: brain malformations are common and few patients have idiopathic disease. *J. Clin. Endocrinol. Metab.* 100 (8): 3074–3080.

Useful Information for Patients and Parents

Information for parents about a range of disorders, including diabetes insipidus in multiple languages, may be found on the European Society for Paediatric Endocrinology website in the patient resource section at https://www.eurospe.org/patients (accessed 14 October 2018).

10 Calcium and Bone

Physiology

Introduction

About 99% of the total body calcium is found in the skeleton bound to phosphate and hydroxyl ions in the form of hydroxyapatite. The normal total serum calcium concentration at all ages ranges from 2.2 to 2.6 mmol/L and consists of physiologically active ionized calcium (50%), with the remainder being either bound principally to albumin or globulins (40%), or circulating complexed to citrate, phosphate, or other constituents in the serum (10%). Calcium in intracellular and extracellular fluid is involved in various metabolic processes, including many enzymatic reactions, hormone secretion, and blood coagulation. Calcium metabolism is regulated primarily by vitamin D, parathyroid hormone (PTH) and calcitonin and serum concentrations are influenced by:
- intestinal calcium absorption;
- calcium deposition in bone and mobilization of calcium following bone resorption;
- renal tubular calcium reabsorption.

Approximately 85% of body phosphate is contained within bone hydroxyapatite. Many cellular reactions require either organic or inorganic phosphate. Normal inorganic serum phosphate concentrations drop from 1.3–2.3 mmol/L in infancy to 0.8–1.5 mmol/L at the end of puberty. About 15% of circulating phosphate is protein bound. Free phosphate is required together with ionized calcium for normal bone mineralization.

Vitamin D

Vitamin D is either ingested in the diet or synthesized in the skin following ultraviolet irradiation from sunlight. Circulating vitamin D (Figure 10.1) is metabolized in the liver to 25-hydroxyvitamin D and then in the kidneys to either a metabolically active form (1,25-dihydroxyvitamin D) or an inactive form (24,25-dihydroxyvitamin D). 1,25-dihydroxyvitamin D synthesis is stimulated by hypocalcaemia, PTH and hypophosphataemia.

Circulating vitamin D exerts its target organ effect by binding to an intracellular vitamin D receptor. Vitamin D stimulates the activity of osteoclast-like cells but suppresses that of osteoblast-like cells and, in the presence of PTH, mobilizes calcium from bone. 1,25-dihydroxyvitamin D stimulates intestinal calcium absorption but whether it influences renal handling of calcium and phosphate is less clear. Vitamin D receptors have been located in many other tissues in the body, suggesting a wider role for vitamin D than just regulation of calcium metabolism.

Practical Endocrinology and Diabetes in Children, Fourth Edition. Malcolm D.C. Donaldson, John W. Gregory, Guy Van Vliet, and Joseph I. Wolfsdorf.
© 2019 John Wiley & Sons Ltd. Published 2019 by John Wiley & Sons Ltd.

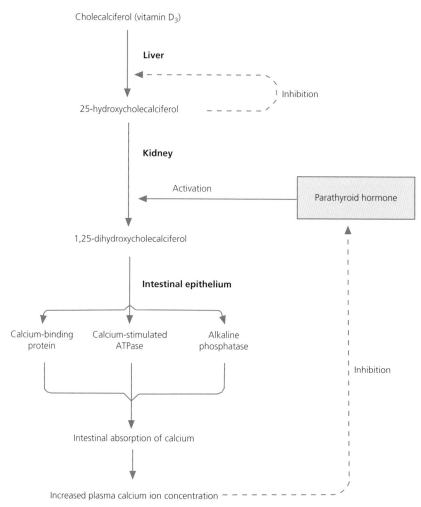

Cholecalciferol (vitamin D₃)

Liver

25-hydroxycholecalciferol

Inhibition

Kidney

Activation

Parathyroid hormone

1,25-dihydroxycholecalciferol

Intestinal epithelium

Calcium-binding protein   Calcium-stimulated ATPase   Alkaline phosphatase

Inhibition

Intestinal absorption of calcium

Increased plasma calcium ion concentration

Figure 10.1 Vitamin D metabolism.

Parathyroid hormone

The PTH gene has been localized to the short arm of chromosome 11. PTH is synthesized as a pre-pro-hormone in the four parathyroid glands. Pre-pro-PTH is converted to pro-PTH as it is transported across the rough endoplasmic reticulum and is stored in secretory granules in the form of the mature 84 amino-acid peptide PTH. PTH release is stimulated by hypocalcaemia and inhibited by hypercalcaemia acting through a specific calcium-sensing (G-protein coupled) receptor on the plasma membrane of the parathyroid cell. This has the capacity to sense small changes in circulating calcium concentrations and to couple this information to intracellular pathways that modify PTH secretion.

The primary function of PTH is to prevent hypocal-caemia. Within minutes, changes in PTH secretion affect renal tubular function, increasing calcium absorption and phosphate excretion, and osteoclastic bone resorption. Over a period of one to two days, by stimulating the synthesis of 1,25-dihydroxyvitamin D, PTH also increases intestinal calcium absorption.

PTH produces its target cell effect by binding to a membrane-bound receptor which stimulates guanine nucleotide-binding protein (G-protein) mediated production of cyclic adenosine monophosphate (cAMP) from adenosine triphosphate (ATP). This, in turn, stimulates activation of protein kinase A and phosphorylation of intracellular enzymes leading to the physiological action of PTH.

Calcitonin

Calcitonin is produced in the 'C' or parafollicular cells of the thyroid gland. Calcitonin is encoded by a gene also located on the short arm of chromosome 11 and is synthesized in the form of a large precursor molecule. Tissue-specific processing may lead to an alternative calcitonin gene product, calcitonin gene-related peptide, which is a potent vasodilator.

Calcitonin secretion is stimulated by calcium and some gastrointestinal hormones (gastrin, cholecystokinin, and glucagon). The primary function of calcitonin is unclear as it appears to have a relatively minor role in calcium metabolism. It reduces serum calcium concentrations by direct inhibition of PTH and 1,25-dihydroxyvitamin D-mediated osteoclastic bone resorption. Calcitonin also increases the urinary excretion of calcium and phosphate but facilitates the absorption of nutrition-derived calcium into blood.

Bone metabolism

Bone has two main functions – (i) forming the rigid skeleton; and (ii) having a central role in calcium and phosphate homeostasis. Macroscopically, there are two types of bone:

1 *Trabecular (cancellous, spongy) bone* is found in the metaphyseal areas of long bones, vertebrae, and most flat bones. It accounts for about 20% of the skeleton and is metabolically very active, having an important role in calcium and phosphate metabolism.

2 *Cortical bone* is found in the diaphyses of the long bones and is relatively metabolically inactive.

Bone consists of:
- an organic matrix – mostly collagen;
- an inorganic mineral phase – hydroxyapatite;
- osteoblasts which synthesize and mineralize the organic bone matrix;
- osteoclasts which resorb bone and are then replaced by osteoblasts which produce new bone;
- osteocytes which are osteoblasts which have become embedded within mineralized bone and which may play a part in sensing mechanical strain or controlling rapid mineral exchange between bone and serum without bone matrix degradation.

Bone growth and reshaping take place throughout childhood and adolescence. Longitudinal growth of the long bones occurs by enchondral bone formation (Figure 10.2). In this process, cartilage cells (chondrocytes) proliferate in columns and undergo hypertrophic differentiation within the growth plate. Chondrocyte proliferation is regulated locally by the interaction of fibroblast growth factor with its receptor fibroblast growth factor receptor-3 (FGFR3). Activating mutations of the *FGFR3* are responsible for achondroplasia and hypochondroplasia. Hypertrophic differentiation of the chondrocyte is regulated by a negative feedback loop involving the cytokine parathyroid hormone-related peptide (PTHrP) and a signalling molecule known as 'Indian hedgehog'. The hypertrophic

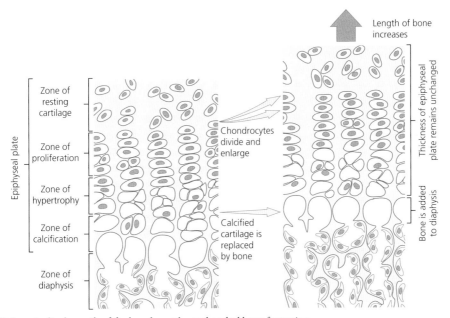

Figure 10.2 Longitudinal growth of the long bones by enchondral bone formation.

Table 10.1 Factors which influence peak bone mass.

Influence	Increased bone mass	Decreased bone mass
Genetic	Afro-Caribbeans	Caucasians
		Orientals
Hormones	Calcitonin	Parathyroid hormone
	Oestrogen	Vitamin D
	Growth hormone	Glucocorticoids
Cytokines	Transforming growth factor β	Interleukin 1
		Tumour necrosis factor α
Nutrition	Calcium	Anorexia
	Obesity	Malabsorption
Mechanical	Exercise	Inactivity

chondrocytes become surrounded by a matrix in which calcium is laid down. Newly calcified cartilage then condenses to become surrounded by osteoblasts which produce calcified osteoid. This calcified tissue is resorbed and replaced by bone trabeculae. By contrast, growth in width and thickness occurs by the process of intramembranous bone formation. This process occurs at the periosteal surface, without a cartilage matrix and with bone resorption taking place at the endosteal surface.

By contrast, bone remodelling is the lifelong process by which skeletal tissue is being continuously resorbed and replaced to maintain skeletal integrity, shape, and mass. In healthy individuals, the balance between bone formation and bone resorption is finely tuned. Bone mass increases progressively through childhood and adolescence until the maximum is attained in young adult life (so-called 'peak bone mass') around 30 years old. Thereafter, a net loss of bone mass occurs as bone resorption exceeds the synthesis of new bone in later life. The amount of peak bone mass is a major risk factor for fractures in old age and is influenced by genetic factors, hormones, nutrition, and mechanical strain (Table 10.1).

Hypocalcaemia

Aetiology

The causes of hypocalcaemia may be subdivided into those which present in infancy and those which present in older children, as shown in Table 10.2. PTH-deficient hypoparathyroidism may be familial (autosomal dominant, recessive or X-linked recessive), caused by activating mutations of the calcium-sensing receptor gene or associated with other abnormalities, such as Addison's disease or deafness. Non-familial PTH-deficient hypoparathyroidism (e.g. in association with DiGeorge's syndrome) may present in infancy and be transient or persistent. In older children, it may be idiopathic, iatrogenic (e.g. following surgical removal of the parathyroids), or secondary (e.g. severe hypomagnesaemia).

Pseudohypoparathyroidism is caused by resistance to the action of PTH. This is known as Albright's hereditary osteodystrophy (AHO) when associated with the dysmorphic features described in Table 11.5 and Figure 11.4. The PTH resistance of AHO is most commonly associated with decreased G-protein activity in cell membranes (type 1a), which may also affect other G-protein coupled receptors (e.g. adrenocorticotrophic hormone (ACTH), thyroid-stimulating hormone (TSH), luteinizing hormone (LH), follicle-stimulating hormone (FSH) and glucagon). The genetics of AHO are complex, with parent-of-origin effects. Maternally inherited inactivating mutations of GNAS cause pseudohypoparathyroidism-type 1a whereas paternally inherited mutations can lead either to pseudopseudohypoparathyroidism (the presence of clinical features of AHO but without biochemical evidence of PTH resistance) or to progressive osseous heteroplasia (ectopic bone formation within skin and muscle). Importantly, because of random monoallelic expression of the allele bearing the mutation that inactivates GNAS, any given hormone resistance may fluctuate over time, i.e. an infant with AHO may have normal calcium and develop severe hypocalcaemia later in life. The parent should therefore be made aware of the signs and symptoms that suggest hypocalcaemia.

Table 10.2 Causes of hypocalcaemia.

Infancy	Childhood
Prematurity	Vitamin D deficiency
Asphyxia	Vitamin D-dependent rickets (types 1 and 2)
Gestational diabetes	Chronic renal failure
Transient or permanent hypoparathyroidism	Hypoparathyroidism
	Pseudohypoparathyroidism
High milk phosphate load	
Hypomagnesaemia	
Parenteral nutrition	
Exchange transfusion	
Chronic alkalosis or bicarbonate therapy	
Maternal hyperparathyroidism	

History and examination

When assessing a child with hypocalcaemia, the following points should be highlighted in the clinical history:

- symptoms suggestive of hypocalcaemia (e.g. paraesthesia, muscle cramps or tetany, seizures, and diarrhoea);
- predisposing risk factors (e.g. intestinal or renal tubular disease) for hypomagnesaemia;
- evidence of endocrine disease affecting other G-protein coupled receptors (e.g. previous thyroxine treatment for a low normal serum T4 concentration with mildly elevated serum TSH concentration);
- symptoms of autoimmune disease;
- previous surgical risk factors (e.g. thyroidectomy or parathyroidectomy);
- a family history of hypoparathyroidism.

If an older child is suspected of having hypocalcaemia, latent tetany may be detected from positive Chvostek's sign (facial twitching in response to tapping of the facial nerve in front of the ear) and Trousseau's sign (carpal spasm within three minutes of inflating a blood pressure cuff above systolic blood pressure; Figure 10.3), or stridor. Extrapyramidal signs from basal ganglia calcification, cataracts, papilloedema, dry skin, coarse hair, brittle nails, and enamel hypoplasia with dental caries are signs suggestive of chronic hypocalcaemia. In contrast to the older child, hypocalcaemia in infancy is associated with relatively non-specific symptoms including tremor, apnoea, cyanosis, and lethargy. Clinical signs suggestive of autoimmune hypoparathyroidism and pseudohypoparathyroidism are shown in Table 10.3 with details of the dysmorphic features of pseudohypoparathyroidism shown in Table 11.5 and Figure 11.4.

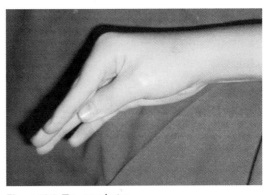

Figure 10.3 Trousseau's sign.

Investigations

If hypocalcaemia is suspected, a blood sample should be taken for the measurement of:

- calcium
- albumin
- phosphate
- magnesium
- alkaline phosphatase
- PTH
- 25-hydroxyvitamin D
- a sample stored for possible measurement of 1,25-dihydroxyvitamin D concentration later, should this be indicated
- a sample stored for possible genetic studies of the GNAS gene to identify variants associated with lack of expression or function of the GNAS complex as occurs in pseudohypoparathyroidism.

The differential diagnosis of biochemical abnormalities of calcium metabolism is shown in Table 10.4.

Table 10.3 Clinical signs to look for on examination.

Clinical sign	Possible diagnosis
Candidiasis Dental enamel and nail dystrophy Alopecia Vitiligo Signs of Addison's disease or hypothyroidism	Autoimmune hypoparathyroidism (polyglandular autoimmune disease type 1)
Short stature Subcutaneous calcification Dysmorphic features	Pseudohypoparathyroidism
Swollen wrists Prominent costochondral junctions (rachitic rosary) and Harrison's sulci Bow-leg or knock-knee Craniotabes Delayed dental eruption and enamel hypoplasia Muscle weakness and tetany	Vitamin D-deficient rickets
Poor growth Bowing of the legs	Hypophosphataemic rickets
Blue sclerae Abnormal dentition Hyperextensible joints Deafness	Osteogenesis imperfecta
Broad and prominent forehead Short turned-up nose with flat nasal bridge Overhanging upper lip Late dental eruption Supravalvular aortic stenosis Peripheral pulmonary stenosis Learning difficulties with emotional lability Mild short stature	Williams syndrome
Alopecia	Vitamin D-dependent rickets type 2

Treatment

Emergency management of acute hypocalcaemia complicated by tetany or a seizure

1 Take initial diagnostic blood sample.

2 Slow intravenous (IV) injection over 5–10 minutes of 10% calcium gluconate:

a *Neonates:* 0.11–0.46 mmol (0.5–2.0 ml or 50–200 mg)/kg body weight for one dose.

b *Child:* 0.11 mmol/kg (maximum 4.5 mmol (20 ml or 2 g)).

3 Maintain IV infusion of 10% calcium gluconate:

a *Neonates:* 0.5 mmol/kg per day (may be necessary for a few days).

b *Children aged one month to one year:* 1 mmol/kg per day (usual maximum 8.8 mmol).

c *Children aged 2–17 years:* 8.8 mmol over 24 hours.

4 Once acute symptoms are resolved, treatment should be changed to oral preparations and adjusted according to response:

a *Neonates:* 0.25 mmol/kg four times daily.

b *Children aged one month to four years:* 0.25 mmol/kg four times daily.

c *Children aged 5–11 years:* 0.2 mmol/kg four times daily.

d *Children aged 12–17 years:* 10 mmol four times daily.

Care must be taken when IV calcium is administered as extravasation of calcium into subcutaneous

Table 10.4 Differential diagnosis of disorders of vitamin D and parathyroid hormone (PTH) metabolism.

Diagnosis	Ca$_2$	PO$_4$	PTH	25-OHD	1,25-(OH)$_2$D
Vitamin D-deficient rickets	LN	↓	↑	↓	↓, N, ↑
Vitamin D-dependent rickets					
Type 1 (deficiency of 1α-hydroxylation)	↓	↓	↑	N, ↓	↓
Type 2 (resistance to 1,25-(OH)$_2$D)	↓	↓	↑	N, ↓	N, ↑
X-linked hypophosphataemic rickets	N	↓	N	N	↓, N
Hypophosphataemic rickets with hypercalciuria	N	↓	N	N	↑
Tumour-induced rickets	N	↓	N	N	↓
Renal osteodystrophy	N, ↓	↑	↑		N, L
Primary hyperparathyroidism	↑	↓	↑	N	N, ↑
Hypoparathyroidism	↓	↑	↓	N	↓, N
Pseudohypoparathyroidism	↓	↑	↑	N	↓, N
Vitamin D intoxication	↑	N	↓	↑	N, ↑
Hypercalcaemia in granulomatous disorders	↑	N	↓	N	↑

Ca$_2$, calcium; PO$_4$, phosphate; 25-OHD, 25-hydroxyvitamin D; 1,25-(OH)$_2$D, 1,25-dihydroxyvitamin D; ↑, high; N, normal; ↓, low; LN, low–normal.
Source: From Ranke (1992).

tissues around the injection site can lead to tissue necrosis; transfer to oral medication as soon as possible is advised. Long-term maintenance treatment of hypocalcaemia requires vitamin D given as alfacalcidol (neonates 50–100 ng/kg daily, children aged 1 month to 11 years 25–50 ng/kg daily and children aged 12–17 years 1 μg daily) or calcitriol (children aged 1 month to 11 years initially 15 ng/kg daily, increased by 5 ng/kg daily to a maximum of 250 ng and children aged 12–17 years 250 ng daily increased by 5 ng/kg daily (maximum step 250 ng) every 2–4 weeks to a usual dose of 0.5–1.0 μg daily). These preparations are recommended because of their short half-life and rapid cessation of action should toxicity occur. Vitamin D may need to be given in combination with calcium. Frequent monitoring of serum calcium concentrations is required shortly after starting treatment – weekly, if there is concern about the response to therapy. Once the patient has demonstrated a satisfactory response, serum calcium concentration and the urinary calcium:creatinine (UCa:Cr) ratio should be measured every three months thereafter, aiming to keep UCa:Cr <0.7 mmol/mmol. Regular renal ultrasounds should also be performed to monitor for calcification.

In children with hypoparathyroidism (particularly those due to mutations of the calcium-sensing receptor gene), the aim of therapy is to achieve low normal serum calcium concentrations (2.0–2.25 mmol/L) [8.0–9.0 mg/dL] while avoiding urinary calcium:creatinine ratios greater than 0.7 mmol/L/mmol/L [0.16 mg/dL/mg/dL]. In those with pseudohypoparathyroidism, the resistance to PTH primarily affects the proximal renal tubule and not renal handling of calcium. Therefore, to avoid adverse bone sequelae, treatment should suppress PTH levels to the normal range, which may require maintenance of serum calcium concentrations towards the upper end of the normal range (2.25–2.5 mmol/L) [9.0–10.0 mg/dL]. In contrast to the management of primary hypoparathyroidism, there is less concern in pseudohypoparathyroidism about potential risks of adverse renal effects of hypercalciuria.

Rickets

Aetiology
Mechanisms for rickets:
- vitamin D deficiency or resistance
- calcium deficiency
- phosphate deficiency
- acidosis.

Rickets is caused by delayed matrix mineralization at the growth plate resulting in excessive accumulation of uncalcified cartilage and bone (osteoid) matrix. The most common causes of rickets are those associated with vitamin D deficiency. They present most frequently at times of rapid growth which may occur in infancy or in puberty, particularly in children with increased skin pigmentation. Vitamin D deficiency may be a result of dietary insufficiency, malabsorption (e.g. coeliac disease) or inadequate exposure to sunlight. There is a need for a greater clinical awareness of vitamin D-deficient rickets in Western industrialized societies as the current prevalence, particularly in infancy and adolescence, seems higher than is often appreciated even in relatively sunny countries. To prevent rickets, it is recommended that food be supplemented with 400 units (10 μg) of vitamin D daily for all children aged under four years and adolescents, particularly girls with darker skins. Children who consume more than 500 ml of infant formula milk do not need vitamin D supplementation as the milk is already fortified. Rickets of prematurity is thought to be caused by calcium and/or phosphate deficiency rather than vitamin D deficiency.

Hypophosphataemic rickets is an X-linked dominant disorder which causes a failure of phosphate resorption in the proximal renal tubule. It is usually due to an inactivating mutation in the PHEX gene, which results in abnormal PHEX-mediated up-regulation of FGF23 activity. Vitamin D-dependent rickets is very rare and is caused either by deficiency of 1a-hydroxylation of 25-hydroxyvitamin D (type 1) or resistance to 1,25-dihydroxyvitamin D (type 2). The classification of the different forms of rickets and their biochemical characteristics are shown in Table 10.4.

In severe renal failure, deficiency of 1α-hydroxylase causes impaired 1,25-dihydroxyvitamin D synthesis which, in conjunction with increasing serum phosphate concentrations, leads to hypocalcaemia and secondary hyperparathyroidism with bone disease (renal osteodystrophy).

Both rickets and osteomalacia (defective mineralization of osteoid tissue) are common in the many causes of Fanconi's syndrome and type 2 renal tubular acidosis. The metabolic bone disease is caused by a combination of phosphaturia-induced hypophosphataemia, hypercalciuria, abnormal vitamin D metabolism, and renal insufficiency.

History and examination

If a child presents with rickets, then the following details should be elicited:
- symptoms suggestive of associated disease (e.g. renal failure, malabsorption);
- dietary history of food intake, such as dairy products, which are rich in calcium and vitamin D;
- risk factors for inadequate exposure to sunlight;
- family history of rickets.

The child should undergo careful clinical examination, including documentation of growth and pubertal status. The clinical signs to look for on examination are shown in Table 10.3.

Investigations

Rickets causes abnormal bone mineralization which may be evident on X-ray. Additional radiological features commonly include a characteristic widening of the growth plate with cupping, splaying and fraying of an irregularly margined metaphysis (Figure 10.4). The characteristic clinical signs of vitamin D-deficient and hypophosphataemic rickets are detailed in Table 10.3 and Figure 10.5 and Figure 10.6.

The lowered renal threshold for resorption of phosphate, which is associated with hypophosphataemic rickets, can be calculated from simultaneous serum and urinary biochemical measurements by reference to Kruse et al. (1982) or Shaw et al. (1990), which also contains details of age-appropriate reference ranges.

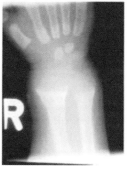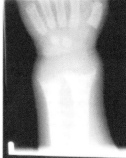

Figure 10.4 X-ray of the wrist of a child with rickets caused by vitamin D deficiency.

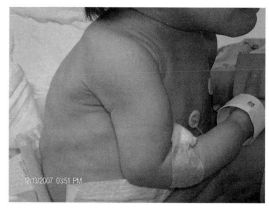

Figure 10.5 Rachitic rosary. Source: Courtesy of Dr Nina Ma.

The presence of glycosuria, amino-aciduria, or a metabolic acidosis with inappropriately alkaline urine is suggestive of a wider defect of tubular function, such as Fanconi's syndrome or renal tubular acidosis.

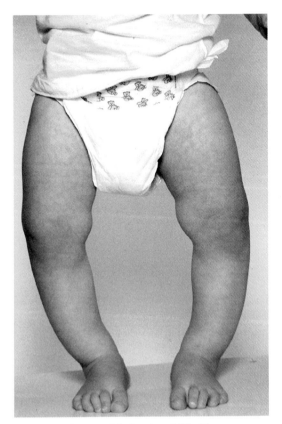

Figure 10.6 Bowing of the legs in a child with hypophosphataemic rickets.

Treatment

Depending on the cause of the rickets, different preparations of vitamin D are required for effective treatment, as shown in Table 10.5. Where renal dysfunction is associated with metabolic bone disease, treatment of the wider systemic metabolic abnormality is required. Detailed guidance for this is beyond the scope of this volume and the reader is advised to consult appropriate textbooks on paediatric nephrology. Children with Fanconi's syndrome may require phosphate therapy, whereas those with renal tubular acidosis require treatment with bicarbonate.

Osteoporosis

Aetiology

Unlike in adults, osteoporosis in childhood is not clearly defined but is caused by reduced bone mass per unit volume with a normal ratio of mineral to matrix. The possibility of osteoporosis should be considered in a child who presents with fractures following minimal trauma in whom there is also evidence of decreased bone mineral density (usually more than three standard deviations below the mean for age, size, and puberty). This may occur as a result of an imbalance between bone formation and bone resorption because of a variety of reasons or as a result of abnormalities of type 1 collagen synthesis (e.g. osteogenesis imperfecta). The causes of decreased bone mineral density, which may predispose to osteoporosis and present in childhood, are shown in Table 10.6.

Table 10.5 Treatment of rickets.

Aetiology	Treatment
Vitamin D-deficient rickets	Calciferol 150 000 units by intramuscular injection, repeated at 1–2 mo OR Cholecalciferol solution total dose of 150 000 units, preferably as a single dose orally or split over 3 d and repeated at 1–2 mo
Rickets of prematurity as a result of phosphate deficiency	Phosphate 1 mmol kg^{-1} daily in 1–2 divided doses by mouth or as an IV infusion
Vitamin D-dependent rickets (type 1)	Calcitriol 0.25–2.0 µg per day
Vitamin D-dependent rickets (type 2)	Calcitriol, large doses (up to 50 µg per day) and long-term high-dose oral or IV calcium
Hypophosphataemic rickets	Phosphate, 2–3 mmol/kg daily in 2–4 divided doses orally (maximum dose 48 mmol in children aged 1 mo–5 yr and 97 mmol in children aged 5–18 yr) AND Calcitriol 15–20 ng/kg per day increased to 30–60 ng/kg per day subdivided into one or two daily doses orally.

Table 10.6 Causes of osteoporosis and other disorders which may lead to decreased bone mineral density.

Pathogenetic basis	Examples
Primary bone disease	Idiopathic juvenile osteoporosis
	Osteogenesis imperfecta
	Osteoporosis pseudoglioma syndrome
Inflammatory	Inflammatory bowel disease
	Rheumatoid arthritis
Endocrine	Cushing's syndrome or disease
Drugs	Glucocorticoids
Others	Immobility
	Acute lymphoblastic leukaemia
	Thalassaemia
	Homocystinuria
	Post transplant
Causes of decreased bone mineral content (osteopenia) not necessarily severe enough to cause or osteoporosis	Anorexia, malnutrition
	Coeliac disease
	Hypopituitarism
	Hypogonadism (e.g. Turner's syndrome)
	Hyperparathyroidism
	Renal failure
	Chronic liver disease
	Thyrotoxicosis
	Burns
	Methotrexate

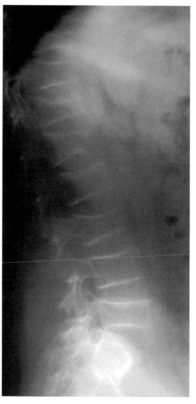

Figure 10.7 X-rays showing vertebral compression in a child with osteoporosis.

History and examination

Osteoporosis may present with obvious signs of a long bone fracture following minimal trauma or with back pain and deformity because of underlying vertebral compression fractures (Figure 10.7). Clinical assessment and investigations should aim to exclude the causes of decreased bone mineral density shown in Table 10.6. If a child presents with osteopenia, then the following details should be elicited:

- symptoms suggestive of associated disease (e.g. renal disease, malabsorption, inflammatory bowel disease);
- features suggestive of growth failure or pubertal delay;
- past medical history of fractures in the absence of significant underlying trauma;
- medication (e.g. steroids);
- family history of osteoporosis or fractures;
- immobility.

Clinical examination should include a careful assessment of growth, nutritional state, pubertal development, and the clinical signs of osteogenesis imperfecta listed in Table 10.3. The presence of unexplained bone tenderness and pain, particularly in the spinal region, and in association with a spinal deformity, such as a kyphosis or scoliosis, might suggest previously unsuspected fractures. These may occur with severe osteoporosis or osteogenesis imperfecta.

Distinguishing between osteogenesis imperfecta and idiopathic juvenile osteoporosis may prove difficult. Osteogenesis imperfecta should be considered in the presence of the clinical signs listed in Table 10.3. A skull X-ray for the presence of wormian bones and a blood sample for genetic testing (e.g. the type 1 collagen genes COL1A1 or COL1A2) may assist in the diagnosis of osteogenesis imperfecta (for classification, see Table 10.7). Idiopathic juvenile osteoporosis may be suggested by X-ray evidence of metaphyseal compression fractures at the knee. Histomorphometric examination of bone biopsy material may also help distinguish between these two conditions.

Investigations

Bone mineral density may be measured by dual energy X-ray absorptiometry (DEXA) scanning of the lumbar spine or hip. This method involves minimal

Table 10.7 Classification of osteogenesis imperfecta.

Type	Phenotype	Gene	Mode of inheritance
I	Mild, blue sclera, early deafness, mild stunting	COL1A1	Autosomal dominant
II	Severe, death in infancy	COL1A1, COL1A2	Autosomal dominant
III	Progressively deforming, infantile blue sclerae	COL1A1, COL1A2	Autosomal dominant
IV	Deforming, normal white sclerae	COL1A1, COL1A2	Autosomal dominant
V	Similar to IV but 'mesh-like' bone	IFITM5	Autosomal dominant
VI	Similar to IV but 'fish-scale' bone	SERPINF1	Autosomal recessive
VII	Severe to lethal	CRTAP	Autosomal recessive
VIII	Severe to lethal	LEPRE1	Autosomal recessive
IX	Severe	PPIB	Autosomal recessive

radiation exposure and is based on the measurement of the attenuation of X-rays of differing energy intensity as they pass through bone. However, these characteristics are influenced by the width of bone through which the X-rays pass, which in children may vary as a consequence of age, body size, or puberty, in addition to illness. Interpretation of the data needs to take these factors into account and appropriate paediatric reference values must be used to interpret the results. It is recommended that bone mineral density should only be measured in children with risk factors for low bone density associated with low trauma or recurrent fractures, back pain, spinal deformity or loss of height, change in mobility status, or malnutrition.

Newer techniques for obtaining volumetric measures of bone mineral density that are not constrained by the limitations of DEXA, such as quantitative computed tomography, are now becoming available.

Treatment

The following measures may help in the treatment of osteoporosis:

- adequate analgesia for fractures;
- physiotherapy, splints and orthopaedic intervention, and occupational therapy where necessary;
- optimal dietary calcium and vitamin D intake with supplements where necessary;
- effective treatment of underlying disease;
- if osteoporosis is steroid-induced, reduce daily glucocorticoid dosage as much as possible, consider alternate day therapy or use those with minimal side effects (e.g. deflazacort);
- induction of puberty with low-dose testosterone or oestrogen if pubertal delay present (see Chapter 5);
- calcitonin has been suggested in a few small studies to be beneficial in children with osteopenia;
- bisphosphonates (e.g. pamidronate) have been used

in childhood, mostly to treat osteogenesis imperfecta. Despite residual uncertainty about their long-term safety, there is growing evidence that they benefit children by reducing the pain associated with mini-fractures, increasing bone mineral density and facilitating physical rehabilitation and mobility. There seem to be few side effects in the short to medium term apart from a transient rise in body temperature, fever, and influenza-like symptoms during the initial course of infusions. It is advised to optimize dietary calcium and vitamin D intake during therapy to reduce to a minimum the risks of developing hypocalcaemia. Furthermore, after prolonged use, consideration should be given to tapering the dose down gradually to avoid the development of an abrupt junction between bone formed whilst receiving bisphosphonate therapy and that formed thereafter, as this may represent a point of weakness at increased risk of fracture.

Hypercalcaemia

Aetiology

Hypercalcaemia occurs when the serum calcium concentration exceeds 2.65 mmol/L. The causes of hypercalcaemia are shown in Table 10.8.

Mild idiopathic hypercalcaemia of infancy presents with symptoms between the ages of two and nine months, but resolves spontaneously by the age of four years. When severe, it may present in the neonatal period in association with the dysmorphic features of Williams syndrome (Table 10.3 and Figure 10.8). Hypercalcaemia is associated with granulomatous disease (e.g. sarcoidosis and tuberculosis) as a result of the conversion of 25-hydroxyvitamin D to 1,25-dihydroxyvitamin D in granulomatous cells.

Table 10.8 Causes of hypercalcaemia.

Neonatal or infantile onset	Gestational maternal hypocalcaemia
	Idiopathic hypercalcaemia of infancy
	Subcutaneous fat necrosis
	Williams syndrome
	Neonatal primary hyperparathyroidism
	Preterm or intrauterine growth retarded-associated phosphate depletion
	Vitamin D intoxication (most commonly iatrogenic, e.g. during treatment of hypoparathyroidism)
Childhood onset	Parathyroid adenoma
	Isolated familial hyperparathyroidism
	Multiple endocrine neoplasia type 1
	Multiple endocrine neoplasia type 2A
	Familial hypocalciuric hypercalcaemia
	Hypercalcaemia in granulomatous disorders
	Acute lymphoblastic leukaemia
	Immobilization

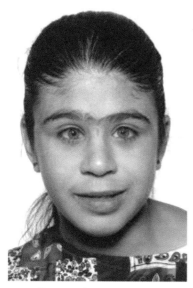

Figure 10.8 Williams syndrome.

Neonatal hypercalcaemia

Neonatal primary hyperparathyroidism is a serious disorder caused by homozygous mutations of the calcium-sensing receptor gene, the product of which regulates PTH secretion. It causes anorexia, hypotonia, chest deformities, and respiratory distress. It is associated with a high mortality in the neonatal period and, to be successfully treated, requires urgent parathyroidectomy. Similar heterozygous mutations are responsible for autosomal dominant, familial hypocalciuric hypercalcaemia.

Hypercalcaemia in childhood

Primary hyperparathyroidism as seen in association with pituitary adenomas and gastrinomas or other pancreatic tumours (multiple endocrine neoplasia type 1) or in association with medullary thyroid cancer and phaeochromocytoma (multiple endocrine neoplasia type 2A) is exceptional in the paediatric age group. These two groups of disorders are inherited in an autosomal dominant fashion and all offspring of affected individuals should be screened for these endocrinopathies. The presence of elevated serum concentrations of PTH will distinguish hyperparathyroidism from hypercalcaemia caused by vitamin D intoxication, idiopathic infantile hypercalcaemia, granulomatous disease, and malignancy.

History and examination

When assessing a child with possible hypercalcaemia, the following points should be highlighted in the clinical history:
- symptoms suggestive of hypercalcaemia (e.g. weakness, anorexia, nausea and vomiting, abdominal pain, constipation, polyuria, and polydipsia);
- symptoms suggestive of tuberculosis or sarcoidosis;
- vitamin D therapy;
- a family history of multiple endocrine neoplasia.

Investigations

If hypercalcaemia is suspected, a blood sample should be taken for the measurement of:
- calcium
- phosphate
- PTH
- 25-hydroxyvitamin D
- a sample should be stored for possible measurement of 1,25-dihydroxyvitamin D concentration later, should this be indicated.

The differential diagnosis of biochemical abnormalities of calcium metabolism is shown in Table 10.4.

Treatment

The treatment of hypercalcaemia involves promoting a low-calcium diet and where relevant, stopping vitamin D, calcium supplements and other drugs, such as thiazides, which increase calcium concentrations. Patients should be encouraged to drink plenty of fluids. If significant dehydration is present, this should be corrected with IV 0.9% saline. Prednisolone may be helpful if hypercalcaemia is secondary to sarcoidosis or vitamin D intoxication. If hypercalcaemia persists, bisphosphonate therapy may help by inhibiting mobilization of calcium from the skeleton. A parathyroid adenoma may be located by careful ultrasound examination and treated by surgical removal of the affected gland. Hyperparathyroidism caused by diffuse hyperplasia requires surgical removal of all four glands.

When to involve a specialist centre

- Hypoparathyroidism.
- Hypophosphataemic rickets.
- Osteoporosis which is of sufficient severity that treatment with bisphosphonates is to be considered.
- Osteogenesis imperfecta.
- Osteoporosis secondary to other underlying disorders (e.g. inflammatory bowel disease, rheumatoid arthritis, or Cushing's syndrome or disease) should have the treatment of their underlying disease discussed with the relevant specialists.
- Hyperparathyroidism.

Transition

Many causes of hypocalcaemia, rickets, and hypercalcaemia are transient and resolve in childhood without the need for referral onto adult services. However, where the underlying cause has potential implications into adult life (e.g. hypoparathyroidism or pseudohypoparathyroidism), then referral through local transition arrangements should be organized. Of note, even if well and currently asymptomatic, children known to be at risk of multiple endocrine neoplasia require referral to adult services for the organization of ongoing monitoring. Where there is an underlying genetic cause for a disorder of bone or calcium biochemistry which may have implications for future offspring, organization of genetic counselling may be particularly important.

Given the importance of bone mineral accretion into the third decade of life, teenagers undergoing monitoring for osteopenia should also be referred.

Discussion may need to take place between paediatric and adult specialists regarding the interpretation of successive bone mineral density scan reports, given that paediatric practice involves interpreting data for body size (using Z-scores) whereas the tendency in adult practice is to interpret data relative to peak bone mass (T scores).

Future developments

- Administration of sufficiently high doses of phosphate to children with hypophosphataemic rickets remains problematic and alternative therapeutic strategies are required, such as monoclonal antibodies directed against FGF23 to prevent the development of bone deformity in these children.
- The cause of idiopathic juvenile osteoporosis remains to be established. A diagnostic test for this is greatly needed to assist clinicians in the investigation and management of children presenting with fractures associated with severe osteoporosis.
- More information is required about the long-term safety of bisphosphonate treatment and on alternative strategies for the treatment of severe childhood osteoporosis.
- Clarification of the molecular basis of primary hyperparathyroidism will enable earlier detection of this disorder and of multiple endocrine neoplasia type 1. The discovery of the calcium-sensing receptor offers the promise of alternative therapeutic strategies for the treatment of hyperparathyroidism.

Controversial points

- Does the severity of osteopenia in the growing child predict the future fracture risk as in postmenopausal women?
- Do girls with Turner syndrome have an increased risk of osteopenia over and above that caused by inadequately treated hypogonadism?
- Do androgens have a direct effect on bone mineralization which is independent of their conversion to oestrogens?
- Is bisphosphonate treatment indicated for the treatment of osteopenia in the absence of fractures?
- Is bisphosphonate treatment in young children without risk to future bone health?
- What are the frequency and aetiology of fractures in infancy not due to non-accidental injury?

Potential pitfalls

• Diagnostic confusion between vitamin D deficiency and hypoparathyroidism as the cause of hypocalcaemia in infancy. Careful interpretation of serum concentrations of phosphate, PTH, and vitamin D should help distinguish between the two conditions.

• Over-aggressive treatment of hypoparathyroidism increasing the risks of nephrocalcinosis from hypercalciuria.

• Unnecessary measurement of bone mineral density in a child at relatively low risk of developing osteoporosis.

• Incorrect diagnosis of osteoporosis based only on X-ray findings reportedly suggestive of osteopenia or from failure to take into account a child's small size when interpreting a dual energy X-ray measurement of bone mineral density.

• Failure clinically to suspect vertebral compression fractures. These should be considered in any child with osteoporosis who complains of backache or stiffness or who has evidence of even relatively minor spinal shape deformity.

• Diagnostic confusion between osteogenesis imperfecta and non-accidental injury as the cause of fractures in a young child. Where the diagnosis is unclear, these children should be referred for further evaluation by clinicians with expertise in child protection and bone disease.

• Failure to appreciate that most causes of hypercalcaemia in infancy are benign, self-limiting, and respond well to conservative management.

Case histories

Case 10.1
A two-year-old boy was referred for further assessment of his increasingly bowed legs. His mother was known to have hypophosphataemic rickets. X-rays show bowing of the femoral shafts but no radiological evidence of rickets. The following blood measurements were obtained:

Calcium 2.37 mmol/L [9.50 mg/dL]
Phosphate 1.13 mmol/L [3.50 mg/dL]
Alkaline phosphatase 805 IU/L (reference range 100–400 IU/L)
PTH 1.3 pmol/L [12.35 pg/ml] (reference range 0.9–5.5 pmol/L)

Questions and Answers

1 Is this child likely to have X-linked hypophosphataemic rickets?

This boy has a 50% chance of inheriting rickets from his mother. With an X-linked dominant disorder, he would be expected to be more severely affected than his mother. In the presence of his bone deformity, the absence of biochemical evidence of hypophosphataemia is surprising.

2 What additional investigations may clarify the diagnosis?

A simultaneous blood and urine sample should be obtained for the measurement of phosphate and creatinine so that the renal threshold phosphate concentration can be calculated (Kruse et al. 1982; Shaw et al. 1990). In this patient, the diagnosis of X-linked hypophosphataemic rickets was confirmed by the demonstration of a markedly decreased tubular reabsorption of phosphate (55%) and a renal threshold phosphate concentration of 1.4 mmol l^{-1}.

Case 10.2
A nine-year-old girl was admitted with severe back pain after she had fallen over her dog. She had sustained a previous fracture of her wrist following significant trauma. Her weight was above the 99th centile, height on the 50th centile, and she had early breast development.

X-rays demonstrated multiple wedge collapse fractures of several thoracic and lumbar vertebrae and widespread osteopenia. Initial investigations demonstrated the following:

Calcium 2.45 mmol/L [9.82 mg/dL]
Phosphate 1.32 mmol/L [4.10 mg/dL]
Alkaline phosphatase 264 IU/L (reference range 100–400 IU/L)
PTH 4.2 pmol/L [40 pg/ml] (reference range 0.9–5.5 pmol/L)
25-hydroxyvitamin D 12.4 ng/ml [39.9 pg/ml] (reference range 8–50 ng/ml)
C-reactive protein <1 mg/L
Normal renal, liver, and thyroid function tests, and negative anti-endomysial antibodies

Questions and Answers

1 What further clinical observations would be of interest?

It would be helpful to know if she had evidence of blue-coloured sclerae, joint hyperextensibility, or abnormal hearing which might suggest osteogenesis imperfecta. Given her obesity, it might also be important to assess for other signs suggestive of Cushing's syndrome.

2 What additional investigations are required?

A dual energy X-ray absorptiometry scan confirmed the severity of the osteopenia with a lumbar spine bone mineral content of −2.79 SD and femoral neck −3.65 SD. Three 24-hour urine collections demonstrated normal cortisol excretion rates which excluded Cushing's syndrome.

3 What is the differential diagnosis?

This girl is most likely to have either idiopathic juvenile osteoporosis or, possibly, osteogenesis imperfecta.

Case 10.3

A three-month-old boy presented to a peripheral unit with cyanosis during feeding. No abnormalities were found on clinical examination and these episodes did not reoccur thereafter. Investigations at presentation showed the following:

Serum calcium 2.72 mmol/L [10.9 mg/dL]
Serum phosphate 1.73 mmol/L [5.37 mg/dL]
Urinary calcium:creatinine ratio 0.91 mmol/mmol[1] creatinine (normal <0.7 mmol/mmol creatinine)

Serial blood samples over the next six months continued to demonstrate mild hypercalcaemia. Although he remained clinically well, he was referred for further assessment.

Questions and Answers

1 What other investigations are indicated?

The infant should undergo measurement of PTH and vitamin D status. A renal ultrasound is useful to check for nephrocalcinosis. The parents should undergo measurement of their serum calcium, phosphate, and PTH concentrations, and if abnormalities are present, discussion with geneticists regarding mutational screening of genes involved in the calcium sensing receptor or PTH is indicated. The absence of any dysmorphic features makes a diagnosis of Williams syndrome relatively

unlikely though this can be formally excluded by screening for mutations of the elastin gene.

2 What treatment is worth considering and when?

In the presence of persistent hypercalcaemia, particularly when associated with symptoms, a calcium and vitamin D restricted diet should be offered.

3 Investigations following referral did not demonstrate any additional abnormal findings and the serum calcium concentration normalized at the age of one year. What is the likely diagnosis?

The absence of any abnormal findings on investigation and spontaneous resolution of the hypercalcaemia would be consistent with a diagnosis of idiopathic infantile hypercalcaemia.

Case 10.4

A two-year-old Pakistani girl was referred with bowing of her legs. She experiences no difficulties walking and is said to have a good diet with plenty of dairy products. Initial blood tests demonstrate the following:

Calcium 2.43 mmol/L [9.7 mg/dL]
Phosphate 1.66 mmol/L [5.15 mg/dL]
Alkaline phosphatase 330 IU/L (reference range 100–300 IU/L)
25-OH cholecalciferol <7.0 ng/ml (reference range (>30 ng/ml)
PTH 10.8 pmol/L (reference range 0.9–5.4 pmol/L)

Questions and Answers

1 What features in the clinical history should be explored?

Enquiry should be made into how long this child was breast-fed and whether the mother's vitamin D status is known. Also, the presence of symptoms of malabsorption should be explored. In this case, mother received treatment during pregnancy for vitamin D deficiency and breast-fed till 23 months with no recent assessment of her vitamin D status.

2 What other investigations are indicated?

An X-ray of her legs is indicated to see if there are radiological signs of rickets.

3 What treatment is required?

She requires vitamin D treatment.

Case 10.5

A four-month-old girl with a known ventriculo-septal defect and failure to thrive was admitted with diarrhoea after starting antibiotics for a chest infection. She was also receiving Amiloride and Furosemide. She was found to have hypocalcaemia and blood tests demonstrated the following:

Calcium 1.97 mmol/L [7.9 mg/dL]
Phosphate 2.61 mmol/L [8.1 mg/dL]
Alkaline phosphatase 270 IU/L (reference range 100–300 IU/L)
PTH 2.6 pmol/L (reference range 0.9–5.4 pmol/L)
Urine calcium:creatinine ratio 0.95 mmol/mmol creatinine

Questions and Answers

1 What other investigations does she require?

She requires fluorescence *in situ* hybridization (FISH) studies for a microdeletion of chromosome 22q11 and, given her clinical history, measurement of her T-cell subsets.

2 What is the likely diagnosis?

Despite the presence of normal T-cell subsets, a microdeletion of chromosome 22q11 was confirmed, consistent with a diagnosis of DiGeorge's syndrome and primary hypoparathyroidism.

3 What treatment may be required?

She may require alfacalcidol therapy to maintain serum calcium around 2.0–2.2 mmol/L with ongoing monitoring of her urinary calcium losses to ensure that therapy does not put her at risk of nephrocalcinosis.

Significant Guidelines/Consensus Statements

Fewtrell, M.S., British Paediatric and Adolescent Bone Group (2003). Bone densitometry in children assessed by dual x ray absorptiometry: uses and pitfalls. *Arch. Dis. Child.* 88: 795–798.

Lewiecki, E.M., Gordon, C.M., Baim, S. et al. (2008). International Society for Clinical Densitometry 2007 adult and pediatric official positions. *Bone* 43: 1115–1121.
Munns, C.F., Shaw, N., Kiely, M. et al. (2016). Global consensus recommendations on prevention and management of nutritional rickets. *J. Clin. Endocrinol. Metab.* 101: 394–415.
Wagner, C.L. and Greer, F.R., American Academy of Pediatrics Section on Breastfeeding & American Academy of Pediatrics Committee on Nutrition (2008). Prevention of rickets and vitamin D deficiency in infants, children, and adolescents. *Pediatr.* 122: 1142–1152.

References

Kruse, K., Kracht, U., and Göpfert, G. (1982). Renal threshold phosphate concentration (TmPO4/GFR). *Arch. Dis. Child.* 57: 217–223.
Shaw, N.J., Wheeldon, J., and Brocklebank, J.T. (1990). Indices of intact serum parathyroid hormone and renal excretion of calcium, phosphate and magnesium. *Arch. Dis. Child.* 65: 1208–1211.

Further Reading

Al Zahrani, A. and Levine, M.A. (1997). Primary hyperparathyroidism. *Lancet* 349: 1233–1238.
Kruse, K. (1992). Vitamin D and parathyroid. In: *Functional Endocrinologic Diagnostics in Children and Adolescents*, 1e (ed. M.B. Ranke), 153–167. Mannheim: J & J Verlag.
Levine, M.A. (2012). An update on the clinical and molecular characteristics of pseudohypoparathyroidism. *Curr. Opin. Endocrinol. Diabet. Obes.* 19: 443–451.
Marini, J.C. (2003). Do bisphosphonates make children's bones brittle or better? *N. Engl. J. Med.* 349: 423–426.
Ranke, M.B. (1992). *Functional Endocrinologic Diagnostics in Children and Adolescents*. Mannheim: J&J Verlag.
Reid, I.R. (ed.) (1997). *Baillière's Clinical Endocrinology and Metabolism: Metabolic Bone Disease*. London: Ballière Tindall.
Singh, J., Moghal, N., Pearce, S.H.S., and Cheetham, T. (2003). The investigation of hypocalcaemia and rickets. *Arch. Dis. Child.* 88: 403–407.
Warner, J.T., Cowan, F.J., Dunstan, F.D.J. et al. (1998). Measured and predicted bone mineral content in healthy boys and girls aged 6–18 years: adjustment for body size and puberty. *Acta Paediatr.* 87: 244–249.
Wharton, B. and Bishop, N. (2003). Rickets. *Lancet* 362: 1389–1400.
Zipitis, C.S. and Akobeng, A.K. (2008). Vitamin D supplementation in early childhood and risk of type 1 diabetes: a systematic review and meta-analysis. *Arch. Dis. Child.* 93: 512–517.

Key Weblink

www.nos.org.uk The National Osteoporosis Society is a UK-based charity dedicated to the diagnosis, prevention and treatment of osteoporosis (accessed 14 October 2018).

Useful Information for Patients and Parents

National Osteoporosis Society, Camerton, Bath, BA2 0PJ, UK. Tel: 08454 500230. Website: www.nos.org.uk. Contains useful information about osteoporosis (accessed 14 October 2018).

National Osteoporosis Foundation, 1232 22nd Street NW, Washington, DC 20037, USA. Tel: 1 (800) 231 4222. Website: www.nof.org. Contains helpful information about bone health in adolescence (accessed 14 October 2018).

11 Obesity

Physiology

Definition

In childhood, obesity may be assessed in different ways. Measurement of weight alone is inadequate, given the influence of height on weight. Although obesity may be clinically obvious if the child's weight centile is greater than the height centile, the severity of obesity is better defined by the use of the body mass index (BMI) in which

$$BMI = weight(kg) / (height(m))^2$$

It should be noted that although excess BMI is good at identifying excess weight, it does not distinguish between fat and lean tissue and in unusual circumstances (e.g. heavy-weight sports) may not indicate excess fat. Alternatively, body fatness can be assessed from direct measurements of subcutaneous skinfold thickness using skinfold thickness callipers or from measurement of waist circumference. Given the normal variations of BMI, skinfold thickness and waist circumference through childhood, reference to centile charts is required for interpretation of the data. The utility of skinfold thickness and waist circumference measurements is limited by the practical difficulties of obtaining these measurements accurately and so measurement of BMI is currently the best clinical method for identifying and monitoring obesity in childhood.

There are no universally agreed definitions of obesity in childhood as there are few data correlating specific definitions with future health risks. In practice in the United Kingdom, children with a BMI above the age- and sex-specific 91st centile can be defined as overweight and those above the 98th centile as clinically obese (see Appendix 1 for sex-specific BMI centile reference charts). Throughout the industrialized world, there is clear evidence of a rapid increase in the prevalence of obesity in children and adults, with older children more affected than infants and those from Hispanic and non-Hispanic black communities in the United States more affected than non-Hispanic whites. In the United States, more than 20% of 12–19-year-old children have a BMI that exceeds the 95th centile (the US definition of obesity).

Aetiology

An increased risk of obesity is associated with genetic, environmental (Table 11.1), and pathological factors (Table 11.2). It is likely that a combination of an increasingly sedentary lifestyle combined with an excessive calorie intake for need is principally responsible for the rapid increase in the prevalence of obesity noted in recent decades.

Obese children under three years of age without obese parents are at low risk of obesity in adulthood. However, in older children, the presence of obesity becomes an increasingly important predictor of adult

Practical Endocrinology and Diabetes in Children, Fourth Edition. Malcolm D.C. Donaldson, John W. Gregory, Guy Van Vliet, and Joseph I. Wolfsdorf.
© 2019 John Wiley & Sons Ltd. Published 2019 by John Wiley & Sons Ltd.

Table 11.1 Non-pathological risk factors for obesity.

Risk factor	Examples
Genetic	Obesity in either or both parents
	Early adiposity rebound
Environmental	Socio-economic deprivation
	Single child
	Single parent
Diet-related	Bottle-fed in infancy
	High fat diet
	Disorganized eating patterns
Activity-related	Physical inactivity
	Increased television watching
	Short sleep duration

Table 11.2 Pathological causes of excess body weight.

Cause	Examples
Syndromes	Laurence–Moon–Biedl syndrome
	Down's syndrome
	Prader–Willi syndrome (Figure 11.2)
Single gene mutations	*Melanocortin-4 receptor*
	Proopiomelanocortin
	Leptin
	Leptin receptor
	GNAS (pseudohypoparathyroidism)
Hypothalamic damage	Trauma
	Tumours, e.g. craniopharyngioma
	Post encephalitis
Endocrine abnormalities	Growth hormone deficiency
	Hypothyroidism
	Cushing's syndrome
	Hyperinsulinism
Immobility	Spina bifida
	Cerebral palsy
Impaired skeletal growth	Achondroplasia
Drugs	Insulin
	Steroids
	Antithyroid drugs
	Sodium valproate
	Antipsychotics e.g. risperidone

obesity, regardless of whether the parents are obese or not, with more than two-thirds of children who are obese aged 10 years or older becoming obese adults. Parental obesity more than doubles the risk of adult obesity in young children. Twin studies have suggested a heritability of fat mass of 40–70%.

Regulation of body fat

The normal amounts of body fat change through childhood, as can be seen from the BMI centile charts (see Appendix 1). Infants gain fat, as a consequence of increasing adipose cell size, relatively rapidly until the age of one year, but then slim down until the age of approximately six years as adipose cells reduce in size. From this point onwards, there is a steady increase in body fat into young adult life (the so-called 'adiposity rebound') associated with increases in adipose cell numbers. There is little difference in the amount of body fat in infant girls and boys. However, after infancy, subcutaneous fat increases more rapidly in girls, particularly during puberty when males demonstrate greater centralization of body fat stores.

Obesity occurs when energy intake chronically exceeds energy expenditure. In obese children there are wide variations in energy intake and not all obese children eat excessively. The high calorie density and fat content of the modern diet are associated with an increased risk of obesity.

The hypothalamus has a central role in the regulation of energy balance, integrating neuronal, hormonal, and nutrient messages from within the body and transmitting signals which lead to the sensations of hunger or satiety (Figure 11.1). The hypothalamus also influences energy expenditure via autonomic nerve function and the regulation of pituitary hormone release. Many hypothalamic neurotransmitters have been shown to influence energy intake (Table 11.3).

Energy expenditure consists of the following three components:

1 Resting metabolic rate is the energy expended at rest for the maintenance of basic cellular activities, excluding maintenance of body temperature, and it accounts for 60–70% of total energy expenditure. Fat-free mass is metabolically more active than fat mass. Obese individuals have increased amounts of both body fat and fat-free mass and therefore most obese individuals have increases in their *absolute* resting metabolic rates because of their increased fat-free mass.

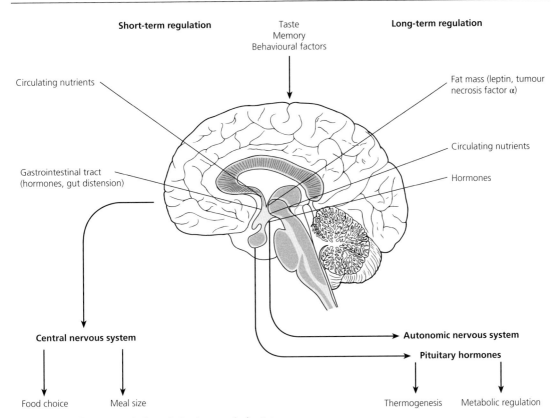

Figure 11.1 Influences on the hypothalamic control of satiety.

2 Thermogenesis is the energy expended in response to digestion and absorption of food, temperature changes, emotional influences or drugs which influence the physiological responses to such stimuli. It accounts for about 10% of total energy expenditure. It is unlikely that variations in thermogenesis are clinically important in the energy balance of the obese individual.

3 Energy expended in physical activity in children varies widely both on an individual daily basis and between individuals and accounts for 20–30% of total energy expenditure. Although obese children may be relatively physically inactive, they have an increase in the energy cost of weight-bearing activities and therefore do not demonstrate marked reductions in this component of energy expenditure when compared to normal-weight children.

As a consequence of these influences on energy expenditure, in most obese children, *absolute* total energy expenditure is increased. However, there is evidence that a low *relative* metabolic rate (i.e. adjusted for body size) predisposes to weight gain.

Complex interactions exist between signalling pathways that control energy intake and satiety and those that regulate fat mass. Adipose tissue may influence the hypothalamic regulation of the energy balance through the secretion of leptin, a hormone which crosses the blood–brain barrier and suppresses the production of neuropeptide Y within the hypothalamus, leading to reduced appetite and increased energy expenditure. However, most obese children have increased leptin concentrations in proportion to their increased body fat mass. Disorders of leptin synthesis or action (leptin receptor mutations) are very rare and account for few cases of obesity.

Preliminary examination and investigation

History

Most children with obesity do not have an underlying pathological cause and have so-called 'simple obesity', also known as exogenous obesity. Such children

Table 11.3 Factors which influence the central nervous system regulation of energy intake.

Factors which increase food intake	Factors which decrease food intake
Noradrenaline	Serotonin
Opioids (e.g. dynorphin and β-endorphin)	Dopamine
Ghrelin	Cholecystokinin
Galanin	Corticotrophin-releasing factor
Neuropeptide Y	Neurotensin
Melanin-concentrating hormone	Bombesin
Agouti-related peptide	Calcitonin gene-related peptide
Orexins A and B (hypocretins 1 and 2)	Thyrotropin-releasing hormone
Growth hormone-releasing hormone	Amylin
	Adrenomedullin
	Peptide YY$^{3-36}$
	Leptin
	Glucagon
	Glucagon-like peptide 1
	α-Melanocyte stimulating hormone
	Cocaine- and amphetamine-related peptide
	Somatostatin

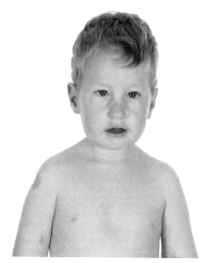

Figure 11.2 Prader–Willi syndrome. Source: M. Donaldson, Glasgow.

usually demonstrate rapid growth and physical development. By contrast, children who are obese, short, and growing slowly are much more likely to have an endocrine abnormality or, if associated with dysmorphic features and intellectual impairment, a syndromic cause to their obesity. A careful history and examination are required to distinguish the few children with significant underlying pathology causing their obesity from those who have 'simple obesity'. The history should include the following details:

- *Birth weight:* if increased, this suggests an underlying mechanism, such as hyperinsulinism, which may have started in utero.
- *Age of onset of obesity:* early onset of obesity (before the age of two years) or while exclusively breast-fed is more suggestive of a genetic or syndromic cause.

- *Presence of congenital abnormalities or symptoms suggestive of a syndrome:* e.g. initial feeding problems requiring nasogastric tube feeds and hypotonia with certain dysmorphic features might suggest Prader–Willi syndrome (Figure 11.2).
- *Detailed feeding and dietary history:* it is often useful to go through a typical day's diet. Ravenous appetite and lack of satiety suggest a rare genetic cause of obesity.
- *Information about levels of physical activity.*
- *The extent to which the obesity may be having adverse effects on the child:* if these are particularly psychosocial or related to school. Also the extent of the desire of the child and parents for the child to lose weight and the extent and success of previous interventions to achieve weight control.
- *Medication.*
- *Symptoms of hypothalamo–pituitary pathology:* e.g. headache, visual symptoms or previous history of trauma or encephalitis.
- *Symptoms suggestive of endocrine abnormality* (Table 11.2).
- *Presence of polydipsia and polyuria:* these are indicative of type 2 diabetes.
- *Family history of obesity.*

Examination

On examination, the child should undergo an accurate assessment of height and weight with measurements plotted on height, weight, and BMI centile charts. Height measurements should be compared with the target height range derived from the mid-parental height centile, as those who are relatively short for their genetic background are more likely to have a syndromic or endocrine cause for their obesity, whereas those who are relatively tall are more likely to suffer from simple obesity. Further assessment of the severity of the obesity can be made from the measurement of waist circumference or triceps and subscapular skinfold thickness, although these measurement techniques require training and are difficult to perform in very obese individuals. Not all pathological causes of obesity will be self-evident and careful clinical examination is required to identify signs suggestive of certain disorders or complications of obesity. It is particularly important to note the presence of acanthosis nigricans most commonly seen in the axillae or neck (see Figure 1.9), as this may indicate evolving insulin resistance and an increased risk of developing type 2 diabetes. Key signs to note on clinical examination are shown in Table 11.4. The clinical features of syndromes, which may present with obesity, are summarized in Table 11.5.

Complications

The main adverse effects of obesity are summarized in Table 11.6. In childhood, acute medical complications of simple obesity are usually few and minor. The combination of insulin resistance, hypertension, hypertriglyceridaemia, and a low concentration of high-density lipoprotein (HDL) cholesterol (so-called 'metabolic syndrome') used to be rarely seen in childhood, although in the United States, nowadays, one in four overweight children in the age group 6–12 years has impaired glucose tolerance and 60% of these have at least one risk factor for heart disease. There are particular concerns about the increased prevalence of obesity and its metabolic complications in ethnic minority groups in both Europe and North America. Furthermore, being overweight in childhood has been shown to be a major risk factor for the development of the metabolic syndrome and coronary artery disease in adult life. Long-standing obesity leads to children being tall for their age, relative to genetic height potential, and to an advanced bone age (so that adult height is not increased). Why excess body fat has this effect is unclear. Obese children may also have an impaired self-image and for boys this may be complicated by a marked suprapubic fat pad leading to the penis being buried in fat and, as a result, appearing very small.

Table 11.4 Clinical signs to look for on examination.

Clinical sign	Possible diagnosis
Acanthosis nigricans	Type 2 diabetes (insulin resistance)
Hypertension	Syndrome X (metabolic syndrome)
Dysmorphic features (see Table 11.5)	Laurence–Moon–Biedl syndrome (Figure 11.3) Prader–Willi syndrome (Figure 11.2) Pseudohypoparathyroidism (Figure 11.4) Beckwith–Wiedemann syndrome
Impaired visual fields	Intracranial tumour, e.g. craniopharyngioma
Papilloedema or optic atrophy	
Tall stature or increased height velocity	Simple obesity, hyperinsulinism
Short stature or decreased height velocity	Growth hormone deficiency, hypothyroidism, Laurence–Moon–Biedl syndrome Prader–Willi syndrome Pseudohypoparathyroidism
Cranial midline defects (e.g. cleft lip and palate)	Growth hormone deficiency
Truncal obesity	
Goitre	Hypothyroidism
Prolonged ankle tendon reflexes	
Proximal myopathy	Cushing's syndrome
Hypertension	
Truncal obesity	
Abnormal gait	Spina bifida Cerebral palsy

Investigations

The following investigations should be considered in those in whom there is clinical concern regarding an underlying pathological cause or a possible metabolic complication of obesity:

- An assessment of glucose tolerance, fasting blood glucose or, occasionally, an oral glucose tolerance test.
- Increased fasting serum insulin and decreased sex-hormone-binding globulin concentrations may confirm the presence of insulin resistance.

Table 11.5 Clinical features of common syndromic causes of obesity (Figures 11.2–11.4).

System	Prader–Willi syndrome	Laurence–Moon–Biedl syndrome	Pseudohypo-parathyroidism
Facial	Narrow forehead Olive-shaped eyes Antimongoloid slant Epicanthic folds Squint Carp mouth Micrognathia Abnormal ear lobes	Squint	Round facies Short neck
Skeletal	Short stature Small hands and feet Clinodactyly Syndactyly Scoliosis Dislocated hips	Short stature Polydactyly Clinodactyly	Short stature Shortened fourth metacarpals and metatarsals
Neurosensory development and behaviour	↓ IQ Hypotonia and feeding problems in infancy Insatiable appetite Uncontrollable rage	↓ IQ Retinitis pigmentosa	↓ IQ
Endocrine	Hypogonadotrophic hypogonadism Type 2 diabetes	Hypogonadotrophic hypogonadism Diabetes insipidus	PTH-resistant hypocalcaemia
Other		Renal anomalies	Subcutaneous calcifications

- Lipid profile.
- Thyroid function tests (TFTs) (serum thyroxine [T4] and thyroid-stimulating hormone [TSH] concentrations). However, in the absence of clinical evidence of hypothyroidism such as decreased linear growth, TSH should NOT be measured. Indeed, the mild hyperthyrotropinemia often seen in exogenous obesity is not causally related to it and disappears if weight loss is achieved.
- Liver function tests.
- Three 24-hour urinary cortisol estimations.
- Bone age.
- Serum luteinizing hormone (LH), follicle-stimulating hormone (FSH), oestradiol, 17-hydroxy progesterone, androstenedione, and testosterone concentrations and a pelvic ultrasound in a girl with hirsutism or menstrual irregularity thought to be at risk of having polycystic ovarian syndrome. The need for additional investigations will depend on the level of clinical concern.

- In cases of suspected or proven hypothyroidism, Cushing's syndrome, hyperinsulinism or growth hormone (GH) deficiency, consult the relevant chapters in this volume for further investigations.
- If Laurence–Moon–Biedl syndrome is suspected, referral to a geneticist may be of help in identifying the relevant dysmorphic features and referral to an ophthalmologist for detailed retinal examination, including electroretinography, is important. Renal function should be assessed.
- Prader–Willi syndrome can be confirmed molecularly by methylation studies of chromosome 15q11-13.
- If pseudohypoparathyroidism is suspected, measure serum calcium, phosphate and parathyroid hormone (PTH) concentrations. In the case of a low serum calcium and elevated phosphate and PTH, the diagnosis may be confirmed by demonstration of inactivating mutations of the *GNAS* gene which encodes the G protein stimulatory, alpha subunit which is located on the long arm of chromosome 20.

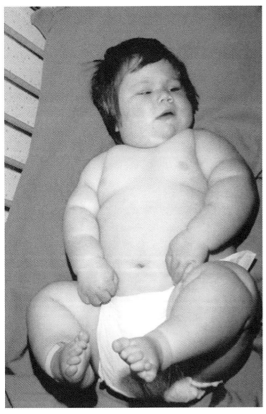

Figure 11.3 Polydactyly in a child with Laurence–Moon–Biedl syndrome.

Table 11.6 Complications of simple obesity.

System	Adverse effect
Metabolic and endocrine	Hyperinsulinaemia
	Impaired glucose tolerance
	Type 2 diabetes
	Hyperlipidaemia
	Metabolic syndrome
	Advanced pubertal development
	Polycystic ovarian disease
	Non-alcoholic steatohepatitis (NASH)
	Cholelithiasis
Cardiovascular	Hypertension
Respiratory	Breathless on exertion
	Obstructive sleep apnoea
	Pickwickian syndrome
Skeletal	Knock knee or bow legs
	Slipped capital femoral epiphysis
Skin	Furunculosis
	Intertrigo
Neurological	Idiopathic intracranial hypertension
Psychological	Poor self-image
	Bullying
	Behavioural problems
	Anxiety
	Depression

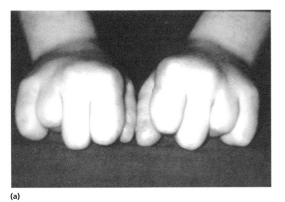

(a)

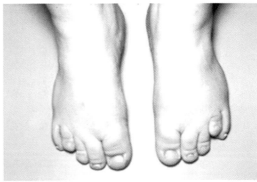

(b)

Figure 11.4 Shortening of the fourth metacarpal (a) and metatarsal (b) in pseudohypoparathyroidism.

• In syndromes associated with hypogonadism, investigation of the pituitary–gonadal axis should be considered in those who have genital hypoplasia, markedly delayed puberty or inadequate development of secondary sex characteristics (see Chapter 5).

Treatment

Young infants frequently appear fat and a spontaneous reduction in body fat occurs as part of the normal changes in body composition with increasing age. In general, therefore, it is rare that a slimming regimen needs to be considered in the young child. However, investigations to exclude a pathological cause of obesity should be undertaken in all infants with severe, early onset obesity. If calorie restriction is deemed necessary in infancy, the aim should be maintenance of body weight rather than weight loss, as the latter may lead to specific dietary (e.g. vitamin) deficiencies or growth failure.

For many obese children, weight loss down to an 'ideal body weight for height' is probably unrealistic. Nevertheless, more modest weight reduction, or even prevention of further weight gain, may produce significant long-term health benefits. Such goals, which are more likely to be achievable, should be considered when planning individual therapeutic regimens. Unfortunately, there is almost no published evidence for any effective treatment for childhood obesity.

Older children with simple obesity should be encouraged to try and control their weight gain by:
• educating about the nature of obesity and its long-term consequences;
• realistic assessment of the ease and likely benefits of slimming regimens;
• healthy eating (e.g. regular family meal times, avoidance of excessive 'snacking', fried foods, added fats and sugars, and high energy drinks, while encouraging foods with high fibre content) with modest calorie restriction and advice from a dietician where necessary;
• increasing habitual physical activity (e.g. walking rather than taking transport to school, participation in games or sports that the child enjoys, restricting television or computer games);
• psychological support (e.g. regular attendance at a dedicated clinic with dietetic support, group therapy, such as Weight Watchers, with the emphasis on mutual support, promotion of positive self-esteem and enhancing motivation to change life-style factors).

Once a child has developed significant obesity, both weight loss and long-term maintenance of an improved body weight become difficult to achieve. Encouragement for children with simple obesity is best provided by frequent visits (e.g. three-monthly) by the patient to a clinic or support service with motivated and interested staff. Multidisciplinary services involving community paediatricians, general practitioners, dieticians, psychologists, or psychiatrists may help to improve the outcome. However, there is no point in continuing to encourage attendance in obese patients who do not adhere to suggested interventions and who do not achieve significant weight loss, although intermittent clinical follow-up to monitor for early signs of the complications of obesity may still be necessary.

Although medical therapy, including inhibitors of nutrient absorption from the gut (e.g. acarbose, guar gum, and pancreatic lipase inhibitors), appetite suppressants (e.g. amphetamine derivatives and serotoninergic agents) and agents which increase energy expenditure (e.g. T4 and adrenergic agonists), have been used in the treatment of obesity in adults, there is little experience of their use and efficacy in childhood. Side effects may be problematic and their use is not currently recommended in children. There has also been recent interest in the potential benefits of metformin though results of randomized trials have proved disappointing and treatment of obesity in the absence of type 2 diabetes with metformin is not routinely advised.

There is increasing interest in the value of bariatric surgical interventions, such as laparoscopic gastric banding or the Roux-en-Y gastric bypass procedure in extremely obese children. When undertaken in children, dramatic amounts of weight loss can be achieved although such children will require careful monitoring for side effects in specialist clinical services.

Where excessive weight is the consequence of an underlying endocrinopathy, treatment of hormone deficiency with the relevant hormone replacement (e.g. GH or T4) should result in a decrease in body fat. There is evidence that Prader–Willi syndrome is associated with hypothalamic dysfunction, including impaired GH secretion. GH therapy (0.25 mg/kg per week to a maximum of 2.7 mg daily) is now widely used for the improvement of growth and body composition in children with Prader–Willi syndrome, providing there is no evidence of upper airway obstruction or severe obesity (weight exceeding 200% of ideal for height) and pre-treatment sleep studies do not demonstrate any evidence of sleep apnoea. Specific medical or surgical interventions for hyperinsulinism or Cushing's syndrome will also lead to significant weight loss.

When to involve a specialist centre

• Children with suspected hypothalamic tumours or endocrine causes of obesity should be managed in consultation with centres with expertise in the relevant neurosurgical investigations and paediatric endocrinology.

• Children with obesity of such severity that significant adverse cardio-respiratory consequences are suspected may need referral to a specialist unit for a detailed cardiorespiratory assessment, including sleep studies.

• Children with sufficiently severe obesity that drug treatment or surgery is to be considered should be referred to a specialist centre for further evaluation.

Future developments

• High-quality randomized controlled trials of lifestyle interventions which aim to prevent or treat obesity in childhood by altering eating behaviour or patterns of physical activity are required.

• A clarification of the role and benefits of pharmacological interventions in obese children.

• An evaluation of the risks and benefits of surgery to treat childhood obesity.

• Clarification of the value and ideal structure of an 'obesity service'.

• Further research should clarify the role and relationship between the multiple neurotransmitters known to influence hypothalamic function in the hope that a compound will be discovered which may have a significant effect on satiety without adverse side effects.

Transition

Obese teenage patients who have significant comorbidities, such as type 2 diabetes or other metabolic abnormalities or those experiencing significant adverse effects on cardio-respiratory function, will require referral to adult services in their mid-to-late teenage years. Seeing these patients in a joint clinic staffed by both adult and paediatric specialists may be especially helpful to the paediatrician as it is likely that his/her adult colleagues will have much greater experience of a range of therapeutic interventions relevant to the management of the obese individual, some of which may be of value in the teenage age group.

Controversial points

• How extensively should tall, obese children with no dysmorphic features be investigated?

• How relatively important are genetic and environmental risk factors for obesity in childhood?

• What is the future risk of obesity in adult life for an obese young child?

• Is childhood-onset obesity a risk factor for adverse metabolic consequences in adult life, independent of the presence of obesity in adult life?

• Are children who become obese, less active than those who do not?

• Do children from obese families, who are at increased risk of obesity, have an inherited decrease in their metabolic rates?

Potential pitfalls

• Failure to recognize the diagnostic importance of distinguishing between obese children who are growing fast and those who have decreased linear growth.

• Excessive and unrealistic expectations of the likely success of interventions to treat childhood obesity, especially when both parents are already obese.

• Over-investigation for a non-existent pathological cause of obesity in an otherwise well, rapidly growing child.

• Encouraging obese children to achieve dramatic short-term weight loss is unlikely to be successful in achieving satisfactory regulation of longer-term weight.

• Excessive weight loss may lead to impaired growth.

• Delayed diagnosis of type 2 diabetes or its misdiagnosis as type 1 diabetes in an obese child with minimal symptoms and absence of ketonuria when hyperglycaemia is finally documented.

• Failure to diagnose clinically significant disturbances of respiratory function during sleep.

Case histories

Case 11.1

A 12-year-old boy presented with obesity. He had been floppy and a poor feeder as an infant with recurrent fits until the age of seven years.

On examination, he had developmental delay and special educational needs. His height was on the 50th centile and weight well above the 97th centile. The following measurements were obtained on a basal blood sample:

Calcium 1.95 mmol/L [7.82 mg/dL]

Albumin 41 g L [4.1 g/dL]

Phosphate 1.90 mmol/L [5.9 mg/dL]

Creatinine 78 μmol/L [0.9 mg/dL]

Alkaline phosphatise 202 IU/L (reference range 100–400)

PTH 14.5 pmol L (reference range 0.9–5.5) [138 pg/ml (reference range 10–65)]

25-OH-cholecalciferol 16.1 ng/ml (reference range 8–50)

Free T4 11 pmol/L (reference range 9.8–23.1) [0.88 ng/dL (reference range 0.8–2.4)]

TSH 5.7 mU/L (reference range 0.35–5.5)

Questions and Answers

1 What do these results demonstrate?
Hypocalcaemia with hyperphosphataemia, raised PTH concentration and borderline TFT results.

2 What is the most likely diagnosis?
Pseudohypoparathyroidism is the most likely diagnosis.

3 What additional investigations may clarify the diagnosis?

The diagnosis may be confirmed by DNA analysis. Because hormone resistance may vary over time, serum TSH should be measured regularly, although clinical hypothyroidism is rare.

Case 11.2

A one-year-old girl was referred with massive obesity. She had been the product of a normal delivery at 41 weeks' gestation, birth weight 4.28 kg. She was noted to have polydactyly of both hands and a bifid left fifth toe. She was breast-fed from birth, with solids introduced at nine months. There was no evidence of retinal pigmentation. Her general intelligence quotient (excluding locomotor skills) was 89. Initial serum biochemical investigations demonstrated the following:

Creatinine, electrolytes and glucose normal

Calcium 2.24 mmol/L [9.0 mg/dL]

Phosphate 1.33 mmol/L [4.1 mg/dL]

Free T4 14.9 pmol/L [1.2 ng/dL]

TSH 1.82 mU/L

Insulin-like growth factor (IGF-I) 5.7 nmol/L (reference range 5.0–33.6) [44 ng/dL (normal range (38–257)]

Questions and Answers

1 What is the most likely diagnosis?

Laurence–Moon–Biedl syndrome is the most likely diagnosis.

2 What additional investigations may be of assistance?

Further evaluation of her retinal function demonstrated no visual evoked potential or electroretinogram response to flash. An abdominal ultrasound examination did not demonstrate any associated renal abnormalities.

Case 11.3

A 10-year-old boy was referred for assessment of his overweight. His birth weight was 3.7 kg and after initial feeding difficulties he demonstrated early onset of excessive weight gain. He is progressing well in school and has no history of polydipsia or polyuria. At referral, he is tall (height + 2.6 SDS [standard deviation score]) with a BMI of 30.6 kg m^{-2}. He had no dysmorphic features and was pre-pubertal. Blood pressure was 126/70 mmHg and he had acanthosis nigricans on his neck and axillae.

Questions and Answers

1 What investigations are indicated?

The presence of acanthosis nigricans suggests he is developing insulin resistance and it would be advisable to measure fasting blood glucose and lipids and/or HbA1C if not fasting to ensure he has not developed type 2 diabetes and other metabolic complications. Although his early feeding difficulties would raise the possibility of Prader–Willi syndrome, his lack of dysmorphic features and normal school progress make it unlikely that DNA testing would produce an abnormal result.

2 What is the most likely diagnosis and prognosis?

Given his tall stature and lack of dysmorphic findings, the most likely diagnosis is 'simple obesity'. He should be supported in efforts to lose weight as he is likely to be at high risk of developing type 2 diabetes in the future.

Case 11.4

A 15-year-old girl was referred with amenorrhoea of two years' duration following one year of a regular menstrual cycle. In recent years, she had encountered increasing problems of excess weight gain. Her height was on the 50th centile and weight 5 kg above the 99.6th centile.

Since menarche, she had been troubled with acne and excessive body and facial hair. Initial blood tests demonstrated the following:

LH 6.7 U/L

FSH 4.7 U/L

Oestradiol 214 pmol/L

Testosterone 3.1 nmol/L

Free T4 14.7 pmol/L (reference range 9.8–23.1)

TSH 1.86 mU/L (reference range 0.35–5.5)

Prolactin 154 mU/L

Sex hormone binding globulin 24.8 nmol/L (reference range 19.8–122 nmol/L)

DHEAS 3.7 μmol/L (reference range 1.8–10.0)

17-OH-progesterone 6.3 nmol/L (reference range 2.0–6.0)

Androstenedione 18.0 nmol/L (reference range < 3.6)

Questions and Answers

1 What is the most likely diagnosis?

The development of secondary amenorrhoea in the context of obesity, acne, and hirsutism makes a diagnosis of polycystic ovarian syndrome likely. Although an elevated androstenedione concentration raises the possibility of congenital adrenal hyperplasia, the minimally raised 17-OH-progesterone and normal testosterone concentrations make this unlikely.

2 What additional investigations may be of assistance?

A pelvic ultrasound examination showed ovarian cysts consistent with a diagnosis of polycystic ovarian syndrome.

3 What treatment may be advised?

This girl should be advised to lose weight if at all possible. In the longer term, this may lead to reduced hirsutism though in the short term, local cosmetic approaches will be required. The use of combined oral contraceptives containing the anti-androgen cyproterone acetate may help reduce hair growth and acne and there has been much interest in the possibility that metformin may be beneficial in this condition although this remains unlicensed for this indication at present.

Case 11.5

A seven-year-old girl of Pakistani origin was referred with obesity (BMI 27.9 kg/m²) and acanthosis nigricans affecting her neck and axillae. A fasting blood sample demonstrated a plasma glucose of 4.3 mmol/L, rising to 7.6 mmol/L two hours following an oral glucose tolerance test. Despite dietetic and lifestyle advice, she continued to gain weight and on examination has developed hepatomegaly. One year later, a fasting blood sample demonstrates the following:

HbA1c 7.1%

Triglyceride 1.4 mmol/L (reference range 0.4–1.6)

Cholesterol 4.1 mmol/L (reference range 2.5–5.2)

HDL-cholesterol 0.8 mmol/L (reference range 0.9–2.0)

Aspartate transaminase 47 IU/L (reference range 5–45)

Questions and Answers

1 What is the interpretation of these data?

The rising HbA1c concentration suggests that this girl has now developed type 2 diabetes. A suppressed HDL-cholesterol concentration suggests she is also at risk of developing wider features of the multimetabolic syndrome. The presence of hepatomegaly and a rising aspartate transaminase concentration suggests she may also be showing evidence of non-alcoholic steatohepatitis.

2 What additional investigations may be of assistance?

A hepatic ultrasound is indicated. This confirmed the presence of an enlarged, echogenic liver in keeping with fatty infiltration.

3 What treatment should be advised?

The failure of dietary advice to help her control her weight gain and the development of evidence of type 2 diabetes are indications for a trial of metformin treatment. If this fails to improve matters, then sulphonylurea or insulin therapy may be required.

Further Reading

Caprio, S., Daniels, S.R., Drewnowski, A. et al. (2008). Influence of race, ethnicity, and culture on childhood obesity: implications for prevention and treatment: a consensus statement of Shaping America's Health and the Obesity Society. *Diabetes Care* 31: 2211–2221.

Daniels, S.R., Greer, F.R., and Committee on Nutrition (2008). Lipid screening and cardiovascular health in childhood. *Pediatr.* 122: 198–208.

Daniels, S.R., Jacobson, M.S., McCrindle, B.W. et al. (2009). American Heart Association Childhood Obesity Research Summit: executive summary. *Circul.* 119: 2114–2123.

Livingstone, M.B., McCaffrey, T.A., and Rennie, K.L. (2006). Childhood obesity prevention studies: lessons learned and to be learned. *Public Health Nutrition* 9: 1121–1129.

Mattsson, N., Rönnemaa, T., Juonala, M. et al. (2007). The prevalence of the metabolic syndrome in young adults: the Cardiovascular Risk in Young Finns Study. *J. Intern. Med.* 261: 159–169.

Mead, E., Atkinson, G., Richter, B. et al. (2016). Drug interventions for the treatment of obesity in children and adolescents. *Cochrane Database of Systematic Reviews* (11): CD012436. https://doi.org/10.1002/14651858.CD012436.

National Clinical Guideline Centre (UK) (2014). *Obesity: identification, assessment and management of overweight and obesity in children, young people and adults: partial update of CG43*. London: National Institute for Health and Care Excellence (UK).

Oude Luttikhuis, H., Baur, L., Jansen, H. et al. (2009). Interventions for treating obesity in children. *Cochrane Database of Systematic Reviews* (1): CD001872. https://doi.org/10.1002/14651858.CD001872.pub2.

Scottish Intercollegiate Guidelines Network (SIGN) (2003). *Management of Obesity in Children and Young People*. Edinburgh.: SIGN,.

Styne, D.M., Arslanian, S.A., Connor, E.L. et al. (2017). Pediatric obesity-assessment, treatment, and prevention:
an Endocrine Society Clinical Practice Guideline. *J. Clin. Endocrinol. Metab.* 102: 709–757.

Viner, R.M., White, B., Barrett, T. et al. (2012). Assessment of childhood obesity in secondary care: OSCA consensus statement. *Arch. Dis. Child. Educ. Prac.* 97: 98–105.

Key Weblinks

www.healthforallchildren.co.uk Source of the UK-WHO 2009 growth charts and body mass index centile charts (see Appendix 1) (accessed 13 October 2018).

www.mendprogramme.org MEND (Mind, Exercise, Nutrition…Do it!) is a childhood family-based obesity programme developed at Great Ormond Street Hospital in London, dedicated to reducing global childhood and family overweight and obesity levels through the provision of free healthy living programmes (accessed 13 October 2018).

Useful Information for Patients and Parents

The Child Growth Foundation is a UK-based charity relating to children's growth including the prevention of obesity. Website: www.childgrowthfoundation.org (accessed 13 October 2018).

The National Obesity Forum is an independent UK charity working to improve the prevention and management of obesity. Website: www.nationalobesityforum.org.uk (accessed 13 October 2018).

12 Endocrine Effects of Cancer Treatment

Pathophysiology

There has been a remarkable increase in the survival rates of children with most malignancies during the past 50 years. This improvement has resulted from the use of sophisticated regimens of multi-agent chemotherapy, frequently combined with radiotherapy and surgery. Treatment of childhood cancer is intensive and associated with effects on a number of organs, of which the endocrine system is particularly vulnerable. The risk of late endocrine effects in survivors is related more to the treatment received than to the nature of the underlying malignancy. Organs related to endocrine function or growth which are susceptible to the effects of cancer treatment are shown in Table 12.1.

Chemotherapy

Cytotoxic chemotherapy may damage normal developing cells and the damage is dependent on the type and dose of chemotherapeutic agent used. The germinal epithelium in the testis is highly susceptible to alkylating agents, such as cyclophosphamide. Similarly, the potential for normal ovarian function may be impaired with intensive chemotherapy. Many regimens include high-dose glucocorticoids, which induce iatrogenic Cushing's syndrome.

Radiotherapy

Radiotherapy, used either alone or in combination with chemotherapy or surgery, is effective in treating a number of childhood cancers. However, the 'price of cure' may be high in terms of endocrine function and growth. The potential for damage is related to the dose of radiotherapy delivered, the protocol of delivery, and the site of the primary lesion. Direct damage to the growth plates may also result from spinal or total body irradiation.

Damage to the hypothalamo–pituitary axis is relatively common following irradiation of tumours of the brain, face, orbit, and adjacent areas. The thyroid is susceptible to head and neck irradiation. Similarly, the prepubertal testis – often the site of relapse in leukaemia – is highly susceptible to direct radiotherapy.

Surgery

Surgery may represent an additional risk factor for these children. Any neurosurgery in the area of the hypothalamo–pituitary axis may impair signalling between these glands which may present relatively acutely but transiently (e.g. postoperative diabetes insipidus) or in the longer term (e.g. 'hypothalamic' obesity). Self-evidently, surgery which involves removal of substantial proportions of a gland may also place the child at risk of subsequent endocrine deficiency.

Practical Endocrinology and Diabetes in Children, Fourth Edition. Malcolm D.C. Donaldson, John W. Gregory, Guy Van Vliet, and Joseph I. Wolfsdorf.
© 2019 John Wiley & Sons Ltd. Published 2019 by John Wiley & Sons Ltd.

Table 12.1 Organs related to endocrine function or growth which are susceptible to damage from cancer treatment.

Hypothalamic–pituitary axis
  Growth hormone
  Adrenocorticotrophic hormone
  Luteinizing hormone/follicle-stimulating hormone
  Thyroid-stimulating hormone
  Antidiuretic hormone (vasopressin)
Thyroid
Testis
Ovary
Spine
Long bones
Growth plates
Breast tissue
Fat mass

Investigation and management of late endocrine effects

The combined oncology–endocrine clinic

Figure 12.1 describes all the people who should be involved in a 'late effects' clinic. The specific organizational structure will vary among institutions, but oncologists should be encouraged to work closely with paediatricians and paediatric endocrinologists to establish a joint clinic aimed at identification, investigation, and management of late endocrine effects. The principal aim of the oncologist is to treat and monitor the status of the patient's primary disorder. The endocrinologist can support this process by contributing knowledge and experience of potential

and actual endocrine and growth dysfunctions. Monitoring of growth and puberty is an essential function of this clinic.

Referral to the late effects clinic

Late referral to this clinic can lead to considerable delay in diagnosis of treatable endocrine effects. Consequently, *all patients* who have received radiotherapy in childhood *to any organ* should be referred one year after completion of treatment. In this way, growth monitoring can identify early growth failure and potential abnormalities of puberty. Patients treated with chemotherapy, which can cause potential endocrine dysfunction, should also be referred. Any oncology patient with concerns about growth, puberty, or changes in body composition, for example, obesity, can benefit from early referral to this clinic.

Investigation and monitoring of patients

Procedures which may be undertaken either in or associated with the late effects clinic are shown in Table 12.2.

Specific endocrine and growth abnormalities associated with cancer treatment

Cancer treatment may affect the function of a number of specific endocrine organs and tissues related to growth. Frequently, several organ systems are affected in the same patient. The major endocrine organs at risk and growth abnormalities are described individually.

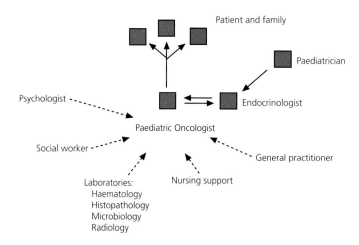

Figure 12.1 Suggested model for a late effects clinic.

Table 12.2 Procedures in or associated with the joint oncology–endocrine clinic.

Clinic attendance – every 4–6 mo
Growth monitoring
   Height
   Height velocity
   Sitting height
   Weight
   Bone age
   Body mass index
Pubertal development staging (including testicular volume)
Hormone measurements
Basal levels: FT4, TSH, cortisol, testosterone, oestradiol, LH, FSH, prolactin, IGF-I
Dynamic tests: GH stimulation tests, low-dose ACTH stimulation test, GnRH test
Thyroid: careful palpation and ultrasound if a nodule is suspected
Pelvic ultrasound in girls if puberty is precocious or delayed
DEXA scan for bone mineral density and body composition

Abnormal linear growth

Growth can be impaired by:
- direct effect of radiotherapy on the spine;
- damage to the hypothalamo–pituitary axis with resulting growth hormone (GH) deficiency;
- gonadal damage with sex steroid deficiency, resulting in delayed pubertal growth;
- effect of radiotherapy and chemotherapy on the growth plates.

Spinal irradiation

Spinal irradiation, as given for conditions such as medulloblastoma (Figure 12.2) and germinoma, will seriously affect spinal growth, particularly when radiotherapy is given in early childhood. Spinal growth is an essential component of the adolescent growth spurt. Consequently, short stature with disproportion because of shortness of the trunk is frequently seen in these patients.

GH deficiency (GHD)

Damage to the hypothalamo–pituitary axis resulting in growth hormone deficiency (GHD) can occur following radiotherapy given in:
- high doses (>3000 cGy) as curative therapy for brain, orbit or adjacent tissue tumours;

- doses of 1800–2400 cGy as prophylaxis for central nervous system (CNS) leukaemia;
- doses of 750–1600 cGy as total body irradiation.

The prevalence and severity of GHD are related to the total dosage of radiotherapy and the fractionation schedule. The same total dosage given in a larger number of smaller fractions is likely to be less damaging. Radiotherapy regimens for brain tumours and tumours of the face and orbit, which deliver doses >3000 cGy to the hypothalamic–pituitary axis, will almost always result in GH deficiency. This is usually present by two years after treatment.

The frequency of overt GHD following prophylactic CNS irradiation and after total body irradiation is variable. However, several studies have reported a prevalence of up to 50%. In addition, the physiological increment in GH secretion at puberty does not occur.

Diagnosis

A high index of suspicion is important when children at risk of GHD are seen in the late effects clinic. Children should undergo GH stimulation testing at the earliest suspicion of a subnormal height velocity. For an interpretation of the results, see Chapter 3. The pubertal status must always be assessed and considered when interpreting the growth curve. Puberty will stimulate growth and, particularly when precocious, can mask coexistent GH deficiency. Of note, precocious boys who have received alkylating agent may not show the expected increase in testicular volume, so that sequential plasma testosterone levels (preferably at 8.a.m.) are required.

Treatment

The same principles apply to the treatment of irradiation-induced GH deficiency as with other aetiologies. There is no evidence that GH therapy increases the risk of recurrence of the malignancy after remission has been induced.

Direct damage to growth plate and long bones

Radiotherapy is a well-recognized cause of direct damage to gonads and bone. Sex steroid deficiency will be discussed in section 'Gonadal Damage'. Growth failure in the absence of direct spinal irradiation or GH deficiency has also been described. The mechanism of this apparent effect of chemotherapy is not clear. It is possible that the growth plates in the spine and long bones are susceptible to damage from intensive chemotherapy.

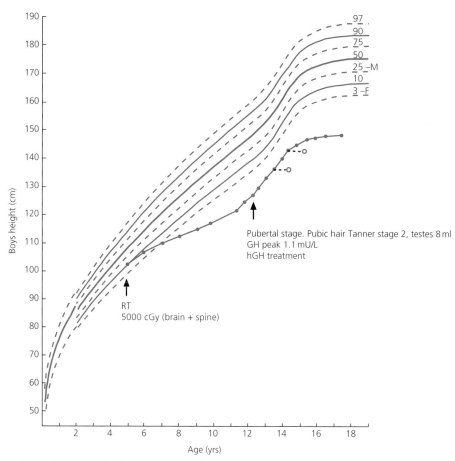

Figure 12.2 Growth following radiotherapy to brain and spine for medulloblastoma. Note the severe height loss because of spinal irradiation, the rather early puberty and the adult height much lower than target, despite GH treatment. RT, radiotherapy.

Abnormal pituitary function

The GH axis is most vulnerable to early damage by radiotherapy. Comparatively, other anterior pituitary hormones are resistant, but central hypogonadism, hypoadrenalism, and hypothyroidism (in order of decreasing frequency) may occur throughout life.

Early puberty following cranial irradiation

This phenomenon was first reported in the 1980s and is now a recognized complication, particularly in girls. Children who received cranial irradiation, particularly at a young age, have a significantly earlier onset of puberty with respect to chronological age and bone age.

The combination of GH deficiency and early puberty severely reduces growth potential. In this situation, puberty should be suppressed using gonadotrophin-releasing hormone (GnRH) analogue therapy to allow maximum benefit from GH replacement.

Gonadal damage

Gonadal damage in childhood can occur following chemotherapy or radiotherapy. There are specific differences affecting the testis and ovary, so each will be described separately.

The testis
Chemotherapy

The use of chemotherapeutic regimens which include alkylating agents, such as cyclophosphamide, chlorambucil, and the nitrosoureas, in addition to procarbazine, vinblastine, cytosine arabinoside, and possibly *cis*-platinum, are likely to cause damage to germinal epithelium, resulting in azoospermia and infertility in adult life. This has been reported particularly in leukaemia and Hodgkin's disease. Chemotherapeutic regimens are now being modified with the aim of minimizing this complication. Elevation of basal follicle-stimulating hormone (FSH) is a useful guide to damage of the germinal epithelium. Testosterone production from Leydig cells is generally not affected.

Radiotherapy

The testis is vulnerable to radiation damage, which in turn depends on the total dosage and dose per fraction. Following total body irradiation (dose 1200–1500 cGy) for leukaemia in prepubertal children, Leydig cell function is not affected but azoospermia may occur. After direct testicular irradiation, testosterone production is also severely reduced.

Consequently, it is important to assess testicular size and function in order to define the need for testosterone replacement. Long-term androgen therapy may be indicated to ensure satisfactory pubertal development and normal testosterone levels in adult life.

The ovary
Chemotherapy

The ovary is apparently more resistant to damage than the testis. Normal fertility and endocrine function can be expected in adult survivors of childhood leukaemia treatment. Intensive chemotherapeutic regimens for conditions such as Hodgkin's disease may confer more risk of ovarian dysfunction. High plasma FSH and low AMH (anti-Müllerian hormone) indicate ovarian damage.

Radiotherapy

The ovary is susceptible to damage from radiotherapy. Direct radiotherapy, or indirect radiotherapy as in total body irradiation, can cause ovarian failure with impairment of ovulation and possible subnormal sex steroid secretion. Vulnerable patients need to be carefully assessed by the endocrinologist and normal pubertal development ensured.

Thyroid abnormalities

After radiotherapy that includes the thyroid area, three main types of thyroid abnormalities may occur: hypothyroidism, benign thyroid nodules, and thyroid cancer. After treatment for Hodgkin's disease with 3000–5000 cGy to the neck, patients should have their plasma thyroid-stimulating hormone (TSH) regularly measured and T4 replacement should be started as soon as TSH rises to above normal.

Total body irradiation and cranial irradiation are also associated with hypothyroidism, which is often partly central and partly primary, and should therefore be evaluated by measuring both TSH and fT4.

Elevation of TSH for long periods of time may confer greater risk of malignancy in the irradiated gland. Thyroid nodules may develop after a long interval and are more likely to be malignant in patients with a history of low dose external radiation. Patients should be reminded to have their neck carefully examined clinically once a year throughout life and any palpable nodule should be promptly evaluated by ultrasound.

Adrenal abnormalities

Although rare, adrenocorticotrophic hormone (ACTH) deficiency may be a late complication of high-dose (>3000 cGy) cranial irradiation and should be considered if other anterior pituitary hormones are deficient.

Abnormalities of body composition

Survivors of childhood leukaemia and brain tumours often become obese. While surgery and radiotherapy in the hypothalamo–pituitary region may predispose to this condition, other factors likely also play a role. In the longer term, obesity and decreased physical activity are risk factors for the development of the 'metabolic syndrome' in adult life. Counselling about this late effect and lifestyle modification to prevent or minimize it is important.

Impaired bone mineralization may also occur during childhood and can be demonstrated on dual energy X-ray absorptiometry (DEXA) scanning. Chronic illness, reduced exercise, glucocorticoid therapy, direct effects of other chemotherapeutic agents on osteoblasts, GH deficiency, impaired sex steroid secretion at puberty, and suboptimal vitamin D intake are all potential factors contributing to reduced bone mineralization. The prompt and accurate diagnosis and treatment of endocrine deficiencies will help to normalize bone mineralization, hence diminishing the risk of osteoporosis in adult life.

When to involve a specialist centre

Many long-term survivors of childhood cancer who have received treatment known to place them at significant risk of endocrine late effects will remain under follow-up review in a specialized department. Transfer in late adolescence to a health care facility with expertise in late effects is critical, even for those few patients in whom none has been identified in the paediatric age (see section 'Transition').

Future developments

• The challenge for oncologists is to develop future treatments which are effective for the treatment of the primary neoplasm but cause minimal late effects.
• More specific and targeted radiotherapy techniques are being developed.
• Prior to cancer therapy, adolescent males should be offered the chance to collect and bank sperm. Cryopreservation of gonadal tissue should be discussed with the parents of younger boys and girls.

Transition

Any patient who is receiving hormone replacement or is known to be at high risk of developing endocrine dysfunction, such that they require regular endocrine testing, should be seen in a clinical service that allows transition of care from a paediatrician to an adult physician with endocrine expertise. In addition, those demonstrating evidence of osteopenia or osteoporosis will require referral to an adult 'osteoporosis service'. It is also helpful for patients at risk of infertility to be seen for a consultation by adult specialists with expertise in infertility treatment, so that they are counselled about the options available to them later in their adult lives.

Controversial points

• Ethical, practical, and financial issues of harvesting and cryopreservation of gametes prior to treatment causing gonadal damage.
• Possible protection of gonads from chemotherapeutic or radiotherapeutic damage by endocrine therapy, i.e. GnRH suppression of the pituitary–gonadal axis.
• Management of menstruation in patients likely to develop heavy bleeding.

Potential pitfalls

• Failure to appreciate that a suboptimal growth response to GH replacement in children with GHD previously treated with cranio-spinal radiotherapy may reflect radiotherapy-induced growth plate damage of the spine.
• Importance of regular clinical staging of puberty (and of plasma testosterone in boys) to ensure that

GHD coexistent with precocious puberty is not missed.
• Failure to appreciate that absence of endocrine deficiency soon after radiotherapy does not mean that endocrine deficiency will not develop later. Hence, the need for long-term follow-up in patients who received cranial irradiation in excess of 1800 or 2400 Gy.

Case histories

Case 12.1
A three-year-old boy was diagnosed to have a rhabdomyosarcoma of the left maxillary antrum. He received radiotherapy to the tumour (5046 cGy) and chemotherapy. There has been no recurrence of the tumour. At the age of five years, his growth started to slow down. He was not referred to the joint oncology–endocrine clinic until the age of 7.4 years, by which time his height was far below the 3rd centile and his height velocity was 3.6 cm per year.

Questions and Answers
1 What investigations are indicated?

The growth curve was carefully analysed and basal hormone measurements were performed (see Table 12.2). Biochemistry was normal. The peak GH level on two stimulation tests was <5 µg/L, indicating GHD. GH replacement increased height velocity to 8.4 cm per year in the first year.

2 What should be followed during treatment?

At the age of 14 years, his FT4 was 5.8 pmol/L (normal range 57–170) and his TSH was 1.6 mU/L (normal range 0.4–5.0). This indicates central hypothyroidism and replacement with T4 100 µg per day was started.

3 Does he have gonadotrophin deficiency in addition to his GH and TSH deficiencies?

At the age of 15 years, his pubertal stage was G1P3 with a testicular volume of 2 ml bilaterally. Basal plasma testosterone was <0.3 nmol/L and luteinizing hormone (LH) and FSH were not elevated. This indicates hypogonadotropic hypogonadism, which is likely to be permanent, and monthly injections of testosterone enanthate was started at progressively increasing doses. Growth, virilization, and testis volume need to be monitored. Overall diagnosis is multiple pituitary hormone deficiencies secondary to irradiation of a rhabdomyosarcoma in close proximity to the hypothalamic–pituitary axis.

Case 12.2

A 13.5-year-old boy previously treated for acute lymphoblastic leukaemia, including testicular disease, was referred for assessment because of concerns about his lack of puberty. He had received testicular radiotherapy four years earlier and had completed chemotherapy a year before referral. On clinical examination, his pubertal stage is G1P2 with 2 ml testes bilaterally. Blood tests showed the following:

FSH 23.1 mU/L

LH 5.8 mU/L

Testosterone <0.3 nmol/L

Questions and Answers

1 What prognosis for testicular function should he and his parents be given?

Given his previous history of testicular irradiation, it is highly probable that he has primary hypogonadism. His elevated plasma FSH concentration, despite his otherwise prepubertal state and small testicular volumes, suggests that his future fertility will be severely impaired. Although Leydig cells are more resistant to the adverse effects of radiotherapy, his rising plasma LH concentration and undetectable testosterone level also suggest that Leydig cell function is impaired.

2 How should his puberty be managed?

Although not all boys will have entered puberty at the age of 13.5 years, given his past history and evidence of likely gonadal damage, induction of puberty with low doses of testosterone, steadily increased towards adult replacement levels over three years should there be no evidence of testicular growth, would be indicated. Once full virilization has been completed, or earlier in the unlikely event of increasing testicular volumes, testosterone therapy should be temporarily discontinued to allow repeat biochemical evaluation of gonadal function to confirm that long-term testosterone therapy is required.

Case 12.3

A 15-year-old boy with Down's syndrome presents with increasing polyuria and polydipsia while receiving 6-mercaptopurine as maintenance chemotherapy for acute lymphoblastic leukaemia. Previously, he had experienced marked hyperglycaemia while receiving chemotherapy, including dexamethasone, and had required insulin therapy and metformin on several occasions though this had been discontinued between courses of glucocorticoids due to normalization of blood glucose levels. He is overweight and has acanthosis nigricans. His father has type 2 diabetes. His HbA1c had increased from 6.2% to 7.0%.

Questions and Answers

1 What is his likely diagnosis and what is the prognosis?

The previous history was strongly suggestive of glucocorticoid-induced diabetes mellitus. However, given his overweight, clinical signs of insulin resistance, and family history, the recurrence of signs of diabetes when not receiving glucocorticoid therapy suggests he is developing type 2 diabetes, which is likely to persist and require longer-term therapy.

2 How should he be managed?

The current picture strongly suggests insulin resistance to be the underlying problem. His urine or blood should be checked to confirm the absence of significant ketosis and he should be started on metformin therapy. Should this fail to normalize his blood glucose concentrations, then insulin therapy may need to be considered.

Case 12.4

A six-year-old girl is referred with concerns about her growth following treatment two years earlier for a metastatic pinealoblastoma, which included chemotherapy and craniospinal radiotherapy. On examination, her height is falling across the centiles and she has evidence of increased central adiposity. Blood testing in the clinic demonstrated the following:

TSH 8.8 mU/L

Free T4 13.5 pmol/L (1.05 ng/dL)

Cortisol 234 nmol/L (8.48 µg/dL)

IGF-I 29.8 nmol/L (normal range 6.8–38.9)

Questions and Answers

1 What is the interpretation of these blood tests?

Although this girl is at risk of hypopituitarism, these initial results suggest the presence of mild primary hypothyroidism, presumably secondary to the effect of her spinal radiotherapy on the thyroid gland. The random plasma cortisol is within the normal range for unstressed early morning samples. Her plasma (IGF-I) concentration is also normal although it should be interpreted with caution in the context of obesity in which the effects of hyperinsulinism on IGF-I levels may mask evolving GHD.

2 How should she be managed?

She should be started on T4 replacement and doses adjusted at monthly intervals to bring TSH levels to within the normal range. Significant growth failure and weight excess are relatively unusual features of hypothyroidism when biochemically mild, as in this case. The latter findings may be more suggestive of GHD and if they do not resolve following normalization of thyroid function, then formal GH stimulation testing should be performed. In this case, a formal diagnosis of GHD was confirmed less than a year later.

Case 12.5

An eight-year-old girl had been diagnosed with a medulloblastoma and spinal metastases at age five years. She was treated with chemotherapy and radiotherapy (40 Gy to the whole CNS, 15 Gy to the primary tumour site and 55 Gy boost to the spinal metastases). A few months earlier, a diagnosis of primary hypothyroidism had been made and she had been started on T4 treatment. On examination, she now has a height velocity of only 1.5 cm per year and is in mid-puberty with Tanner stage 3 breast development. Blood testing demonstrated the following:

Free T4 23.5 pmol/L (1.83 ng/dL)
TSH 0.07 mU/L
Cortisol 346 nmol/L (1.25 µg/dL)
IGF-I 6.8 nmol/L (normal range 12.9–64.0)

Questions and Answers

1 What is the interpretation of her growth pattern at present?

Her present height velocity is extraordinarily low, particularly given her precocious pubertal development. It is likely that she has both GHD and impaired spinal growth due to the direct adverse effects of radiotherapy on the vertebral growth plates.

2 What investigations are indicated?

Formal GH testing confirmed the presence of severe GHD.

3 What treatment may be required?

GH replacement is likely to significantly increase height velocity, though 'catch-up' growth may be limited by a poor spinal response due to local radiotherapy-induced damage to the vertebrae. Precocious puberty is not uncommon following treatment for medulloblastoma and should be confirmed biochemically to be gonadotrophin-dependent. Further pubertal development can then be suppressed using gonadotrophin-releasing hormone (GnRH) agonist treatment to maximize adult height in response to GH replacement.

Significant Guidelines/Consensus Statements

Children's Oncology Group (2008) Long-term follow-up guidelines for survivors of childhood, adolescent, and young adult cancers. www.survivorshipguidelines.org (accessed 14 October 2018).
NHS Improvement. Survivorship: living with and beyond cancer www.improvement.nhs.uk/cancer/SurvivorshipLivingWithandBeyondCancer/tabid/65/Default.aspzx (accessed 14 October 2018).
Skinner R, Wallace WHB, Levitt GA (2005) Therapy based long term follow up: practice statement. www.ukccsg.org.uk/public/followup/PracticeStatement/index.html (accessed 14 October 2018).

Further Reading

Bhakta, N. et al. (2017). The cumulative burden of surviving childhood cancer: an initial report from the St Jude Lifetime Cohort Study (SJLIFE). *Lancet* 390: 2569–2582.

Wallace, H. and Green, D. (2004). *Late Effects of Childhood Cancer*. London: Arnold.

Wallace, W.H. and Thomson, A.B. (2003). Preservation of fertility in children treated for cancer. *Arch. Dis.Child.* 88: 493–496.

Wallace, W.H.B. and Kelnar, C.J.H. (2009). *Endocrinopathy after Childhood Cancer Treatment*. Basel: Karger.

Key Weblink

www.childgrowthfoundation.org The Child Growth Foundation is a UK-based charity which supports children with growth and endocrine disorders and their families (accessed 14 October 2018).

Useful Information for Patients and Parents

www.bsped.org.uk/patients/serono/index.htm and http://www.eurospe.org/patient/English/index.html are links providing downloadable booklets endorsed by the British Society for Paediatric Endocrinology and Diabetes and European Society for Paediatric Endocrinology, respectively, which provide information for children and their families about a range of endocrine problems encountered after treatment of childhood malignancies (accessed 14 October 2018).

http://www.lwpes.org contains a number of links to organizations suggested by the Lawson Wilkins Paediatric Endocrine Society (accessed 14 October 2018).

www.cclg.org.uk/families/booklet.php?bid=6&3id=31&2id=9 lists several pages on the Children's Cancer and Leukaemia Group website which provide information about endocrine complications of childhood cancer treatment (accessed 14 October 2018).

13 An Endocrinologist's Guide to Genetics in the Age of Genomics

Introduction

Comparative genomic hybridization (CGH) and next-generation sequencing (NGS) have revolutionized genetics and molecular endocrinology. The use of these new technologies is spreading; clinicians nowadays need to understand the basic concepts and techniques of genetics in order to explain them to patients to obtain informed consent. Moreover, NGS delivers such a wealth of data that geneticists also need the help of clinicians to filter results and to find causative mutations related to the phenotype. Therefore, clinicians need an understanding of genetics and an awareness of these new techniques, their invaluable advantages, as well as their inherent limitations.

Basic concepts

A complete list of definitions is provided in Table 13.1. Some concepts useful for understanding the NGS technologies are explained in more detail hereafter.

Genes, exome, and genome

A protein-coding gene is a linear sequence of nucleotides (a segment of deoxyribonucleic acid, DNA) that provides coded instruction for ribonucleic acid (RNA) synthesis and translation to protein. The exons are the coding sequences of a gene, which are interrupted by non-coding sequences, the introns. The human genome contains 3 billion nucleotides or 3080 million base pairs (Mb) with about 26 000 genes which contain 234 000 exons and 208 000 introns (Scherer 2008). On average, there are 8.8 exons and 7.8 introns per gene (Sakharkar et al. 2004). The totality of all exons of the genome is defined as the exome. Although the exome covers 1–2% of all the genome, approximately 85% of the disease-causing mutations arise within these protein-coding regions. The genome is the complete sequence of DNA in an organism. More than 98% of the genome does not code for protein, but it does contain regulatory regions and also several transcribed RNAs (such as long non-coding RNAs), many of which play roles in the regulation of gene function.

Chromosomes

The genome is organized and divided into chromosomes, which are structures within the cells that contain the genetic material (Brooker 2018). The term *chromosome* means 'coloured body' which refers to the appearance of chromosomes after coloration through dyes. Human cells are diploid, which means that they have two sets of 23 chromosomes. The first 22 chromosomes

Practical Endocrinology and Diabetes in Children, Fourth Edition. Malcolm D.C. Donaldson, John W. Gregory, Guy Van Vliet, and Joseph I. Wolfsdorf.
© 2019 John Wiley & Sons Ltd. Published 2019 by John Wiley & Sons Ltd.

Table 13.1 Definition of basic concepts in molecular genetics.

Term	Definition
Base	Nucleic acid. There are five different bases subdivided into two categories, the purine bases, adenosine (A) and guanine (G), containing a double-ring structure; and the pyrimidine bases thymine (T), cytosine (C) and uracil (U), containing a single-ring structure.
DNA	Deoxyribonucleic acid is a nucleoside which contains a base (A, G, T, or C) linked to a sugar backbone, deoxyribose.
RNA	Ribonucleic acid is a nucleoside which contains a base (A, C, U, or C) linked to a sugar backbone, ribose.
Nucleotide	Nucleosides (DNA or RNA) link to one or more phosphate groups (e.g. ADP, ATP) to form nucleotides. Nucleotides are linked together linearly to form a strand of DNA or RNA. Two strands of DNA interact to form a double helix.
Chromosomes	Structures in the living cell that contain genetic material in the form of a double helix folded with proteins that influence its 3D structure and activity.
Chromatid	After replication, the two copies of a chromosome are called chromatids. There are joined by a centromere to form a unit known as sister chromatids or dyad. After cell division, a chromosome contains a set two chromatids (the long and the short arms of the chromosome) or a monad. Consequently, a normal human cell in interphase has 46 chromosomes and 92 chromatids.
Genome	The DNA found in all the chromosomes.
Gene	A single unit of genetic information. Protein-coding genes express their information through transcription (RNA expression from DNA), followed by translation (protein synthesis from copy RNA). The pathway of expression from DNA to RNA to protein is called the central dogma of genetics.
Exons	The protein-coding sequence within a gene.
Introns	The non-coding sequence within a gene, located between exons. Introns are removed during transcription through a process called splicing.
Diploidy	The existence of pairs of chromosomes (2n) in human cells.
Haploidy	The existence of one set of chromosomes (n) in gametes.
Aneuploidy	An odd number of chromosomes (2n +/− n).

are numbered according to their size: chromosome 1 is the largest with 250 Mb and chromosomes 21 and 22 only ~50 Mb. The X chromosome is 155 Mb long and the Y, 58 Mb. Gene density is not equal across the chromosomes, e.g. chromosome 19 contains 26 genes/Mb and the Y chromosome only 3.5 genes/Mb.

Gametogenesis and meiosis

Human cells are diploid. They contain two sets of chromosomes, 23 pairs of chromosomes for a total of 46 chromosomes (Figure 13.1). In contrast, gametes (sperms and egg cells or their precursors) are haploid, which means that gametes contain a total of 23 chromosomes, i.e. half that of normal diploid cells. To produce gametes, normal cells have to reduce the number of their chromosomes by meiosis, the term given to cell division with a reduction of the genetic material. Meiosis is a succession of two cell divisions which

reduce the set of chromosomes from 2 to 1. It is during the first cell division (meiosis I) that crossing-over of the genetic material occurs, followed by disjunction, which is the division of the genetic material through the centrosomes. Non-disjunction refers to a failure of the chromosome set to separate correctly. Non-disjunction in meiosis I is the major source of abnormality in the number of chromosomes in a cell (aneuploidy, see section 'Aneuploidy'), but non-disjunction can also occur in meiosis 2.

Aneuploidy

Aneuploid cells have an abnormal number of chromosomes, and aneuploidy is often associated with human syndromes such as Down's, Klinefelter, or Turner syndromes. Aneuploidy may arise from several cytogenic mechanisms, but in humans meiotic or mitotic non-disjunction is the usual mechanism. Non-disjunction

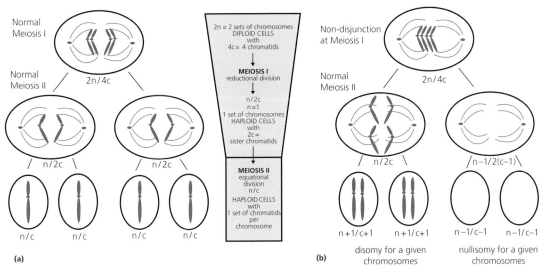

Figure 13.1 (a) schematic view of a normal meiosis for one chromosome pair, each replicated into chromatids (4c) with first division into two cells each containing two sister chromatids (2c) then second division resulting in four cells each containing one set of chromatids (c), also called a monad equivalent to a haploid chromosome. (b) Example of a non-disjunction in meiosis I results in an aberrant number of chromosomes in the gametes so that after the second division, two cells are disomic for the chromosome and two cells are nullisomic.

in maternal meiosis 1 is the most common cause of autosomal trisomy and is associated with maternal age (see Figure 13.1). Of note, aneuploidies are genetic conditions that are often *de novo* (not inherited): thus, while the majority of inherited conditions are genetic, not all genetic conditions are inherited. Even if obvious to geneticists and physicians, this latter point is crucial to explain when counselling parents of children presenting with aneuploidy.

Cytogenetic nomenclature

The International System for Human Cytogenetic Nomenclature (ISCN) is an official standard for human chromosomes. Normal or abnormal chromosome composition in humans is designated as follows:

- the total number of chromosomes, e.g. 46 or 47.
- a comma.
- the sex chromosomal complement: XY in normal males; XX in normal females.
- the specific abnormality, if any, is listed after a second comma.

The normal female chromosomes is thus designated 46,XX and the normal male chromosome is designated 46,XY. An abnormal number of chromosomes is designated first by the total number of chromosomes, the appropriate number of sex chromosomes, and the additional or missing chromosome is identified by + or −, followed by the specific

Table 13.2 Example of chromosome nomenclature following ISCN standard.

Official designation	Description
46,XY	Normal male karyotype
46,XX	Normal female karyotype
47,XXY	Klinefelter syndrome
48,XXYY	Variant of Klinefelter syndrome
45,X	Monosomy X; Turner syndrome
45,X/46,XX	45,X/46,XX mosaicism (Turner mosaicism)
46,X,i(Xq)	A rare type of Turner syndrome with Xp monosomy and Xq trisomy due to an Xq isochromosome
46,X,r(X)	Female with a ring X chromosome
47,XX,+21	Female with trisomy 21
46,X,del(X) (p21)	Terminal deletion of the short arm of X distal to band 21.

responsible chromosome. Thus, a male with trisomy 21 is designated 47,XY,+21. Examples are listed in Table 13.2 and further complementary definitions and explanations of isochromosomes and ring chromosomes are provided in Figure 13.2. For more complex

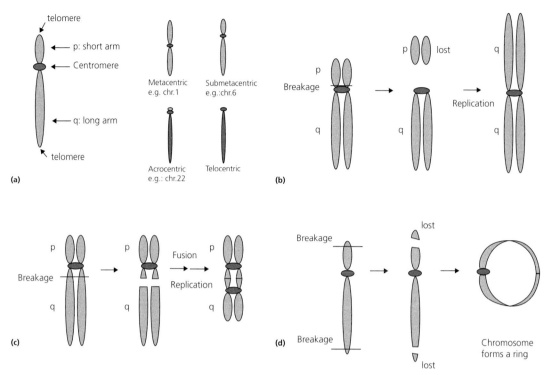

Figure 13.2 (a) The parts of a chromosome: the centromere divides the chromosome into a short arm (abbreviated p) and a long arm (abbreviated q). Normal or abnormal chromosomes can be classified relative to the position of the centromere: metacentric chromosomes with p and q of equal length; submetacentric chromosomes with q slightly greater than p; acrocentric chromosomes with q much greater than p, with a nearly terminal centromere, and telocentric chromosomes with a terminal centromere. (b) Isochromosome (drawn here in metaphase): a chromosome with identical arms. This abnormal chromosome arises when the centromere divides horizontally rather vertically; the telocentric product then replicates to produce a metacentric chromosome. (c) Isodicentric chromosome (drawn here in metaphase): a chromosome with two centromeres arising when breakage occurs in the chromatid arms. (d) Ring chromosome: arising when breakages occur in the telomeric region of the both arms and the telomeres then stick together to form a ring.

cases, we refer to this link of the Human Genome Variation Society (HGVS): http://www.hgvs.org/mutnomen/ISCN.html.

Mutations and mode of inheritance

Mutations
Mutations may be defined as any change in DNA sequence (substitutions, additions, or deletions), which may be inherited or which arise *de novo*. This definition raises some problems: the difference between mutations and variants may be difficult to determine. To link a variant (a genotype) to a range of signs and symptoms (a phenotype), a strong association should be made between the presence of the variant and the disease. This is referred to as *co-segregation* of the genotype with the phenotype.

The different types of mutations are presented in Table 13.3. Of note, germline mutations arise in cells destined to develop into gametes and can be transmitted to offspring while somatic mutations occur in single cells in developing somatic tissue and are not transmitted.

Mutation nomenclature
The HGVS provides recommendations for nomenclature of variants (den Dunnen et al. 2016). All mutations should be described at the most basic level, the DNA level, and in relation to an accepted reference sequence. The reference sequence should be public and clearly described. If the mutation is described at the genomic level, the assembly of the genome used should be specified (e.g. currently the reference genome is hg38). If the mutation is described at the level of coding DNA, the isoform should be specified,

Table 13.3 Different types of mutations.

Type	Effect	Example
Silent mutations	No change of amino acid	CAC → CAT (His to His)
Missense mutations	Change of amino acid	AGC → ATC (Ser to Ile)
Nonsense mutations	Replacement of an amino acid codon by a stop codon	TGT → TGA (Cys to STOP)
Splice site mutations	Create or destroy signals for exon/intron splicing	CTGgtaag → CTGatag (247 + 1G → A)
Frameshift mutations (deletions/insertions)	Triplet codon is read wrongly	
Gene deletion	Complete gene is missing	Protein is missing

e.g. NM_014080.4 is the reference coding sequence for the dual oxidase 2 (DUOX2) gene.

A letter prefix should be used to indicate the type of reference sequence used. The accepted prefixes are:

- 'g' for a genomic reference sequence;
- 'c' for a coding DNA reference sequence;
- 'm' for a mitochondrial reference sequence;
- 'n' for a non-coding DNA reference sequence;
- 'r' for an RNA reference sequence;
- 'p' for a protein reference sequence.

Descriptions at the DNA, RNA, and protein levels are different.

- At the *DNA level*, after the prefix, one number describes the chromosome and the second number describes the 3′-position of the variant on the chromosome. Nucleotides are written in capitals.
  - For *duplication*, after the prefix, two numbers indicate the range of the nucleotides that are duplicated. The numbers are followed by the suffix 'dup'. For example, a duplication in the dystrophin coding sequence responsible for the Duchenne myodystrophy is designated as follows: NM_004006.2:c.20_23dup.
  - For *deletion*, the same rule as for duplication applies, but with 'del' as the suffix.
  - For *inversion*, the same rule as for duplication applies, but with 'inv' as the suffix. Inversion is a sequence change where more than one nucleotide replacing the original sequence come from the reverse complement of the original sequence.
  - For *insertion*, after the prefix, two numbers indicate the flanking region of the insertion site, then the 'ins' suffix defines the insertion and the inserted sequence follows at the end. For example, NM_004006.2: c.169_170InsA means that extra genetic material (here an adenosine) has been inserted between the coding sequence positions 169 and 170 of the dystrophin gene, for which the NM_004006.2 is the reference for this particular gene.

- For other examples of complex variants, the HGVS site provides detailed descriptions (http://varnomen.hgvs.org).
- At the *RNA level*, after the position number, nucleotides are written in lower case.
- At the *protein level*, the amino acids affected in three-letter code are ideally followed by a number and by the predicted consequences after the number. For a *missense* mutation, the description NM_014080.4: p.Pro303Arg means that proline at codon 303 is changed to an arginine in the *DUOX2* coding sequence. For a *silent* mutation, NM_014080.4: p.Pro303=, the '=' means that the nucleotide change causes no change in the amino acid sequence. For a *nonsense* mutation, the stop codon is abbreviated with 'Ter' or the symbol '*', for example: NM_000549.4: c.205C>T; p.Gln69Ter or p.Gln69*, means that a stop codon occurs in the coding sequence of the thyroid-stimulating hormone-beta (*TSHB*) gene.

Mendel's laws

In his work published in 1866, Mendel showed that breeding tall and short pea plants did not produce 'average' offspring plants but either tall or short plants, and in an uneven ratio. From this observation and given that one gene (defined as a unit of heredity influencing one trait) has two copies, Mendel deduced the first law of segregation, which states that the two copies of a gene segregate (or separate) from each other during transmission from parent to offspring. The second law of independent assortment states that two independent genes will randomly assort their alleles during the formation of haploid cells (gametes). The second law implies that genetic recombination can occur during gametogenesis if the independent genes are on the same chromosome.

Pedigree analysis and single-gene mendelian inheritance patterns

A disease might be suspected to be a classical Mendelian condition if the following characteristics are present: (i) the likelihood of having an affected family member is higher than in the general population (increased familial relative risk); (ii) monozygotic (MZ) twins share the disease more often than dizygotic (DZ) twins (MZ concordance for the trait); (iii) the disease is transmitted vertically from parents and is not a communicable (infectious) disease spreading from siblings to others; (iv) genetic disease occurrence is variable in different ethnic groups (cystic fibrosis is rare in Black-African descendants but frequent in North European descendants); (v) genetic diseases have typical ages at onset of symptoms; and (vi) a correlation (co-segregation) between the trait and a chromosomal or genetic alteration and/or similar genotype-phenotype correlation is known in animals. The best- known modes of Mendelian inheritance are autosomal recessive, autosomal dominant, X-linked recessive, and X-linked dominant (Wong 2017). Drawing a pedigree is the first step of the genetic analysis. The conventional symbols used and examples of pedigrees are provided in Figure 13.3.

Autosomal recessive inheritance

In autosomal conditions, the trait occurs *equally in both sexes*. In autosomal recessive condition (such as congenital adrenal hyperplasia), both alleles of the gene have to be mutated to cause a phenotype (biallelic mutations). Therefore, the parents are often unaffected carriers (they have monoallelic mutations) with a 25% risk of their child being affected with each pregnancy.

Autosomal dominant inheritance

In autosomal *dominant* conditions, only one allele is mutated and produces the phenotype. Multiple endocrine neoplasia type 2a (MEN2A) due to receptor tyrosine (*RET*) mutations is an autosomal dominant disease. An affected child has one affected parent and this parent has a 50% chance of his/her children being affected. *De novo* monoallelic mutations may also cause the phenotype; for example, about 80% of cases of achondroplasia arise as *de novo* mutations. For some conditions, individuals with biallelic mutations can present with a more severe phenotype than individuals with monoallelic mutations, e.g. familial hypercholesterolemia due to low-density lipoprotein receptor (*LDLR*) mutations. In dominant conditions,

the penetrance of an allele is a quantitative measure assessed at the population level: if only 70% of the mutated allele carriers present with the trait, the trait (phenotype) is said to be 70% penetrant. However, at the individual level, the phenotype is either present or not. At the individual level, the term expressivity is used to describe the qualitative impact of the mutated allele once the phenotype is present: some mutations resulting in no gene product may lead to a more severe phenotype than a mutation substituting only a single amino.

X-linked inheritance

An example of an endocrine X-linked recessive trait is androgen insensitivity syndrome (AIS), a cause of 46,XY DSD (see Chapter 7). The androgen receptor gene (AR) lies on the X chromosome. Therefore, in AIS, only 46,XY males are affected and their mothers are obligate healthy carriers of the condition. In X-linked dominant conditions, such as hypophosphataemic rickets due to *PHEX* mutations, females with monoallelic *PHEX* mutation are less severely affected than males. With X-linked inheritance, affected mothers will transmit the condition to 50% of their daughters and 50% of theirs sons, whereas affected fathers will transmit the condition to 100% of their daughters but none of their sons. (Figure 13.3)

Alternatives to classical genetics and inherited conditions reference

Uniparental disomy (UPD)

Uniparental disomy (UPD) is the consequence of at least three mechanisms: gamete complementation, monosomy rescue, and trisomy rescue as depicted in Figure 13.4.

Gametogenesis (which is a succession of two meioses) is an error-prone process with the occurrence of nullisomy and disomy or, in other words, with zero copy or two copies of a locus coming from one parent in one gamete. Upon fertilization, gamete complementation will occur: one nullisomic gamete might be complemented by a disomic gamete and will result in UPD, meaning that the two copies of a locus come from one parent. If the two copies from a parent are identical, this is defined as isodisomy in contrast to heterodisomy when the two copies are different.

Duplication of a chromosome rescues a zygote monosomic for this particular chromosome. Trisomy is another abnormal and frequent result of gametogenesis. Reduction of a trisomy to disomy during

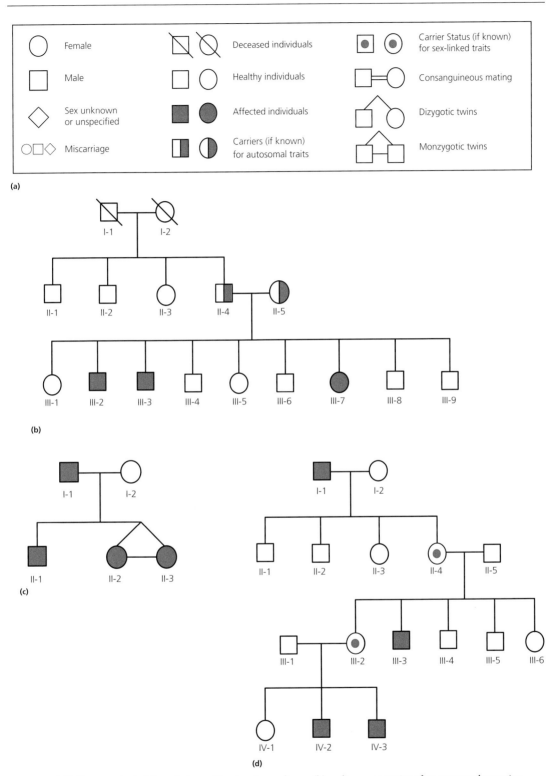

Figure 13.3 Pedigree analysis: (a) symbols used for drawing pedigree; (b) pedigree suggestive of an autosomal recessive condition: parents are not affected and siblings of both sexes are affected; (c) pedigree suggestive of an autosomal dominant disease: direct transmission of a trait from one parent to his/her children; (d) pedigree suggestive of an X-linked recessive disorder: females are obligate carriers of the trait and only males are affected.

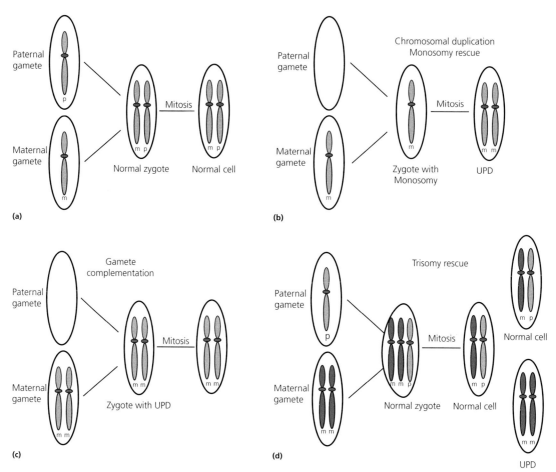

Figure 13.4 Schematic representation of the possible fates of a given chromosome during the process of fertilization: (a) after reductional division (meiosis) the chromosome is present in both parental cells (the gametes) and fertilization results in normal zygote with a copy of each parental chromosome; (b) the chromosome is missing from one parental gamete (nullisomy) but the single parental chromosome is then duplicated – monosomy rescue – resulting in uniparental isodisomy; (c) one parental gamete is nullisomic but the other is disomic, resulting in uniparental disomy (UPD); this is known as gamete complementation; (d) one parental gamete is monosomic (normal) while the other is disomic, resulting in a trisomic zygote. This is followed by loss of one of the extra chromosomes, trisomy rescue, and depending on the parental origin of the remaining two chromosome there is a 1 in 3 possibility of UPD. Source: Modified from Engel and Antonorakis (2002).

the first mitosis of a zygote leaves disomic and tetrasomic cells. Tetrasomy is in general lethal and therefore only the disomic cells will survive.

Genomic imprinting

Genomic imprinting refers to the phenomenon whereby the expression of a gene is influenced by its parental origin. There are up to 150 known imprinted genes and loci (http://igc.otago.ac.nz; http://www.geneimprint.com/site/genes-by-species). Imprinting is often associated with a distinctive methylation mark in the promoter region of imprinted genes: *hypomethylation* of the promoter is associated with expression of the gene whereas *hypermethylation* is associated with repression of gene expression. Of note, the imprinting is tissue-specific in some instances. For example, for the imprinted gene G-protein alpha subunit 1 (*GNAS1*), the transcript is maternally expressed in the pituitary, thyroid, gonads and renal proximal tubule whereas in bone, *GNAS1* shows a random allelic expression. Consequently, pseudohypoparathyroidism type Ia due to maternal inheritance of a *GNAS1* loss-of-function mutation will present with renal parathyroid hormone (PTH) resistance leading to hypocalcaemia whereas this phenotype is absent if the mutation is inherited from the father. The term pseudopseudohypoparathyroidism describes a phenotype of bone dysplasia without PTH resistance and hypocalcaemia. Of note, *activating GNAS* mutations occurring at the *somatic* level, are responsible for the McCune–Albright syndrome (see Chapter 5 on puberty).

An example of the relationship of UPD and imprinting: Prader–Willi syndrome (PWS)

UPD might interfere with imprinting and lead to disomy of alleles whose expression depends on the parent-of-origin. Prader–Willi syndrome (PWD) results from loss of the paternal contribution from a critical area of the long arm of chromosome 15 in the 11–13 region (15q11-q13). Most cases (60–70%) arise from a deletion in the paternal chromosome but maternal disomy of chromosome 15 accounts for up to 30–40%, and 3–5% from changes in methylation profile repressing the paternal expression of genes located on 15q11-q13. Consequently, and whatever the cause of the PWS, the molecular consequence is a change in methylation patterns of imprinted genes on 15q11-q13. This explains why the methylation test is the first test to be ordered when PWS is suspected.

Traditional molecular techniques

Many techniques are required to detect mutations in a distinct region. These include restriction length polymorphisms (RFLP) and denaturing high-performance liquid chromatography (dHPLC). All these techniques need confirmation by Sanger sequencing. Therefore, over time, the polymerase chain reaction (PCR)-based Sanger sequencing has become the gold standard for molecular diagnosis.

Polymerase chain reaction (PCR)

PCR was developed in 1985 by Kary Mullis. After denaturation by raising the temperature, the template DNA is opened, oligonucleotide primers are annealed (bound to) a precise location where they 'prime' the Taq polymerase (an enzyme which copies DNA) which starts to extend the primers. This cycle is repeated 20–30 times. At each cycle of denaturation, annealing, and extension, an exponential amount of DNA between the primers is produced.

PCR-based Sanger sequencing

Frederick Sanger developed this sequencing technique in the 1970s and he received the Nobel Prize in Chemistry in 1980. Sanger sequencing relies on a PCR amplification which is terminated by nucleotide-specific inhibitors. This method is very accurate and remains a valuable validation step to confirm the findings of NGS (see section 'Next Generation Sequencing (NGS) Technology: Whole Exome Sequencing (WES)'). However, its low throughput and high costs render its use outdated for the screening of a large number of genes. Of note, the first sequencing of the human genome of 3.1 billion nucleotides (the Human Genome Project) cost ~US$3 billion ($1 per sequenced base) and took over 13 years (1990–2003) to complete.

Fluorescent *in situ* hybridization (FISH)

Fluorescent *in situ* hybridization (FISH) is a technique used to visualize define nucleic acid sequences in cell preparations by hybridization of complementary oligonucleotide sequences (probes) which are labelled with fluorochrome.

Genomics

Comparative genomic hybridization (CGH)

In 1992, Kalliomiemi, Pinkel, and colleagues designed a method called comparative genomic hybridization (CGH) (Gilissen et al. 2012). Fifteen years later, in 2007, the journal *Science* presented the association of copy number variation (CNVs) assessed by array comparative genomic hybridization (aCGH) with genetic diversity among humans as the discovery of the year. Only a few years later, CGH use had become routine in clinical settings. Briefly, the CGH technique is based on the comparison of an equal amount of fluorescently labelled genomes (e.g. red dye for the case and green dye for a mix of controls). The two samples are combined and then hybridized either on metaphase chromosomes or on arrays (aCGH) where a reference genome is spread on an array at a given resolution; this latter technique being now the standard technique. At each spot of the aCGH, the fluorescence is measured. If a region is present in both the case and the control, the average ratio is 1 (yellow); if the region is deleted, the ratio will be less than 1 (only the green dye of the control is detectable); if a duplication is present, the ratio will be higher than one (red).

Therefore, aCGH has the advantage of detecting insertions and deletions at a higher definition than the classical karyotype. Also, all types of insertion and deletion associated with a condition are detected. For example, even non-classical deletions responsible for the DiGeorge syndrome can be captured with aCGH, which was not the case with the FISH technique used previously. On the other hand, aCGH cannot detect low-grade mosaicism of less than 20%, and if mosaicism is suspected, a classical karyotype remains the investigation of choice. Moreover, aCGH does not detect small insertions and deletions, or equilibrated translocation or inversion, given that the amount of genomic material (and dye) is conserved in all loci.

Next generation sequencing (NGS) technology: whole exome sequencing (WES)

NGS refers to techniques using massing parallel sequencing, one of the most used NGS technology being whole exome sequencing (WES). WES is, in principle, a straightforward technique which consists of three main steps: (i) DNA extraction and fragmentation followed by the capture and amplification of the exome (i.e. all the exons), the component of the genome which encodes proteins; (ii) sequencing of the exome; and (iii) bioinformatic analysis of the raw sequencing data, and its interpretation given the clinical context (Gilissen et al. 2012). Either WES or targeted NGS (see section 'Next Generation Sequencing (NGS) Technology') cover only a small fraction of the genome (1–2% maximum).

Exon capture is performed by gene-specific primers or by capture-based hybridization to a library of probes. The DNA fragments are ligated with adaptors which contain sequencing primers and tags for subsequent data management.

Exome sequencing is performed either by synthesis or by ligation. Sequencing by synthesis is based on the principle that nucleotide incorporation to a sequence emits either pyrophosphate (PPi), derived from adenosine triphosphate (ATP), which can activate luciferase, modify pH or can release fluorescence specific to each nucleotide at a given time. Sequencing by ligation uses primers specific to target sequence for ligation. Consequently, sequencing by ligation is not appropriate for large sequences and is less appealing for true unbiased NGS use.

Data analysis is a four-step process (Figure 13.5). First, the sequencing signal is captured and converted to base call (a process by which the order of

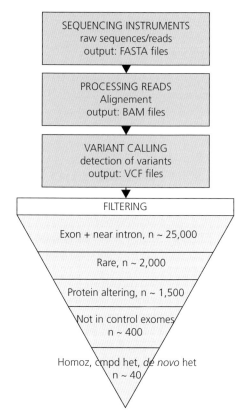

Figure 13.5 Flowchart of whole-exome data analysis. The four steps are: base call (reads), processing reads and alignment, variant calling, and variant filtering. For the last step, the number of variants at each sub-step is indicated.

nucleotides in a template is inferred during a sequencing reaction) and short stretches of sequences called reads (70–150 bp length). At the end of this first step, raw sequence data (reads) are compiled in Fasta files, in which nucleotide sequences are represented using single-letter codes. Second, reads need to be aligned and assembled against the reference genome; aligned reads are then compiled in Bam files (which store sequence data in a binary fashion). At this stage, multiple reads are aligned to a given nucleotide in one exon and this defines the coverage (or depth) in sequencing. For example, a 100x coverage means that, on average, hundreds of reads are aligned at any nucleotide of the sequenced exons. Third, mismatches with the reference sequence are picked up (variants calling), the variants are annotated (information about exact location, relation to other databases, etc.) and compiled in variant call format files (VCF). Finally, filtering and interpretation of variants are performed (Samuels et al. 2014).

Endocrine genetics: from phenotype to genotype

Traditional identification of causative mutations for a disease with a mendelian transmission

Molecular diagnosis through traditional direct sequencing requires the clinician to prioritize a finite number of genes for testing based on a given phenotype. For many endocrine conditions, step-wise flow charts have been developed to prioritize genes for sequencing. However, sequencing one gene after another results in a time-consuming 'diagnostic odyssey'. This step-wise approach has been challenged and is often no longer adequate, considering the improvements in massive parallel sequencing. Of note, even well-defined clinical and biochemical conditions (such as adrenocorticotrophic hormone (ACTH) resistance) have multiple genetic causes and given the falling costs of NGS/WES, exome sequencing is now less expensive and quicker than traditional step-wise sequencing of candidate genes.

Next generation sequencing (NGS) technology

Genomics technologies are now available and affordable and their capacity to interrogate the whole genome quickly for structural variation or for mutations in the coding sequences (the exome) has transformed the molecular diagnosis of genetic endocrine conditions. NGS has two main advantages. First, multiple genes can be sequenced in a one-step process, which has paved the way to the use of panels of genes for some groups of conditions such as the maturity onset diabetes of the young (MODY) panel. Second, NGS is faster and more cost-effective for the sequencing of large genes. For example the Duchenne muscular dystrophy (*DMD*) gene has 2.3 Mb with 79 exons encoding dystrophin and the breast cancer susceptibility 1 and 2 (*BRCA1/2*) gene contains a large exon of >10 kb.

On the other hand, some limitations and pitfalls should be mentioned. Trinucleotide repeats, large insertions or deletions, epigenetic changes, and structural changes are not reliably identified by NGS. Indeed, high guanine-cytosine (GC) content, sequence repeats, and complex secondary DNA structures prevent proper sequencing and, therefore, some genes and/or exons may be insufficiently covered by NGS. Pseudogenes may lead to improper alignment of the reads and decreased sensitivity. Then, reliable clinical interpretation of a large number of variants remains a challenge. At this stage, the help of clinicians having a good knowledge of genes or pathways associated with the reported phenotype is invaluable. Lastly, for some cases, only functional assays will assess whether the candidate genes or mutations have the expected biological impact.

NGS panels for endocrine disorders

The use of an NGS phenotype-based panel has some advantages: (i) only clinically validated genes are usually covered by panels; (ii) the depth and quality of coverage may be better; (iii) increased sequencing depth allows detection of low level mosaicism; and (iv) it mitigates the risk of discovering disease-causing variants in genes unrelated to the primary condition.

However, NGS panels will not lead to discovery of new genes and may prove negative if patients present with atypical or complex phenotypes that prevent the selection of a well-defined panel.

Unbiased NGS sequencing

If traditional sequencing or targeted NGS is negative, the use of an unbiased whole-exome or whole-genome approach is the logical choice. Moreover, with the improvement of methodologies and coverage read depth, it is now possible to detect copy number variations (CNVs) with NGS. The yield of 25–30% solved cases (Yang et al. 2013; Sawyer et al. 2016) with unbiased genome-wide approach for unselected cases (unsolved by the traditional approach) speaks for its use as a first-line genetic test, especially for patients with atypical phenotypes or phenotypes suggesting genetic heterogeneity. This yield can be further improved if a family-based NGS approach is applied.

Family-based NGS analysis

The clinical genetics laboratory offers two approaches regarding WES: the proband-based WES and the trio-WES (a familial trio of the two parents with the index case). This family-based NGS is particularly useful for data analysis and clinical interpretation, and is therefore efficient in finding either de novo variants or compound heterozygous inheritance following the autosomal recessive model. Trio-WES offers a better diagnostic rate compared with proband-WES (35% vs 25%) as well as a better turnaround time. The diagnostic rate further increases to 60% if trio-WES is applied to consanguineous families (Yavarna et al. 2015).

Genetic counselling before NGS

Genetic counselling to obtain a well-informed consent for NGS is an essential prerequisite step (Bick and Dimmock 2011). The parents should be aware of the patterns of inheritance, the concept of penetrance and expressivity, type of variants/mutations (e.g. variants of unknown significance), non-paternity leading to misinterpretations, incidental findings and their impact on family members. An incidental finding which is defined as the discovery of mutation in a gene unrelated to the patient's phenotype (e.g. *BRCA1* gene mutations) is a main issue, and parents can decide whether they want to be informed of these incidental findings. However, in some jurisdictions, only medically actionable conditions of childhood onset are disclosed for paediatric patients. In general, carrier status is not disclosed.

Reporting of NGS results

The variants need to be assessed and reported using standard protocols for clarity. Thus, the American College of Medical Genetics (ACMG; https://www.acmg.net) has released guidelines to standardize the quality of rare variant reporting (Richards et al. 2015). In general, the following essential points need to be clearly stated in an NGS report:

1 The clinical indication for exome testing.
2 A short sentence indicating the most relevant molecular finding.
3 A list of rare variants related to the patient's phenotype. A minimum allele frequency (MAF) of less than 1% defines a rare variant. Variants should be reported using the HGVS nomenclature, as explained in section 'Traditional Molecular Techniques'.
4 Variant pathogenicity should be indicated, as follows: (i) pathogenic; (ii) likely pathogenic; (iii) uncertain significance; (iv) likely benign; and (v) benign. This classification is based on the nature of the variant (null variants: multi-exon deletions, nonsense and/or frameshift mutations in genes where loss of function is known to cause the disease), the literature and clinical databases. Strong arguments for pathogenicity also include: (i) well-established functional assays showing the deleterious effect of the reported variant; (ii) the same amino acid change as an established pathogenic variant; (iii) de novo null variants (maternity and paternity confirmed); and (iv) when prevalence of the rare variant is clearly higher in affected cases when compared to healthy controls.
5 Reports of medically actionable secondary findings.

6 Methodologies and recommendations based on molecular findings. As mentioned in section 'Next Generation Sequencing (NGS) Technology: Whole Exome Sequencing (WES)', WES has some limitations. For example, WES is inaccurate for the diagnosis of triplet nucleotide disorders and an appropriate test should be suggested if such a condition is suspected.

By contrast, the following information is not included in NGS reports:

1 Carrier status (although debate on this issue continues).
2 Variants in a disease gene which are unrelated to the patient phenotype.
3 Benign or likely benign variants.
4 Variants not related to Mendelian disorders but considered as susceptibility variants.

It is obvious that the classification of variants in the pathogenic and/or likely pathogenic variants is a moving target. Moreover, oligogenic causation is becoming the explanation of many phenotypes (Lu et al. 2014), e.g. oligogenic mechanisms explaining isolated gonadotropin-releasing hormone deficiency (Sykiotis et al. 2010). Therefore, the fast-growing knowledge in genetics implies a constant revision of the clinical impact for a given variant, and the re-analysis of existing exome data or resequencing is advised in cases with a family history strongly suggesting a Mendelian disorder.

References

Bick, D. and Dimmock, D. (2011). Whole exome and whole genome sequencing. *Curr. Opin. Pediatr.* 23 (6): 594–600.

Brooker, R.J. (2018). *Genetics: Analysis and Principles*, 6e. New York: McGraw-Hill Education.

den Dunnen, J.T., Dalgleish, R., Maglott, D.R. et al. (2016). HGVS recommendations for the description of sequence variants: 2016 update. *Hum. Mutat.* 37 (6): 564–569.

Engel, E. and Antonorakis, S.E. (2002). *Genomic Imprinting and Uniparental Disomy in Medicine*. New York: Wiley-Liss,.

Gilissen, C., Hoischen, A., Brunner, H.G., and Veltman, J.A. (2012). Disease gene identification strategies for exome sequencing. *Eur. J. Hum. Genet.* 20 (5): 490–497.

Lu, J.T., Campeau, P.M., and Lee, B.H. (2014). Genotype-phenotype correlation – promiscuity in the era of next-generation sequencing. *N. Engl. J. Med.* 371 (7): 593–596.

Richards, S., Aziz, N., Bale, S. et al. (2015). Standards and guidelines for the interpretation of sequence variants: a joint consensus recommendation of the American College of Medical Genetics and Genomics and the Association for Molecular Pathology. *Genet. Med.* 17 (5): 405–424.

Sakharkar, M.K., Chow, V.T., and Kangueane, P. (2004). Distributions of exons and introns in the human genome. *In Silico Biol.* 4 (4): 387–393.

Samuels, M.E., Hasselmann, C., Deal, C.L. et al. (2014). Whole-exome sequencing: opportunities in pediatric endocrinology. *Per. Med.* 11: 63–78.

Sawyer, S.L., Hartley, T., Dyment, D.A. et al. (2016). Utility of whole-exome sequencing for those near the end of the diagnostic odyssey: time to address gaps in care. *Clin. Genet.* 89 (3): 275–284.

Scherer, S. (2008). *A Short Guide to the Human Genome*. New York: Cold Spring Harbor Laboratory Press.

Sykiotis, G.P., Plummer, L., Hughes, V.A. et al. (2010). Oligogenic basis of isolated gonadotropin-releasing hormone deficiency. *Proc. Natl. Acad. Sci. U.S.A.* 107 (34): 15140–15144.

Wong, L.C. (ed.) (2017). *Next Generation Sequencing Based Clinical Molecular Diagnosis of Human Genetic Disorders*. Cham, Switzerland: Springer International Publishing AG.

Yang, Y., Muzny, D.M., Reid, J.G. et al. (2013). Clinical whole-exome sequencing for the diagnosis of Mendelian disorders. *N. Engl. J. Med.* 369 (16): 1502–1511.

Yavarna, T., Al-Dewik, N., Al-Mureikhi, M. et al. (2015). High diagnostic yield of clinical exome sequencing in Middle Eastern patients with Mendelian disorders. *Hum. Genet.* 134 (9): 967–980.

1 Growth Charts and Body Mass Index (BMI) Charts

WHO growth charts 0–4 years, 272	Tanner-Marshall height velocity charts 0–19 years, 282
CDC height and weight charts 2–20 years, 280	WHO-UK BMI charts 2–20 years, 284

Different growth and body mass index (BMI) charts exist in different countries, with some differences between them. In 2010, the United Kingdom-World Health Organization (UK-WHO) growth charts for 0–4 years were introduced. Since 2012, the Royal College of Paediatrics and Child Health (RCPCH) among other organizations has recommended use of the 2–18 year WHO growth charts.

As mentioned in the chapter on Short Stature (see Chapter 3), the authors find that the split format of the WHO charts is not ideal for the monitoring of patients with long-term endocrine problems. They prefer the 1995 Buckler-Tanner 2–18 year growth charts (Castlemead Publications, Hertford SG13 8NP, United Kingdom) for patients in the United Kingdom; the National Center for Health and Statistics Clinical Growth Charts (CDC) 2–20 year growth charts for patients in North America (https://www.cdc.gov/growthcharts/clinical_charts.htm); and the 1985 Tanner and Davies 2–19 year height velocity charts (J Pediatr.

1985 Sep;107(3):317–29 1985) for both United Kingdom and North America.

The authors agree that the WHO 0–4 growth charts (https://www.rcpch.ac.uk/resources/uk-who-growth-charts-0-4-years) are indicated for children aged 0–2 years.

The authors recommend the RCPCH UK-WHO Body Mass Index (BMI) charts (https://www.rcpch.ac.uk/sites/default/files/2018-03/boys_and_girls_bmi_chart.pdf) for BMI assessment in boys and girls aged 0–18 years.

Appendix 1 therefore reproduces the following charts for girls and boys: the WHO 0–4 year and CDC 2–20 year charts for height and weight; the Tanner and Davies 2–19 year charts for height velocity; and the UK-WHO 2–18 year charts for BMI.

Reference

Tanner, J.M. and Davies, P.S. (n.d.). *J. Pediatr.* 107 (3): 317–329.

Practical Endocrinology and Diabetes in Children, Fourth Edition. Malcolm D.C. Donaldson, John W. Gregory, Guy Van Vliet, and Joseph I. Wolfsdorf.
© 2019 John Wiley & Sons Ltd. Published 2019 by John Wiley & Sons Ltd.

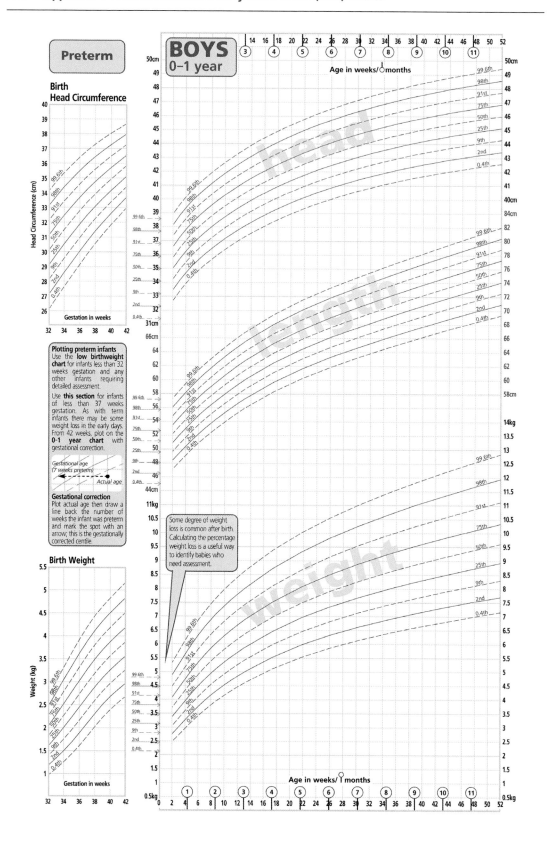

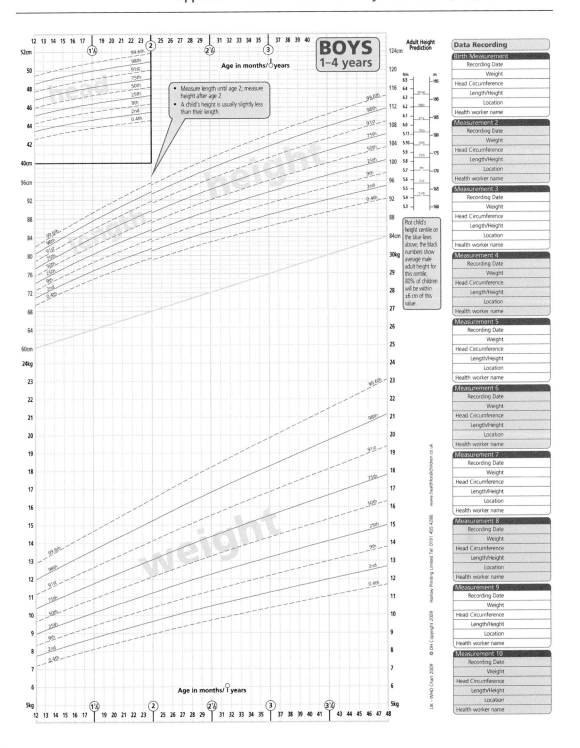

BOYS
1–4 years

Age in months/years

Adult Height Prediction

- Measure length until age 2; measure height after age 2.
- A child's height is usually slightly less than their length.

Plot child's height centile on the blue lines above; the black numbers show average male adult height for this centile; 80% of children will be within ±6 cm of this value.

www.healthforallchildren.co.uk

Harlow Printing Limited Tel: 0191 455 4286

© DH Copyright 2009

UK – WHO Chart 2009

Data Recording
Birth Measurement
Recording Date
Weight
Head Circumference
Length/Height
Location
Health worker name
Measurement 2
Recording Date
Weight
Head Circumference
Length/Height
Location
Health worker name
Measurement 3
Recording Date
Weight
Head Circumference
Length/Height
Location
Health worker name
Measurement 4
Recording Date
Weight
Head Circumference
Length/Height
Location
Health worker name
Measurement 5
Recording Date
Weight
Head Circumference
Length/Height
Location
Health worker name
Measurement 6
Recording Date
Weight
Head Circumference
Length/Height
Location
Health worker name
Measurement 7
Recording Date
Weight
Head Circumference
Length/Height
Location
Health worker name
Measurement 8
Recording Date
Weight
Head Circumference
Length/Height
Location
Health worker name
Measurement 9
Recording Date
Weight
Head Circumference
Length/Height
Location
Health worker name
Measurement 10
Recording Date
Weight
Head Circumference
Length/Height
Location
Health worker name

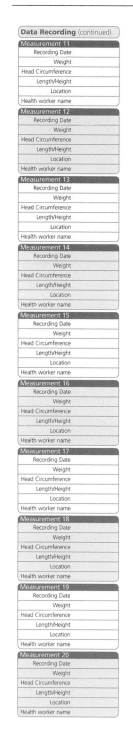

Data Recording (continued)

Measurement 11
Recording Date	
Weight	
Head Circumference	
Length/Height	
Location	
Health worker name	

Measurement 12
Recording Date	
Weight	
Head Circumference	
Length/Height	
Location	
Health worker name	

Measurement 13
Recording Date	
Weight	
Head Circumference	
Length/Height	
Location	
Health worker name	

Measurement 14
Recording Date	
Weight	
Head Circumference	
Length/Height	
Location	
Health worker name	

Measurement 15
Recording Date	
Weight	
Head Circumference	
Length/Height	
Location	
Health worker name	

Measurement 16
Recording Date	
Weight	
Head Circumference	
Length/Height	
Location	
Health worker name	

Measurement 17
Recording Date	
Weight	
Head Circumference	
Length/Height	
Location	
Health worker name	

Measurement 18
Recording Date	
Weight	
Head Circumference	
Length/Height	
Location	
Health worker name	

Measurement 19
Recording Date	
Weight	
Head Circumference	
Length/Height	
Location	
Health worker name	

Measurement 20
Recording Date	
Weight	
Head Circumference	
Length/Height	
Location	
Health worker name	

BOYS UK–WHO
Growth Chart 0–4 years

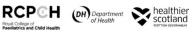

RCPCH
Royal College of
Paediatrics and Child Health
Leading the way in Children's Health

(DH) *Department of Health*

healthier scotland
SCOTTISH GOVERNMENT

Who should use this chart?

Anyone who measures a child, plots or interprets charts should be suitably trained, or be supervised by someone qualified to do so. For further information and training materials see www.growthcharts.rcpch.ac.uk

A growth chart for all children

The UK-WHO growth chart combines World Health Organization (WHO) standards with UK preterm and birth data. The chart from 2 weeks to 4 years of age is based on the WHO growth standard, derived from measurements of healthy, non-deprived, breastfed children of mothers who did not smoke.[1] The chart for birth measurements (32-42 weeks gestation) is based on British children measured around 1990.[2] The charts depict a healthy pattern of growth that is desirable for all children, whether breast fed or formula fed, and of whatever ethnic origin.[3]

Weighing and measuring

When measuring children up to 2 years, remove all clothes and nappy; children older than 2 years should wear minimal clothing only. Always remove shoes.

Weight: use only class III clinical electronic scales in metric setting.

Length: (before 2 years of age). proper equipment is essential (length board or mat). Measurers should be trained.

Height: (from 2 years): use a rigid rule with T piece, or stadiometer. Position head and feet as illustrated with child standing as straight as possible.

Frankfurt st (Plane

Head circumference: use a narrow plastic or paper tape to measure where the head circumference is greatest.

When to weigh

Babies should be weighed in the first week as part of the assessment of feeding and thereafter as needed. Recovery of birthweight indicates that feeding is effective and that the child is well. Once feeding is established, babies should usually be weighed at around 8, 12 and 16 weeks and 1 year at the time of routine immunisations. If there is concern, weigh more often; however, weights measured too close together are often misleading, so babies should be weighed no more than once a month up to 6 months of age, once every 2 months from 6 to 12 months of age, and once every 3 months over the age of 1 year. However, most children do not need to be weighed this often.

Please place sticker (if available) otherwise write in space provided.

Name: _____

NHS/CHI No: [ ][ ][ ][ ][ ][ ][ ][ ][ ][ ]

Hospital No: [ ][ ][ ][ ][ ][ ][ ]

Date of Birth: [ ][ ] / [ ][ ] / [ ][ ][ ][ ]

When to measure length or height

Length or height should be measured whenever there are any worries about a child's weight gain, growth or general health.

Plotting measurements

For babies born at term (37 weeks or later), plot each measurement on the relevant chart by drawing a small dot where a vertical line through the child's age crosses a horizontal line through the measured value. The lettering on the charts ('weight', 'length' etc.) sits on the 50th centile, providing orientation for ease of plotting.

Plot birth weight (and, if measured, length and head circumference) at age 0 on the 0–1 year chart. The coloured arrows at age 0 represent UK birth weight data and show the child's birth centile.

Weight gain in the early days varies a lot from baby to baby, so there are no lines on the chart between 0 and 2 weeks. However, by 2 weeks of age most babies will be on a centile close to their birth centile.

For **preterm infants** a separate low birth weight chart is available for infants of less than 32 weeks gestation and any other infant requiring detailed assessment. For healthy infants born from 32 weeks and before 37 weeks, plot all measurements in the preterm section (to the left of the main 0–1 year chart) until 42 weeks gestation, then plot on the 0–1 year chart using gestational correction, as shown below.

The preterm section can also be used to assess the relative size of infants at the margin of 'term' (e.g. 37 weeks gestation), but these measurements should also be plotted at age 0 on the 0–1 year chart.

Gestational correction

Plot measurements at the child's actual age and then draw a line back the number of weeks the infant was preterm. Mark the spot with an arrow (see diagram): this is the child's gestationally corrected centile. Gestational correction should continue until at least 1 year of age.

Centile terminology

If the point is within 1/4 of a space of the line they are on the centile: e.g. 91st.

If not they should be described as being between the two centiles: e.g. 75th-91st.

A centile space is the distance between two of the centile lines, or equivalent distance if midway between centiles.

Plotting for preterm infants (less than 37 weeks gestation): Draw a line back the number of weeks preterm and mark spot with arrow.

Gestational age (7 weeks preterm)

Actual age

Interpreting the chart
Assessing weight loss after birth
Most babies lose some weight after birth but 80% will have regained this by 2 weeks of age. Fewer than 5% of babies lose more than 10% of their weight at any stage; only 1 in 50 are 10% or more lighter than birth weight at 2 weeks.

Percentage weight loss can be calculated as follows:

Weight loss = current weight–birth weight

$$\text{Percentage weight loss} = \frac{\text{Weight loss}}{\text{Birth weight}} \times 100\%$$

For example, a child born at 3.500kg who drops to 3.150kg at 5 days has lost 350g or 10%; in a baby born at 3.000kg, a 300g loss is 10%.

Careful clinical assessment and evaluation of feeding technique is indicated when weight loss exceeds 10% or recovery of birth weight is slow.

What do the centiles mean?
These charts indicate a child's size compared with children of the same age and maturity who have shown optimum growth. The chart also shows how quickly a child is growing. The centile lines on the chart show the expected range of weights and heights (or lengths); each describes the number of children expected to be below that line (e.g. 50% below 50th, 91% below the 91st). Children come in all shapes and sizes, but 99 out of 100 children who are growing optimally will be between the two outer lines (0.4th and 99.6th centiles); half will lie between the 25th and 75th centile lines.

Being very small or very big can sometimes be associated with underlying illness. There is no single threshold below which a child's weight or height is definitely abnormal, but only 4 per 1000 children who are growing optimally are below the **0.4th centile**, so these children should be assessed at some point to exclude any problems. Those above the **99.6th centile** for height are almost always healthy. Also calculate BMI if weight and height centiles appear very different.

What is a normal rate of weight gain and growth?
Babies do not all grow at the same rate, so a baby's weight often does not follow a particular centile line, especially in the first year. Weight is most likely to track within one centile space (the gap between two centile lines, see diagram). In infancy, acute illness can lead to sudden weight loss and a weight centile fall but on recovery the child's weight usually returns to its normal centile within 2–3 weeks. However, a sustained drop through two or more weight centile spaces is unusual (fewer than 2% of infants) and should be carefully assessed by the primary care team, including measuring length/height.

Because it is difficult to measure length and height accurately in pre-school children, successive measurements commonly show wide variation. If there are worries about growth, it is useful to measure on a few occasions over time; most healthy children will show a stable *average* position over time.

UK children have relatively large heads compared to the WHO standard, particularly after the age of 6 months. After the age of 6 weeks a head circumference below the 2nd centile will be seen in only 1 in 250 children. A head circumference above the 99.6th centile, or crossing upwards through 2 centile spaces, should only cause concern if there is a continued rise after 6 months, or other signs or symptoms.

Why do the length/height centiles change at 2 years?
The growth standards show length data up to 2 years of age, and height from age 2 onwards. When a child is measured standing up, the spine is squashed a little, so their height is slightly less than their length; the centile lines shift down slightly at age 2 to allow for this. It is important that this difference does not worry parents; what matters is whether the child continues to follow the same centile after the transition.

Predicting adult height
Parents like to know how tall their child will be as an adult. The child's most recent height centile (aged 2–4 years) gives a good idea of this for healthy children. Plot this centile on the adult height predictor to the right of the height chart to find the average adult height for children on this centile. Four out of five children will have adult heights that are within 6cm above or below this value.

Weight–height to BMI conversion chart
BMI indicates how heavy a child is relative to his or her height and is the simplest measure of thinness and fatness from the age of 2, when height can be measured fairly accurately. This chart[4] provides an approximate BMI centile, accurate to a quarter of a centile space.

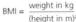

$$\text{BMI} = \frac{\text{weight in kg}}{(\text{height in m})^2}$$

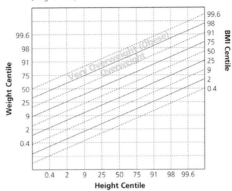

Date:			
Age:			
BMI Centile:			

Instructions for use
1. Read off the weight and height centiles from the growth chart.

2. Plot the weight centile (left axis) against the height centile (bottom axis) on the chart above.

3. If between centiles, read across in this position.

4. Read off the corresponding BMI centile from the slanting lines.

5. Record the centile with the date and child's age in the data box.

Interpretation
In a child over 2 years of age, the BMI centile is a better indicator of overweight or underweight than the weight centile; a child whose weight is average for their height will have a BMI between the 25th and 75th centiles, whatever their height centile. BMI above the 91st centile suggests that the child is overweight; a child above the 98th centile is very overweight (clinically obese). BMI below the 2nd centile is unusual and may reflect undernutrition.

References
1. www.who.int/childgrowth/en
2. Cole TJ, Freeman JV, Preece MA. British 1990 growth reference centiles for weight, height, body mass index and head circumference fitted by maximum penalized likelihood. Stat Med 1998;17:407-29.
3. www.sacn.gov.uk/reports_position_statements/index.html
4. Cole TJ. A chart to link child centiles of body mass index, weight and height. Eur J Clin Nutr 2002;56:1194-9.

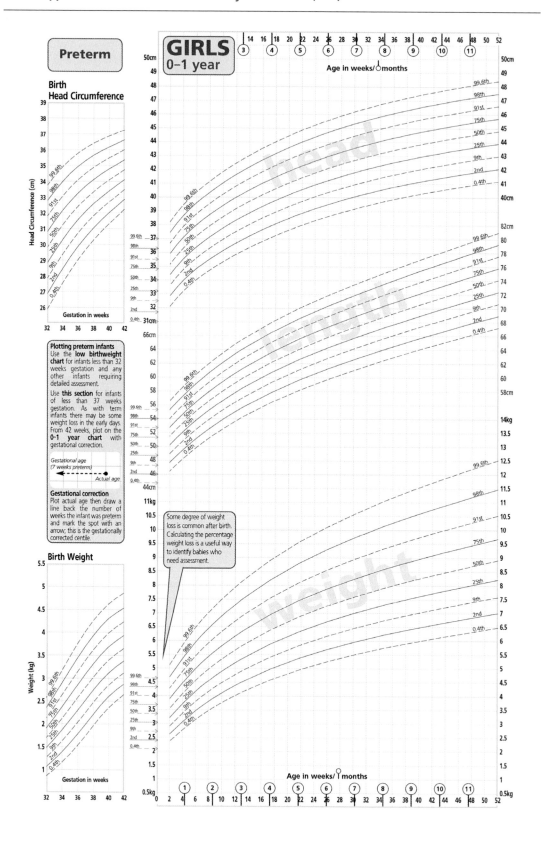

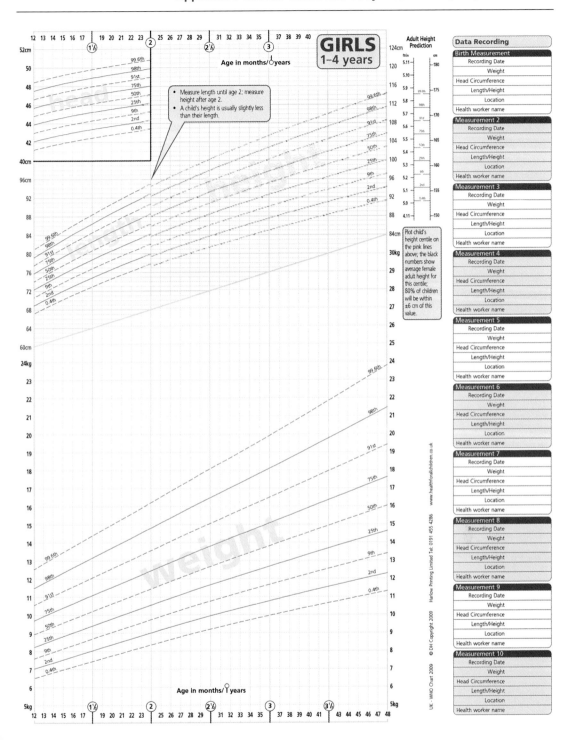

GIRLS
1–4 years

Age in months/○years

Adult Height Prediction

- Measure length until age 2; measure height after age 2.
- A child's height is usually slightly less than their length.

Plot child's height centile on the pink lines above; the black numbers show average female adult height for this centile; 80% of children will be within ±6 cm of this value.

Age in months/○ years

www.healthforallchildren.co.uk

Harlow Printing Limited Tel: 0191 455 4286

© DH Copyright 2009

UK - WHO Chart 2009

Data Recording

Birth Measurement
Recording Date
Weight
Head Circumference
Length/Height
Location
Health worker name

Measurement 2
Recording Date
Weight
Head Circumference
Length/Height
Location
Health worker name

Measurement 3
Recording Date
Weight
Head Circumference
Length/Height
Location
Health worker name

Measurement 4
Recording Date
Weight
Head Circumference
Length/Height
Location
Health worker name

Measurement 5
Recording Date
Weight
Head Circumference
Length/Height
Location
Health worker name

Measurement 6
Recording Date
Weight
Head Circumference
Length/Height
Location
Health worker name

Measurement 7
Recording Date
Weight
Head Circumference
Length/Height
Location
Health worker name

Measurement 8
Recording Date
Weight
Head Circumference
Length/Height
Location
Health worker name

Measurement 9
Recording Date
Weight
Head Circumference
Length/Height
Location
Health worker name

Measurement 10
Recording Date
Weight
Head Circumference
Length/Height
Location
Health worker name

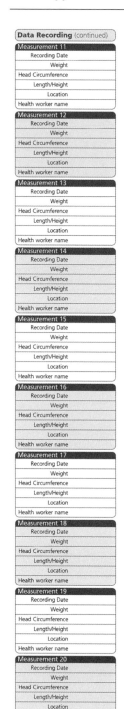

GIRLS UK-WHO

Growth Chart 0–4 years

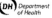 **RCPCH** Royal College of Paediatrics and Child Health

 (DH) *Department of Health*   ✚ healthier scotland

Who should use this chart?

Anyone who measures a child, plots or interprets charts should be suitably trained, or be supervised by someone qualified to do so. For further information and training materials see www.growthcharts.rcpch.ac.uk

A growth chart for all children

The UK-WHO growth chart combines World Health Organization (WHO) standards with UK preterm and birth data. The chart from 2 weeks to 4 years of age is based on the WHO growth standard, derived from measurements of healthy, non-deprived, breastfed children of mothers who did not smoke.[1] The chart for birth measurements (32–42 weeks gestation) is based on British children measured around 1990.[2] The charts depict a healthy pattern of growth that is desirable for all children, whether breast fed or formula fed, and of whatever ethnic origin.[3]

Weighing and measuring

When measuring children up to 2 years, remove all clothes and nappy; children older than 2 years should wear minimal clothing only. Always remove shoes.

Weight: use only class III clinical electronic scales in metric setting.

Length: (before 2 years of age): proper equipment is essential (length board or mat). Measurers should be trained.

Height: (from 2 years): use a rigid rule with T piece, or stadiometer. Position head and feet as illustrated with child standing as straight as possible.

Frankfurt Plane

Head circumference: use a narrow plastic or paper tape to measure where the head circumference is greatest.

When to weigh

Babies should be weighed in the first week as part of the assessment of feeding and thereafter as needed. Recovery of birthweight indicates that feeding is effective and that the child is well. Once feeding is established, babies should usually be weighed at around 8, 12 and 16 weeks and 1 year at the time of routine immunisations. If there is concern, weigh more often; however, weights measured too close together are often misleading, so babies should be weighed no more than once a month up to 6 months of age, once every 2 months from 6 to 12 months of age, and once every 3 months over the age of 1 year. However, most children do not need to be weighed this often.

When to measure length or height

Length or height should be measured whenever there are any worries about a child's weight gain, growth or general health.

Plotting measurements

For babies born at term (37 weeks or later), plot each measurement on the relevant chart by drawing a small dot where a vertical line through the child's age crosses a horizontal line through the measured value. The lettering on the charts ('weight', 'length' etc.) sits on the 50th centile, providing orientation for ease of plotting.

Plot birth weight (and, if measured, length and head circumference) at age 0 on the 0–1 year chart. The coloured arrows at age 0 represent UK birth weight data and show the child's birth centile.

Weight gain in the early days varies a lot from baby to baby, so there are no lines on the chart between 0 and 2 weeks. However, by 2 weeks of age most babies will be on a centile close to their birth centile.

For **preterm infants** a separate low birth weight chart is available for infants of less than 32 weeks gestation and any other infant requiring detailed assessment. For healthy infants born from 32 weeks and before 37 weeks, plot all measurements in the preterm section (to the left of the main 0–1 year chart) until 42 weeks gestation, then plot on the 0–1 year chart using gestational correction, as shown below.

The preterm section can also be used to assess the relative size of infants at the margin of 'term' (e.g. 37 weeks gestation), but these measurements should also be plotted at age 0 on the 0–1 year chart.

Gestational correction

Plot measurements at the child's actual age and then draw a line back the number of weeks the infant was preterm. Mark the spot with an arrow (see diagram): this is the child's gestationally corrected centile. Gestational correction should continue until at least 1 year of age.

Centile terminology

If the point is within 1/4 of a space of the line they are on the centile: e.g. 91st.

If not they should be described as being between the two centiles: e.g. 75th-91st.

A centile space is the distance between two of the centile lines, or equivalent distance if midway between centiles.

Plotting for preterm infants (less than 37 weeks gestation): Draw a line back the number of weeks preterm and mark spot with arrow.

Gestational age (7 weeks preterm) ◀------ ● Actual age

Interpreting the chart
Assessing weight loss after birth
Most babies lose some weight after birth but 80% will have regained this by 2 weeks of age. Fewer than 5% of babies lose more than 10% of their weight at any stage; only 1 in 50 are 10% or more lighter than birth weight at 2 weeks.

Percentage weight loss can be calculated as follows:

Weight loss = current weight–birth weight

$$\text{Percentage weight loss} = \frac{\text{Weight loss}}{\text{Birth weight}} \times 100\%$$

For example, a child born at 3.500kg who drops to 3.150kg at 5 days has lost 350g or 10%; in a baby born at 3.000kg, a 300g loss is 10%.

Careful clinical assessment and evaluation of feeding technique is indicated when weight loss exceeds 10% or recovery of birth weight is slow.

What do the centiles mean?
These charts indicate a child's size compared with children of the same age and maturity who have shown optimum growth. The chart also shows how quickly a child is growing. The centile lines on the chart show the expected range of weights and heights (or lengths); each describes the number of children expected to be below that line (e.g. 50% below 50th, 91% below the 91st). Children come in all shapes and sizes, but 99 out of 100 children who are growing optimally will be between the two outer lines (0.4th and 99.6th centiles); half will lie between the 25th and 75th centile lines.

Being very small or very big can sometimes be associated with underlying illness. There is no single threshold below which a child's weight or height is definitely abnormal, but only 4 per 1000 children who are growing optimally are below the **0.4th centile**, so these children should be assessed at some point to exclude any problems. Those above the **99.6th centile** for height are almost always healthy. Also calculate BMI if weight and height centiles appear very different.

What is a normal rate of weight gain and growth?
Babies do not all grow at the same rate, so a baby's weight often does not follow a particular centile line, especially in the first year. Weight is most likely to track within one centile space (the gap between two centile lines, see diagram). In infancy, acute illness can lead to sudden weight loss and a weight centile fall but on recovery the child's weight usually returns to its normal centile within 2–3 weeks. However, a sustained drop through two or more weight centile spaces is unusual (fewer than 2% of infants) and should be carefully assessed by the primary care team, including measuring length/height.

Because it is difficult to measure length and height accurately in pre-school children, successive measurements commonly show wide variation. If there are worries about growth, it is useful to measure on a few occasions over time; most healthy children will show a stable *average* position over time.

UK children have relatively large heads compared to the WHO standard, particularly after the age of 6 months. After the age of 6 weeks a head circumference below the 2nd centile will be seen in only 1 in 250 children. A head circumference above the 99.6th centile, or crossing upwards through 2 centile spaces, should only cause concern if there is a continued rise after 6 months, or other signs or symptoms.

Why do the length/height centiles change at 2 years?
The growth standards show length data up to 2 years of age, and height from age 2 onwards. When a child is measured standing up, the spine is squashed a little, so their height is slightly less than their length; the centile lines shift down slightly at age 2 to allow for this. It is important that this difference does not worry parents; what matters is whether the child continues to follow the same centile after the transition.

Predicting adult height
Parents like to know how tall their child will be as an adult. The child's most recent height centile (aged 2–4 years) gives a good idea of this for healthy children. Plot this centile on the adult height predictor to the right of the height chart to find the average adult height for children on this centile. Four out of five children will have adult heights that are within 6cm above or below this value.

Weight–height to BMI conversion chart
BMI indicates how heavy a child is relative to his or her height and is the simplest measure of thinness and fatness from the age of 2, when height can be measured fairly accurately. This chart[4] provides an approximate BMI centile, accurate to a quarter of a centile space.

$$BMI = \frac{\text{weight in kg}}{(\text{height in m})^2}$$

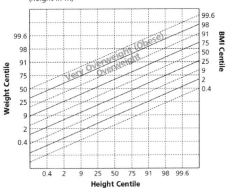

Date:			
Age:			
BMI Centile:			

Instructions for use
1. Read off the weight and height centiles from the growth chart.
2. Plot the weight centile (left axis) against the height centile (bottom axis) on the chart above.
3. If between centiles, read across in this position.
4. Read off the corresponding BMI centile from the slanting lines.
5. Record the centile with the date and child's age in the data box.

Interpretation
In a child over 2 years of age, the BMI centile is a better indicator of overweight or underweight than the weight centile; a child whose weight is average for their height will have a BMI between the 25th and 75th centiles, whatever their height centile. BMI above the 91st centile suggests that the child is overweight; a child above the 98th centile is very overweight (clinically obese). BMI below the 2nd centile is unusual and may reflect undernutrition.

References
1. www.who.int/childgrowth/en
2. Cole TJ, Freeman JV, Preece MA. British 1990 growth reference centiles for weight, height, body mass index and head circumference fitted by maximum penalized likelihood. Stat Med 1998;17:407-29.
3. www.sacn.gov.uk/reports_position_statements/index.html
4. Cole TJ. A chart to link child centiles of body mass index, weight and height. Eur J Clin Nutr 2002;56:1194-9.

2 to 20 years: Boys
Stature-for-age and Weight-for-age percentiles

NAME _____

RECORD # _____

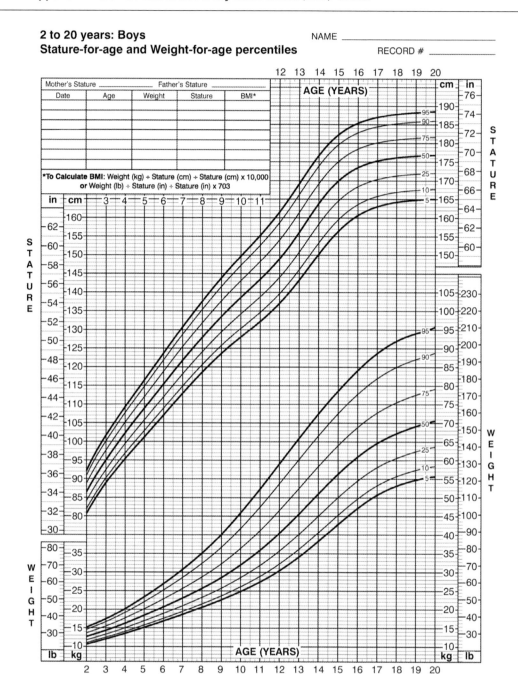

*To Calculate BMI: Weight (kg) ÷ Stature (cm) ÷ Stature (cm) x 10,000
or Weight (lb) ÷ Stature (in) ÷ Stature (in) x 703

Published May 30, 2000 (modified 11/21/00).
SOURCE: Developed by the National Center for Health Statistics in collaboration with
the National Center for Chronic Disease Prevention and Health Promotion (2000).
http://www.cdc.gov/growthcharts

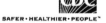

SAFER · HEALTHIER · PEOPLE™

2 to 20 years: Girls
Stature-for-age and Weight-for-age percentiles

NAME _____

RECORD # _____

AGE (YEARS)

Mother's Stature		Father's Stature		
Date	Age	Weight	Stature	BMI*

***To Calculate BMI:** Weight (kg) ÷ Stature (cm) ÷ Stature (cm) x 10,000
or Weight (lb) ÷ Stature (in) ÷ Stature (in) x 703

AGE (YEARS)

Published May 30, 2000 (modified 11/21/00).
SOURCE: Developed by the National Center for Health Statistics in collaboration with
the National Center for Chronic Disease Prevention and Health Promotion (2000).
http://www.cdc.gov/growthcharts

SAFER · HEALTHIER · PEOPLE™

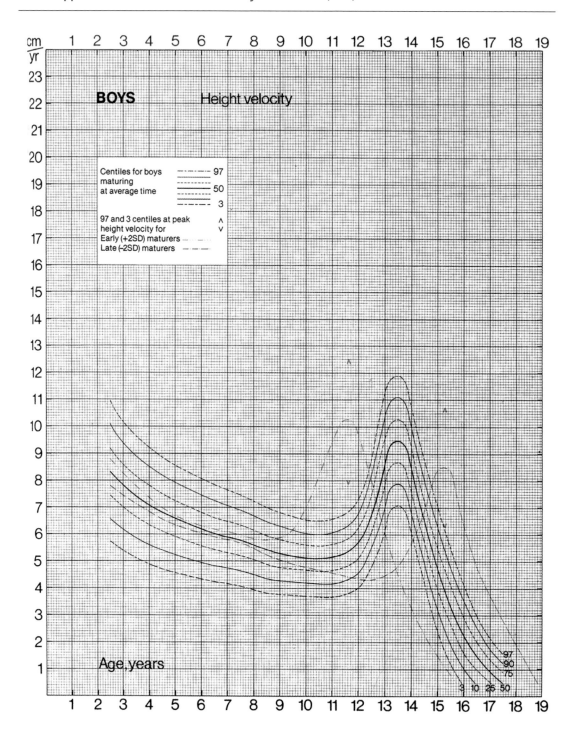

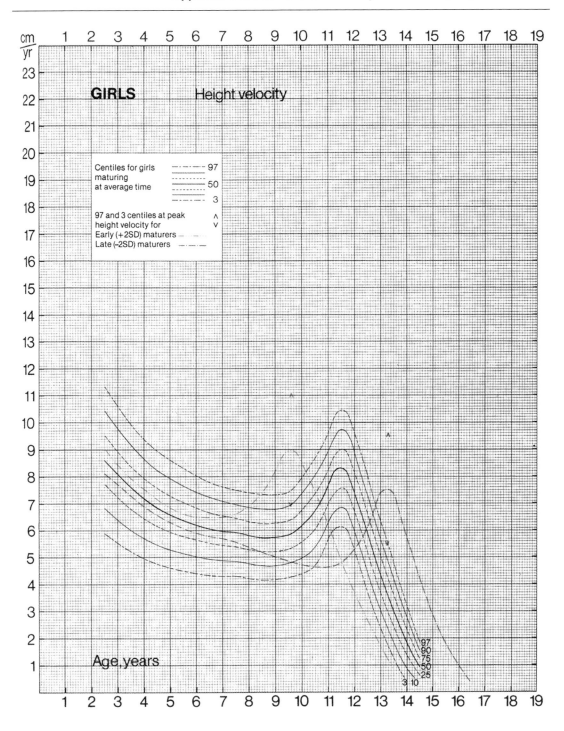

BOYS UK
Body mass index (BMI)
2-20 years

RCPCH
Royal College of
Paediatrics and Child Health
Leading the way in Children's Health

DH *Department of Health*

The BMI centile is a simple and reliable indicator of thinness and fatness in childhood. Where severe over- or underweight is a concern, or where there is a need for monitoring over time, BMI can be calculated and plotted on this chart. It is important also to plot the height and weight separately on the main 2-18 chart. There is also a BMI centile look-up on the standard 2-18 chart for less complex cases.

BMI is calculated by dividing weight (in kg) by the square of height (in metres e.g. 1.32 m, not centimetres e.g. 132 cm).
A simple way to do this on a calculator or mobile phone is:
1. Enter the weight. 2. Divide by height. 3. Divide the result by height.
The result can then be plotted on the chart below.

Overweight and obesity
A BMI above the 91st centile suggests overweight. A child above the 98th centile is very overweight (clinically obese) while a BMI above the 99.6th centile is severely obese. In addition to the usual nine centile lines, the BMI chart displays high lines at +3, +3.33, +3.66 and + 4 SD, which can be used to monitor the progress of children in overweight treatment programmes.

Thinness
A BMI below the 2nd centile is unusual and may reflect undernutrition, but may simply reflect a small build. The chart also displays low lines at -4 and -5 SD for those who are severely underweight. Children whose BMI lies below the 0.4th centile are likely to have additional problems and if not already receiving medical or dietetic attention should be referred.

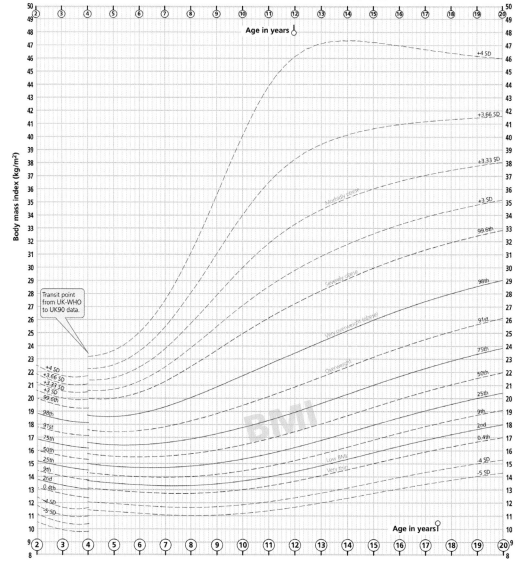

GIRLS UK
Body mass index (BMI)
2-20 years

RCPCH
Royal College of
Paediatrics and Child Health
Leading the way in Children's Health

DH Department of Health

The BMI centile is a simple and reliable indicator of thinness and fatness in childhood. Where severe over- or underweight is a concern, or where there is a need for monitoring over time, BMI can be calculated and plotted on this chart. It is important also to plot the height and weight separately on the main 2-18 chart. There is also a BMI centile look-up on the standard 2-18 chart for less complex cases.

BMI is calculated by dividing weight (in kg) by the square of height (in metres e.g. 1.32 m, not centimetres e.g. 132 cm).
A simple way to do this on a calculator or mobile phone is:
1. Enter the weight. 2. Divide by height. 3. Divide the result by height.
The result can then be plotted on the chart below.

Overweight and obesity
A BMI above the 91st centile suggests overweight. A child above the 98th centile is very overweight (clinically obese) while a BMI above the 99.6th centile is severely obese. In addition to the usual nine centile lines, the BMI chart displays high lines at +3, +3.33, +3.66 and + 4 SD, which can be used to monitor the progress of children in overweight treatment programmes.

Thinness
A BMI below the 2nd centile is unusual and may reflect undernutrition, but may simply reflect a small build. The chart also displays low lines at -4 and -5 SD for those who are severely underweight. Children whose BMI lies below the 0.4th centile are likely to have additional problems and if not already receiving medical or dietetic attention should be referred.

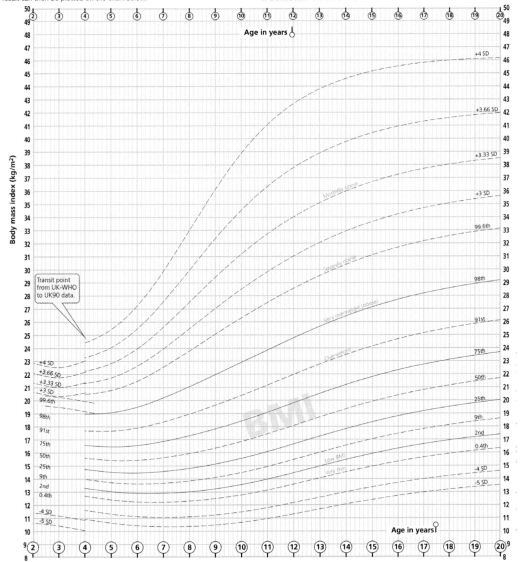

2 Syndrome-specific Growth Charts

Turner syndrome growth charts for girls aged 1–19 years are available from the Child Growth Foundation (2 Mayfield Avenue, London W4 1PW, UK) and are shown in the Appendix. Growth charts for Down Syndrome were jointly produced by the RCPCH and Down Syndrome Medical Interest Group (DSMIG) in 2011 and are available for purchase (https://www.dsmig.org.uk/information-resources/growth-charts/). New Noonan syndrome growth charts are available in Malaquias et al. (2012). New Achondroplasia growth charts are shown in Tofts et al. (2017). These charts are reproduced, with permission.

References

Malaquias, A.C., Brasil, A.S., Pereira, A.C. et al. (2012). *Am. J. Med. Genet.* 158A (11): 2700–2706. https://doi.org/10.1002/ajmg.a.35519.

Tofts, L., Das, S., Collins, F., and Burton, K.L.O. (2017). *Am. J. Med. Genet.* 173 (8): 2189–2200. https://doi.org/10.1002/ajmg.a.38312.

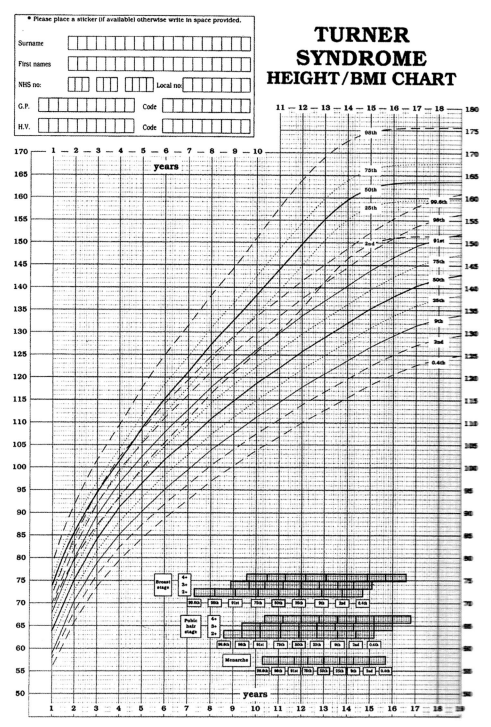

TURNER SYNDROME HEIGHT/BMI CHART

Designed and Published by
© CHILD GROWTH FOUNDATION 1997/1
(Charity Reg. No. 274325)
2 Mayfield Avenue,
London W4 1PW

Printed by and Supplied by

HARLOW PRINTING LIMITED
Maxwell Street ◊ South Shields
Tyne & Wear ◊ NE33 4PU

DATA BOXES FOR INSERTION OF WEIGHT, HEAD CIRCUMFERENCE, LENGTH, HEIGHT AND BMI

Date	Age	Measurement	BMI	Name/Initials
: :	:	:	:	
: :	:	:	:	
: :	:	:	:	
: :	:	:	:	
: :	:	:	:	
: :	:	:	:	
: :	:	:	:	
: :	:	:	:	
: :	:	:	:	
: :	:	:	:	
: :	:	:	:	
: :	:	:	:	
: :	:	:	:	
: :	:	:	:	
: :	:	:	:	
: :	:	:	:	
: :	:	:	:	
: :	:	:	:	
: :	:	:	:	
: :	:	:	:	
: :	:	:	:	
: :	:	:	:	

Date	Age	Measurement	BMI	Name/Initials
: :	:	:	:	
: :	:	:	:	
: :	:	:	:	
: :	:	:	:	
: :	:	:	:	
: :	:	:	:	

How to calculate BMI

Divide weight (kg) by the square of length/height (m²)

example
weight = 25kg
length/height = 1.2m

equation
25 ÷ (1.2 x 1.2)
= 17.4

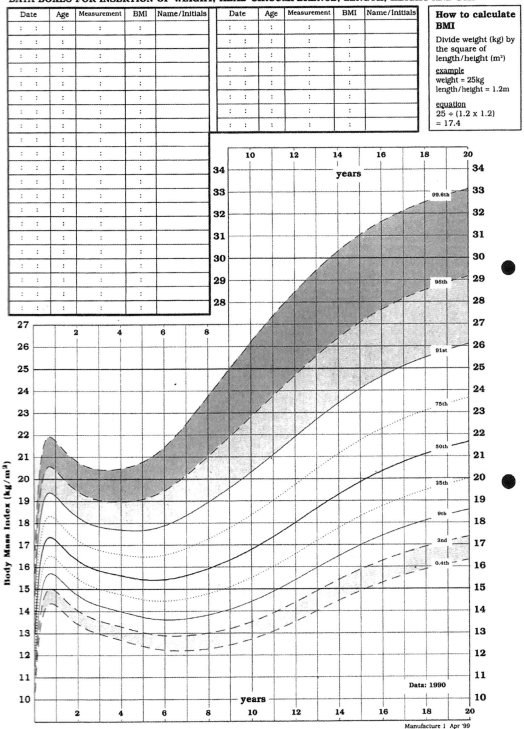

REFERENCES

Growth Curve for girls with Turner Syndrome (AJ Lyon, MA Preece, DB Grant) *ARCH DIS CHILD* 1985; 60: 932-935
Body Mass Index reference curves for the UK, 1990 (TJ Cole, JV Freeman, MA Preece) *Arch Dis Child* 1995; **73**: 25-29

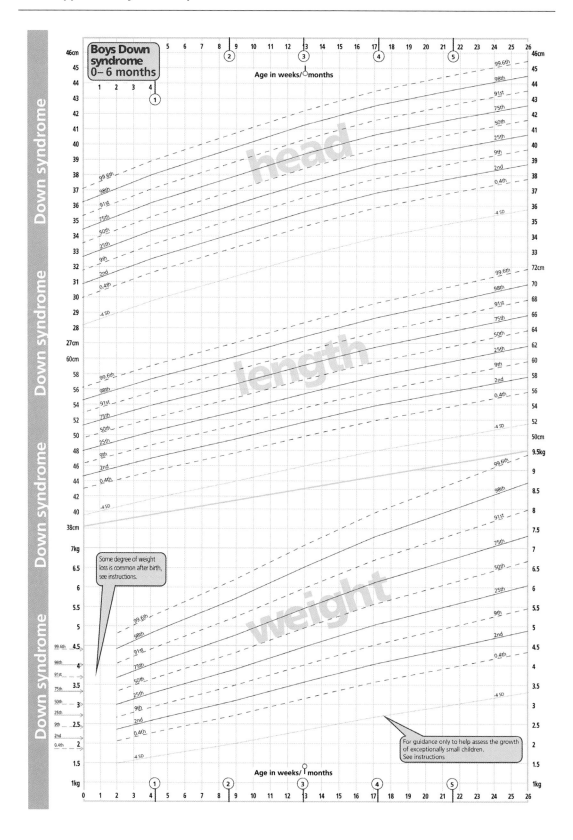

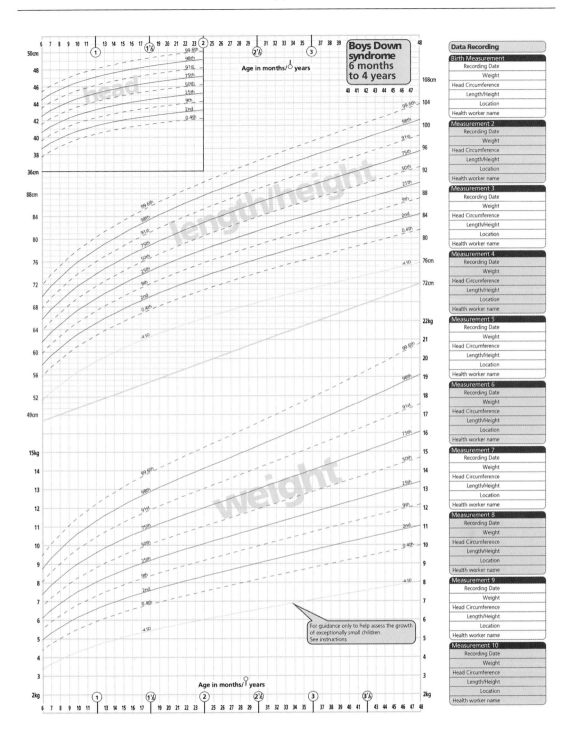

Boys Down syndrome 6 months to 4 years

Age in months/years

For guidance only to help assess the growth of exceptionally small children. See instructions

Data Recording

Birth Measurement
Recording Date
Weight
Head Circumference
Length/Height
Location
Health worker name

Measurement 2
Recording Date
Weight
Head Circumference
Length/Height
Location
Health worker name

Measurement 3
Recording Date
Weight
Head Circumference
Length/Height
Location
Health worker name

Measurement 4
Recording Date
Weight
Head Circumference
Length/Height
Location
Health worker name

Measurement 5
Recording Date
Weight
Head Circumference
Length/Height
Location
Health worker name

Measurement 6
Recording Date
Weight
Head Circumference
Length/Height
Location
Health worker name

Measurement 7
Recording Date
Weight
Head Circumference
Length/Height
Location
Health worker name

Measurement 8
Recording Date
Weight
Head Circumference
Length/Height
Location
Health worker name

Measurement 9
Recording Date
Weight
Head Circumference
Length/Height
Location
Health worker name

Measurement 10
Recording Date
Weight
Head Circumference
Length/Height
Location
Health worker name

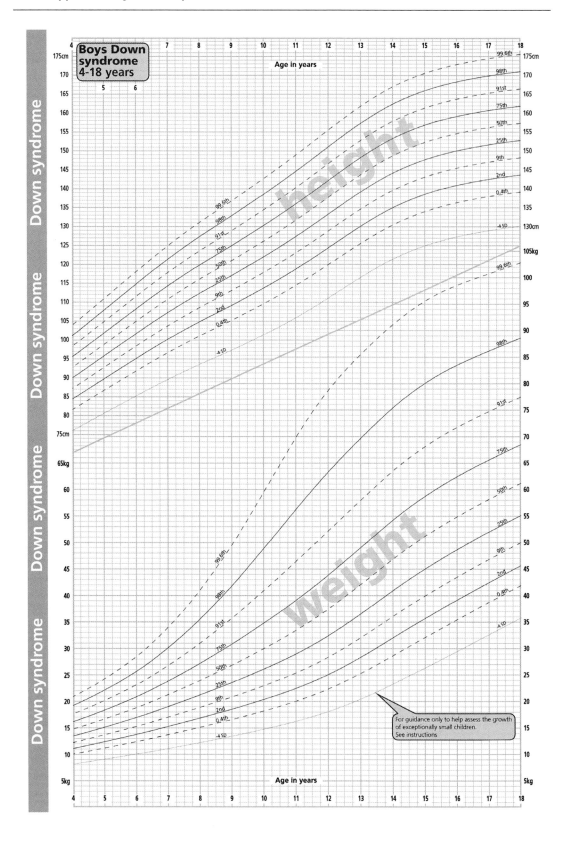

Boys Down syndrome 4-18 years

For guidance only to help assess the growth of exceptionally small children. See instructions

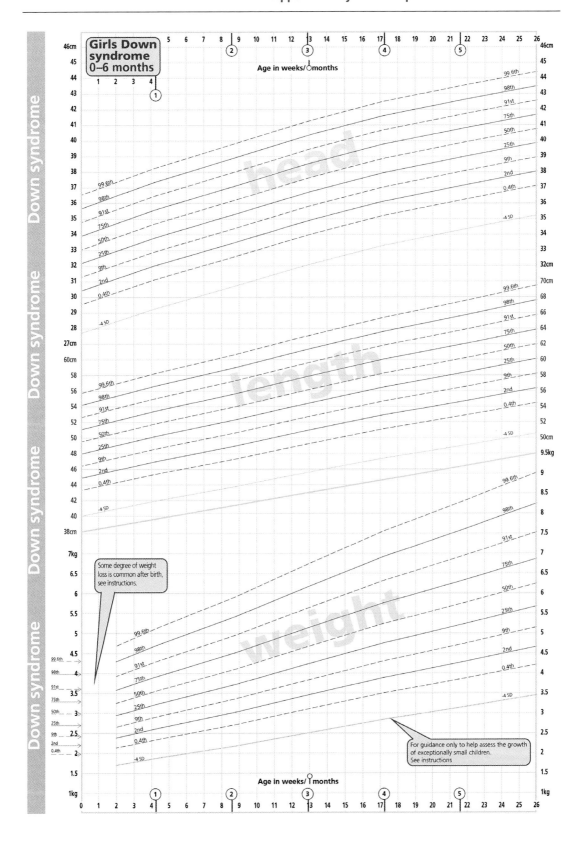

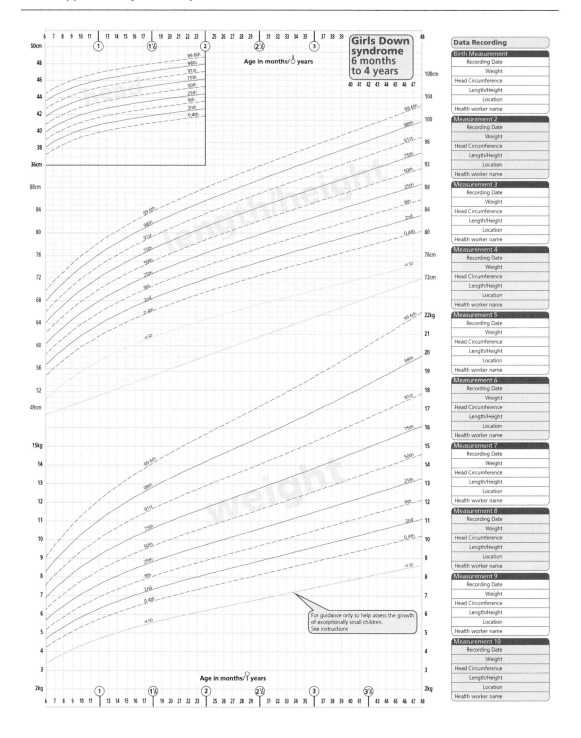

Girls Down syndrome 6 months to 4 years

Age in months/♀ years

For guidance only to help assess the growth of exceptionally small children. See instructions

Data Recording

Birth Measurement
- Recording Date
- Weight
- Head Circumference
- Length/Height
- Location
- Health worker name

Measurement 2
- Recording Date
- Weight
- Head Circumference
- Length/Height
- Location
- Health worker name

Measurement 3
- Recording Date
- Weight
- Head Circumference
- Length/Height
- Location
- Health worker name

Measurement 4
- Recording Date
- Weight
- Head Circumference
- Length/Height
- Location
- Health worker name

Measurement 5
- Recording Date
- Weight
- Head Circumference
- Length/Height
- Location
- Health worker name

Measurement 6
- Recording Date
- Weight
- Head Circumference
- Length/Height
- Location
- Health worker name

Measurement 7
- Recording Date
- Weight
- Head Circumference
- Length/Height
- Location
- Health worker name

Measurement 8
- Recording Date
- Weight
- Head Circumference
- Length/Height
- Location
- Health worker name

Measurement 9
- Recording Date
- Weight
- Head Circumference
- Length/Height
- Location
- Health worker name

Measurement 10
- Recording Date
- Weight
- Head Circumference
- Length/Height
- Location
- Health worker name

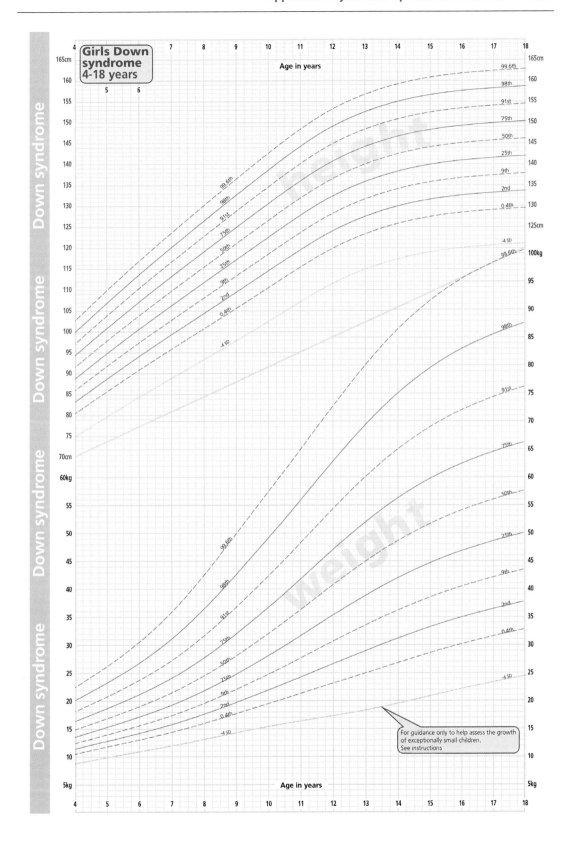

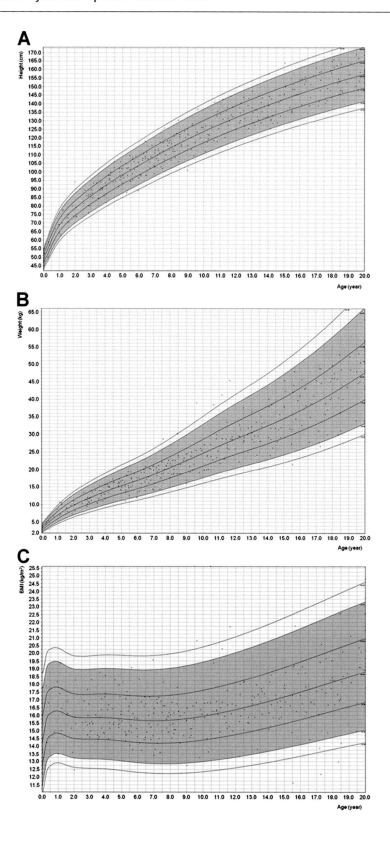

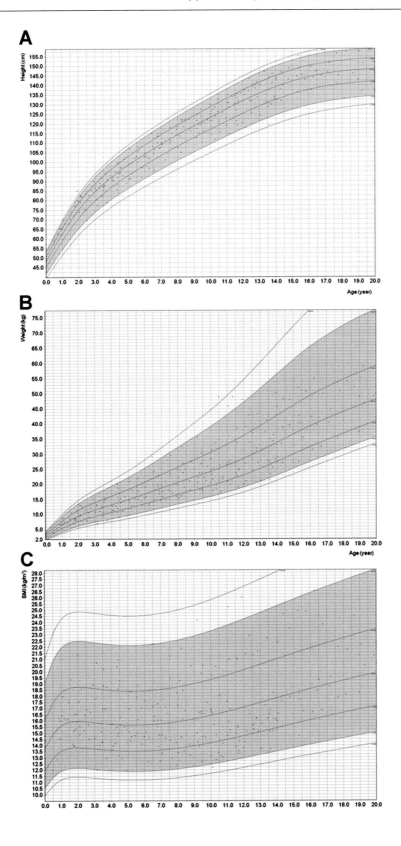

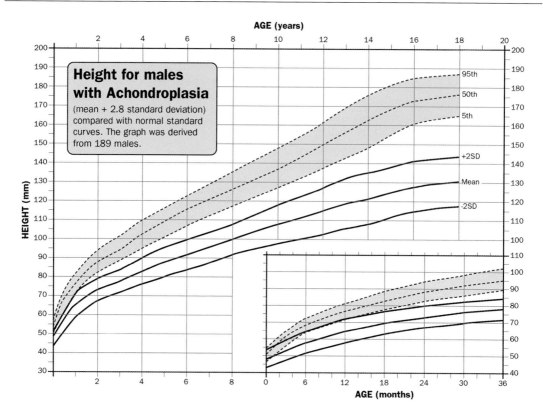

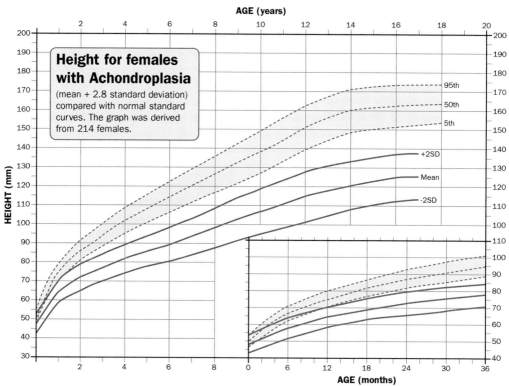

3 Congenital Adrenal Hyperplasia (CAH) Therapy Card

This chart can easily be reproduced and adapted for use in different centres and countries. Families have found them particularly useful in acute situations where the attending doctor may be unfamiliar with CAH.

Instructions for Hospital Doctor

Dear Doctor,

If this child is brought to hospital by the parents as an emergency the following management is advised:

- Insert an I.V. cannula
- Take blood for U's and E's, glucose, and perform any other appropriate tests (e.g. urine culture)
- Check glucostix or dextrostix
- Give _____ mg hydrocortisone intravenously as bolus (unnecessary if parent has already given I.M. hydrocortisone)
- Commence I.V. infusion of 0.45% saline and 5% dextrose at maintenance rate (extra if child is dehydrated). Add potassium depending on electrolyte results.
- Commence hydrocortisone infusion (50mg hydrocortisone in 50ml normal saline via syringe pump) at _____ ml/hour
- **Important!** If blood glucose/glucostix is < 2.5mmol, give bolus of 2ml/kg of 10% dextrose
- If child is drowsy, hypotensive and peripherally shut down with poor capillary return give 20 ml/kg of normal saline stat.

Please contact named consultant at Yorkhill and inform of admission.

Thank you

NHS
Greater Glasgow

CAH THERAPY CARD

The owner of this card has the condition **Congenital adrenal hyperplasia** also known as **CAH** or **Adrenogenital syndrome.**

Name ....

Address ....

....

DoB .... Hospital number ....

Hospital consultant:

Useful telephone numbers:

Hospital switchblade: ....
Ward ....
Dr A ....
Dr B ....
Endocrine Nurse ....
Endocrine Ward ....

GP's name / address / tel no ....

....

....

Front and Back of Card

Practical Endocrinology and Diabetes in Children, Fourth Edition. Malcolm D.C. Donaldson, John W. Gregory, Guy Van Vliet, and Joseph I. Wolfsdorf.
© 2019 John Wiley & Sons Ltd. Published 2019 by John Wiley & Sons Ltd.

Current treatment

Fill in details of the drugs your child is taking, with the dates of any dose changes.

Dose to be taken in

Date	Drug	Tablet size		Morning	Afternoon	Evening

Inside of Card

What to do if your child is unwell

1. In the event of *mild to moderate illness*, e.g. cold, cough, sore throat, flu, tummy upset, double the total daily dose of hydrocortisone and give this doubled dose in 3 equal portions (morning, afternoon and evening) for the duration of the illness.

   The fludrocortisone dose should stay the same.

   i.e Hydrocortisone dose _____ x 3 per day

2. If your child
   - *does not get better* after you have increased the tablets, or
   - *feels drowsy*, or
   - *is unable to take the tablets orally* (e.g. due to continued vomiting),

   the hydrocortisone must be given by injection (intra-muscular).

   Please check that this is not past the expiry date

   The dose of hydrocortisone injection is _____

3. If your child continues to be ill and does not seem to be getting better, telephone the hospital and say that you are bringing him/her up for admission.

   Please bring this card with you and show it to the doctor.

Index

Note: Page references followed by 'f' refer to Figures; those followed by 't' refer to Tables and Boxes

Practical Endocrinology and Diabetes in Children, Fourth Edition. Malcolm D.C. Donaldson, John W. Gregory,
Guy Van Vliet, and Joseph I. Wolfsdorf.
© 2019 John Wiley & Sons Ltd. Published 2019 by John Wiley & Sons Ltd.